Nursing Care Planning

Nursing Care Planning

Second Edition

Dolores E. Little, R.N., M.N.
Professor, School of Nursing,
University of Washington

Doris L. Carnevali, R.N., M.N.
Associate Professor, School of
Nursing, University of Washington

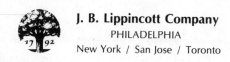

J. B. Lippincott Company
PHILADELPHIA
New York / San Jose / Toronto

Distributed in Great Britain by
Blackwell Scientific Publications, London, Oxford, and
Edinburgh

ISBN 0-397-54184-8

Library of Congress Catalog Card Number 76-6949

Printed in the United States of America

135798642

Library of Congress Cataloging in Publication Data

Little, Dolores E
    Nursing care planning.
    1. Nursing. I. Carnevali, Doris L., joint author.
II. Title. [DNLM: 1. Nursing care. 2. Patient care
planning. WY100 L778n]
RT41.L75   1976   610.73   76-6949

ISBN 0-397-54184-8

This Book is Dedicated to Our "Support Systems":

Bertha Little, whose lifestyle and coping was marked
by so much vitality and
humor—a sustaining force,
even in memory

and

Armando, who copes so well
with a wife who writes

Preface

Much has changed in nursing since the first edition of this book that has dictated a very different approach to the second edition of *Nursing Care Planning*. Nurses, nursing, the consumers, and the environment are changing.

One important change is that nursing is sharply defining its contribution to health care. No longer are medical care and health care synonymous. No longer is nursing seen as being purely a physician extender service. Nurses have identified in practice the contribution they make to health care that is different from the other health care disciplines. Given this clearer definition of nursing's particular orientation and area of accountability, it has been possible and desirable in this edition to be much more specific in translating that nursing component into assessments, diagnoses and treatment plans, as well as evaluation. Following the first edition, for example, we saw a multitude of history or assessment forms. Each institution had its own focus. This time we sought that common core of all nursing assessments regardless of clientele or setting. Beyond this, nurses now are seeing the need for diagnostic taxonomy; at the time of the first edition, many were still wondering if nurses diagnosed. And, at the time of the release of this edition, nurses have few qualms about prescribing nursing therapy; in the first edition we were plugging the idea of nursing orders rather than suggested approaches. This transition to active nursing diagnosis and treatment lends importance to a consideration of nursing's knowledge base and the skills of using that knowledge. This book does not intend to address the substantive knowledge that nurses need, but it has attempted to make more explicit that elusive thinking process that blends data and knowledge into sound diagnosis, prescription, and evaluation. We have attempted to approach a system for nursing diagnoses by examining potential categories of common coping deficits within the nursing field. We have also offered a possible format for organizing nursing knowledge into working diagnostic concepts that are so essential in: the branching logic of nursing assessment, differential diagnosing, and a scientific rationale for prescribing so that one has some assurance of outcomes. In the first edition we were content to discuss the techniques of writing care plans. Here we have attempted the far more difficult task of examining how one must think in order to begin to write or report on plans of care.

Our acknowledgment of the change in the consumers of nursing services will be seen in the word we use to identify them. Consumers are identified as clients rather than patients. A client is defined as one who purchases professional services; a patient is one who is acted upon, one who is expected to endure without complaint. Given a definition of nursing that focuses upon effective daily living and effective coping with the challenges of life related to health, somehow the passivity associated with the concept of "patient" no longer seems appropriate. Therefore, in keeping with our valuing of the consumer as a participant in his health care, at whatever level is possible, we opted to call his role "client." You will note also that we relocated the client and his values from the end of the chapter on values in nursing care plans to the beginning. This also reflects where we are. Beyond that, we have stressed validation of the care planning with the client throughout. In part, this is a reflection, not only of the changes in the consumer, but also in the locale of health care services. Increasingly, nursing is being offered as health care to ambulatory individuals where the power base for change rests entirely with the client—the nurse does not have the opportunity to control his lifestyle as she might in the hospital setting. So, realistically, we must begin, continue, and end with the client and where he is. We alluded to this in the first edition; we have emphasized it explicitly—operationalized it—in this edition.

Our definition of "family" also is a reflection of the changing times. In this edition we refer to the client's close personal network of persons as his family rather than assigning the traditional meaning of parents, spouses, siblings, and offspring.

We could not leave this preface without acknowledging the contribution that thousands of nurses have made to this book. In the years between the first and second editions the authors have been actively involved in giving workshops on nursing care planning to registered nurses in most of the states as well as provinces in Canada and Australia. Nurses have generously shared their expertise, their experiences, their resources, their problems, and their clients with us as we met with them. Their learning needs and their wisdom, as well as the insights we've gained through these contacts have been woven into the very fiber of this edition. We hope they will recognize the ways in which they pushed us to make this edition more challenging, more thought provoking, but more practical as well.

These workshops and our personal experiences have made us increasingly aware of the importance of the climate in the work setting for care planning. Nursing care planning does not occur in a vacuum. Even primary care nurses must interact with nursing colleagues to bring their plans into reality. They must articulate their plans with those of the medical and other professions to have them merge into a total health plan. We have seen edicts about care planning come and go. We have been impressed with care plan systems in which nurses and their leadership genuinely support both a nursing care plan system and their colleagues' efforts at planning and learning. It's difficult at best—this creation and maintenance of the care plan and the care plan system. There are interpersonal challenges as well as skills to be mastered. To this end we've tried to address realistically the interpersonal problems as we have seen them and as our nursing colleagues have made them known to us.

Finally, we must acknowledge that there are changes entering the scene that will have major impact on nursing care planning—changes that we have only touched on here. One that is looming large is problem-oriented records and computerized health records. Since some of our colleagues are effectively addressing this subject extensively in a companion book by Walter, Pardee, and Molbo, *Dynamics of Problem-Oriented Approaches: Patient Care and Documentation,*° we have not dealt with the subject in any depth. We strongly believe that nursing care planning and problem-oriented recording are inseparable. We highly recommend this book to any nurse who needs to see nursing's role in problem-oriented health records.

As in the first edition, we strongly urge readers to thoroughly test for themselves any ideas they find here. No idea is yours until you have tested it in your own clinical environment and found that it works. We learned early that workshops and reading serve a role in expanding our ideas and knowledge, but nursing care planning is a clinical skill. Ultimately it must be learned by the individual through ongoing, critical clinical practice. To this end we would be delighted if you would not read this book through (except perhaps as an overview). Instead, read sections of it selectively as a basis for developing personal modules of learning. Try the activities—they've all been "nurse tested." Use your clinical classrooms to learn the various facets of the care planning skills. Experiment with and evaluate different techniques so that there is no need to climb into a care planning rut. Use your clients and colleagues as your teachers.

Then use your nursing care planning knowledge, skills, and role to heighten your claim to a distinctly colleague role—with each of the other health disciplines. Help clients to recognize what it is that nurses offer so that they will know when to consult nurses as they do other professionals.

Finally, please note that throughout this book we have used the pronoun "she" to refer to the nurse. This was done for convenience and is in no way meant as a slight to our male colleagues whom we welcome in ever growing numbers.

° J. B. Lippincott Co., 1976.

Contents

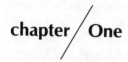

chapter / One

Planning Nursing Care,
an essential nursing function

Nurses diagnose. Nurses prescribe. Nurses have responsibility for planning patient care. Not long ago such statements would have been considered heretical. Yet the acknowledgment that nurses do indeed diagnose, prescribe and plan within their responsibility for health care has resulted in the most dramatic developments in modern nursing.

Until recently most students of nursing have been emphatically taught that diagnosis and prescription are solely the prerogative of the physician. Even some physicians who are advocates of an expanded role for the nurse use the terms "diagnosis" and "treatment" only to describe the doctor's role behaviors, not the nurse's.

It is no wonder, then, that nurses disguised their diagnoses with such phrases as "seems to be" or "appears to be" when actually they knew very well what was going on. Sometimes nurses have diagnosed within a medical area as they witnessed hemorrhage, infection, shock, insulin reaction, the onset of the second stage of labor, Dilantin toxicity, or a comminuted fracture. More than one person is alive today because the nurse did prescribe action for herself or others without waiting for a more official prescription. In less disease-oriented areas, nurses have frequently diagnosed anxiety and fear that was a potent force in the individual's response to health care; they have discovered where learning needs interfere with prevention of illness or convalescence. Here too they have prescribed behavior which is a form of therapy. In most instances the diagnosing and prescribing, however, have been kept at very low-level visibility.

A GRADUAL CHANGE

Since the early 1960s the picture has been changing gradually. Nurses have become increasingly aware of the constant flow of observations, judgments, and modifications they are making. Nor have they been able to overlook the significance of this decision making to their clients' well-being. Nurses noticed that the

1

process they were using to make judgments was the same as that used by physicians to make diagnoses and prescribe treatment. What was the difference in approach? Doctors, it was noted, purposefully and overtly observed, judged, and modified behavior. It was considered an important part of their role. The system was set up to support these functions. Medical education stressed not only the procedural skills of medical care, but the decision making skills and the knowledge used in making sound discriminating decisions and evolving valid criteria for judging the efficacy of their diagnoses and prescriptions.

Nurses finally began to ask themselves, "Are clients being effectively nursed if we behave at a predominately automatic, intuitive level? Do medical diagnosis and treatment cover all aspects of client needs in health and illness? Do the consumers deserve as much expertise in decisions regarding their nursing care as they receive in their medical care? Obviously, nurses decided that there were areas that were not being dealt with in usual medical practice and that their decisions needed to be at least as skilled, as well founded and as critically evaluated as those of their medical colleagues. Thus, the growing interest in nursing diagnosis and treatment and the planning for nursing care.

FORCES SHAPING NURSING PRACTICE

Actually this shift in practice did not occur spontaneously within the nursing profession. There were many external influences. Some of these were: the knowledge explosion, the change from an apprentice to an educational approach in the preparation of nurses, changing of consumer expectations for health care services, rapid expansion of occupations oriented to health care, increasing costs of health care and shifts toward more community based health services.

Knowledge Explosion

The vast expansion of knowledge about human response in health and illness in all of its dimensions—homeostatic mechanisms, pathophysiology, psychosociocultural behavior, genetics, pharmacology. . . . All of these areas have been opened up as research has allowed more insight into the dynamics of situations being encountered. With this additional knowledge nurses could recognize *what* was occurring in a situation and *how* modifications in management of nursing care could affect clients' adaptation to everyday living in the face of current or potential health problems.

Educational Changes

As educational patterns changed within society, candidates for nursing schools came with better preparation, and with the expectations that they would be educated as well as trained. Preparation of nurses began to include more "whys" as well as the formerly stressed "how to's." Questioning became a more

2

popular form of conversation in the nursing world. Reasoning began to replace automatic responses.

The nurses who were products of the newer approach to nursing education were ready to move into a more deliberate style of client care. In fact, it was difficult if not impossible to keep them from assuming accountability in this area.

Consumer Expectations

The concept of consumerism and the increased sophistication of the client have had their impact. Expectations about health care services have changed as the clientele too have become better educated. Television, newspapers, magazines, books, and other forms of communication as well as health-oriented education in schools and increased personal and vicarious experience with health services have given consumers more knowledge and awareness of services that may be desirable or necessary. Prepaid insurance and governmental coverage have in many instances permitted more extensive use of the health care system. Health care is being viewed as a right, not a privilege, everywhere—remote rural area, ghetto, jail, university, or retirement home. Thus, there is a demand for more sophisticated yet humane health care, including nursing care for all segments of the population regardless of geographic locale or income. And there seems to be less passive acceptance of services seen as substandard.

Rising Health Care Costs

Skyrocketing health care costs have dictated that each health care group function at the level of its preparation. Educating nurses to function at one level of competence and then using them at a much lower level, often because of availability or numbers, at last is being seen as an uneconomical use of human resources. It blunts the sharpness of the practitioner's skills and motivation; it inflates the cost to the consumer. Nurses themselves have begun to question the validity of the non-nursing tasks they carried out in the past. Data from activity studies on the use of nurses in both hospitals and clinics or offices could not be ignored. New priorities have begun to appear—nurses nurse clients rather than the desk, the record, the system, or other health care personnel.

Shift Toward More Community Based Health Care Services

The traditional establishment based health care services are no longer the only acceptable approach. A need has been seen to take the services *to* those who require them and to offer the care in a manner compatible with the consumers' values and lifestyle. Gaps in health care, whether absolute, such as the absence of facilities and personnel, or relative, such as broken continuity, have become less acceptable. As a result health care workers, including nurses and nursing students, can be found (often in jeans and sweat shirts instead of uniforms) offering superb health care in mobile clinics, free clinics, hot-line services, mental health group sessions, store front units, residences for ambulatory aging, and a variety of other settings. Often the roles of health care workers in these settings are less formal and may blur traditional disciplinary boundaries. Consumers, too, are involved in both planning and offering the services. There are new patterns and new relationships being built.

Increase in Health-Oriented Occupations

The almost geometric increase in the number of health-oriented occupations has caused nurses, the former jacks-of-all-trades of the health professions, to examine their contribution. They have asked themselves, "What do I do as a nurse that justifies the existence of nursing as a health profession? How does the service I provide to the consumer differ from that of the licensed practical nurse, the respiratory therapist, the social worker, the dietitian, the ward clerk, the doctor, the physician's assistant? This professional and personal soul-searching has contributed to a more discriminating concept of nursing and to a better definition in practice.

NURSING'S RESPONSE

What then is the dramatic change that is occurring in nursing? Basically, there has been an emerging sense of nursing as a separate identity on the health scene, one that did not just pick up delegated pieces left over from other professionals, technicians, or workers, just because they always had done so, or were available at all hours. Instead, nurses began to be aware of the significant contribution they had been making to the individual's and society's health. They found that occupying themselves with non-nursing duties prevented the giving of this service.

Nursing practitioners worked nationally and at the grass roots level to isolate and define their contribution. They looked at their activities, those carried out autonomously, and in them discovered their identity.

Now in the 1970s nursing seems to feel increasingly secure about the major differences between its discipline and any other of the health professional and technical fields. While there are still overlaps in interests and functions the primary focus is identifiably different.

What nurses discovered they were doing when they functioned independently was:

> To help clients and clients' families to cope more effectively with demands of daily living and their desired lifestyle in the face of actual or potential challenges to their health.

From this redefinition of nursing flowed a variety of subsequent responses.

4

Need for a Nursing Data Base

Nursing had always paid at least lip service to the importance of people, but in practice clients were more often seen in terms of interchangeable commonalities, tasks, or locations than as individuals. And as for involvement of individuals in their own care, the tendency was to do to "for" rather than "with," fostering far less individual responsibility. As one consumer of nursing remarked, "They treat patients like delinquent adolescents, lovable but not too bright." Said another, "You're in a factory, in production . . . but nobody's alike so you can't treat all patients the same." And a third, "They were too busy with the administrative details, and the patient could wait until they got the administration out of the way and then take care of him. I blew my cork and told off the nurse."

When the focus of nursing shifts to helping clients in their efforts to cope

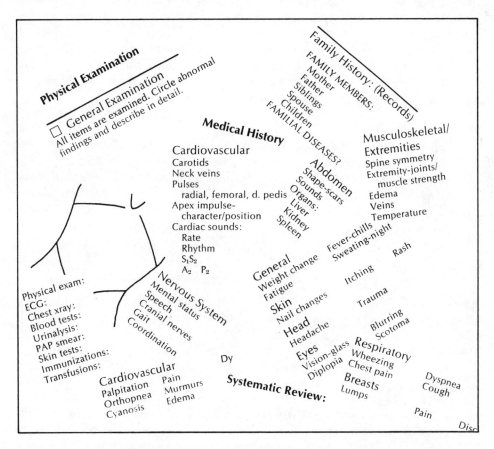

THE MEDICAL PATIENT DATA BASE, A MONTAGE

5

effectively with daily living, the resources and lifestyle of the clientele become important. How can you facilitate what you have not recognized?

Data on the usual daily activities, on strengths and resources available as well as deficits, on values involved and on cultural variations become essential. Unknowing violation of usual lifestyles or patterns, or failure to use existing resources and strengths, now can be considered inadequate nursing. Gradually, the realization has come that nursing needs its own data base, since nursing practice is built on data far different from that collected for medical practice.

For its patient data base, medicine focuses primarily on organ, system, and symptom in order to arrive at diagnosis and prescription. Medical histories and physical examinations yield data that are useful to the nurse in defining the pathology and symptomatology that produce barriers to effective coping, or deficits that require new coping skills or support systems. These data also help to highlight underlying mechanisms involved and thus, are useful in planning nursing care.

But there are still major gaps of information essential to planning *nursing* care. Therefore, the concepts of a nursing history and a functional assessment were born in order to achieve a predictable data base, systematically obtainable, as a foundation for the planning of nursing care.

Nursing Diagnosis

An explicit and distinct focus for nursing also led to the realization that areas of nursing diagnosis are related to, but quite different from, medicine. Where medicine labels symptoms and pathology, nursing describes *the effect of these symptoms and pathology on the activities and style of living, now and in the future. Example:*

If a medical diagnoses were emphysema, the nursing diagnosis might be:

Ineffective coping with nocturnal dyspnea
or (in practical terms)
Shortness of Breath (SOB) → inability to prepare meals and maintain apt.

Nurses have a need now to become as skilled in diagnosing and communicating these problems precisely as their medical colleagues.

Nursing Goals

Nursing goals are directed toward the solution of client problems of effective coping with impaired health, the daily demands of living, and the stresses of illness and treatment.

With the emphysematous patient, if medical treatment can minimize the difficulties in breathing at night, the goal would be to help the client learn to use the physician's prescribed medications or inhalators in such a way as to effectively diminish the dyspnea. Or, if symptoms are not preventable, then the goal might be related to minimizing the fear and anxiety that cause greater difficulty, by helping the person to understand the symptoms and the activities and environment that will be most conducive to coping with the episodes. Where the problem is the client's inability to get out to shop for groceries and prepare meals, the goal may be to enlist community resources, such as Meals-on-Wheels, to make normal nutrition again available.

Nursing Therapy

For a long time there has been a real controversy over whether the nurse is, in fact, a therapist. Today, nurses, and in many instances physicians as well, believe there is no question that nurses are therapists in their own right. The nurse's treatment modalities nearly always include management of the environment, listening and counselling, teaching, introduction or modification of activities, modification of fluid and nutritional aspects, emergency care, provision for safety and security, programming of activities, and occasionally, a medical type of intervention. Nurses, like physicians, within their area of accountability, prescribe and either delegate or personally carry out the activities that are necessary.

Nursing Evaluation

The criteria for evaluating client response to nursing care are also different from those of medicine. Earlier researchers in nursing often tried to measure response to nursing intervention by using medical criteria. It was like using a thermometer to measure an angle; the criteria were not appropriate. With a more definitive statement of client goals within the nursing area it is possible to develop more valid criteria for measuring outcomes. The challenge remains to develop increasingly rigorous nursing criteria comparable to those of other disciplines.

Summary

Nurses, like other health professionals, believe that individuals in our society have a right to the best quality care possible. They realized that nursing could make a more effective contribution if they defined their area of accountability and then systematically implemented and evaluated the resultant care. From these beliefs have come the tangible product: the plan of nursing care, using the nursing process as the vehicle for its development.

HEALTH CARE PLANNING

Health care planning, of which nursing is a part, consists of three obvious concepts—health, care and planning. *Health* can be conceived of as the well-being of individuals and groups as well as those factors which enhance or diminish this well-being. Generally, the following components are associated with a concept of health: physical status and functioning; emotional, intellectual and spiritual status and functioning; socio-cultural and economic factors; and environmental factors. *Care*, in this connotation, might be defined as concerned service. *Planning* is seen as an active decision-making process in which consideration of the relationships between goals, actions and consequences (outcomes) precedes taking action. Health care planners may range from the individual who plans for his own or his family's health, to health workers who plan on a one-to-one basis with clientele, on up to those planning at national and international levels (Robinette, 1970).

EVERYONE INVOLVED IN HEALTH HAS PLANS

One of the many complexities of health care is the reality that each person or group of persons involved in a health problem has a plan and an area of planning. The individual who decides to seek help for a health problem comes with a plan already partially implemented. Those he consults very quickly become involved in planning, whether it be doctor, nurse, neighbor, or government agency or whatever. Each one assesses, diagnoses, prescribes, and evaluates on the basis of his expertise and role.

The Consumer Plans

The consumer (client/patient) has a health care plan. His area of expertise is *his* experience with health problems, earlier coping mechanisms, and knowledge of the resources available to him. Normally he seeks outside assistance in his planning when he desires validation of his own health care plan or when his plan is no longer adequate to deal with the problem(s) he sees himself facing.

Health Professionals Plan

Health care professionals plan for the health of individuals and groups with varying frames of reference. The nutritionist diagnoses problems of nutritional inadequacy and the barriers to restoring balances, then uses knowledge and expertise to try to bring about positive change. The physical therapist deals with problems of musculoskeletal immobility or weakness, the social worker with socio-economic, environmental, and, often, emotional factors in health. And so the list goes.

But what of the two long term major health care providers and their areas of contribution—the doctors and the nurses? For so long, nurses saw their contribution to the client's health as being given through the auspices of the doctor; the nurse facilitated the doctor's medical therapy. With newer role shifts, how do the planning functions differ?

Medical Plans. Viewing physicians in terms of their education, their areas of

8

research, their publications, the content of their conversations about clients and the actions and priorities they prescribe as they plan for medical care, it can be seen that their operationally defined service primarily focuses on pathophysiology or pathopsychology. They plan for the activities needed to diagnose these conditions with precision. Their treatment plans predominantly involve medications and/or surgical intervention. In practice they *primarily, but not exclusively,* plan for the diagnosis, treatment and prevention of pathology.

Nursing Plans. In situations where nurses actually are planning for *nursing* care, not merely carrying out a prescribed medical treatment, the nurse's primary focus is to help the client to participate in living as effectively as possible. A pain medication given is not just a shot or a pill correctly administered, but a means of helping the person to become more comfortable so as to enhance coping with living in the face of suffering. For the nurse, plans are *primarily,* but not exclusively, involved with the client's coping behavior and resources as well as those of persons who are significant to him.

An Example of Medical and Nursing Plans. Let's take the example of an individual who has just had exploratory surgery. The findings: inoperable cancer. The doctor has begun prescription of pain-relieving medications. The client now faces the unenviable and lonely task of living the rest of his days with increasing dysfunction and, eventually, the knowledge of imminent death. The nurse, whether the contact is in the hospital, office or home, develops a plan that is as well founded and as appropriately individualized as the one which the doctor uses to manage the client's subsequent responses to increasing pathology. Both will be closely related.

One of the nurse's primary concerns will be with the way in which the client and his family may be expected to cope with dying in the stages that have been identified—denial, anger, bargaining, grief, and acceptance (Kübler-Ross, 1971). To function effectively, the nurse will need to diagnose the stage at which the client and the family currently wish to function, then plan actions which support their changing patterns over time (Heusinkveld, 1972).

In addition to helping the client and the family cope, intellectually and emotionally, the nurse will also be planning with them the modification needed in activities of daily living and in the environment as functional abilities change. Living with pain is almost always a problem to the person dying of cancer and to those around him. Understanding, supplies and technical skills may all be needed to provide some measure of comfort. Anorexia and nausea also present ongoing challenges each day. Dressings, skin care, grooming, elimination—any and all may require nursing assistance. Symptoms will need to be interpreted to the client and to his family, particularly when an individual chooses to die at home; they need to know what to expect and what to do when health care personnel are not immediately available.

The family may need help to marshal their resources and obtain enough relief from the constant trauma of participating in the dying of a loved one so that they too will have the stamina and endurance needed. Even following the death, the nurse might be involved in assisting relatives to cope with the grief, guilt, and mourning that ensue.

For both the doctor and the nurse, the overall goal is to support the client and those around him to experience death in the way they wish or need to do so. To achieve this goal, each health professional will not only plan separately, but will facilitate the other's planning for achieving the client/family goals.

Summary. The health care resources needed by individuals and groups to maintain their health and well-being vary over time. Often self care is quite adequate. At other times, one or more of the health care disciplines assume portions of the responsibility. When nurses are involved, their contributions need to be as well conceived and as skilled as those of any other practitioner.

THE MANDATE FOR NURSING CARE PLANNING

It is unfortunate that the legal and professional mandate for planning nursing care preceded the nurses' vision of its significance. Small wonder that capable, hard-working nurses who were primarily taught the skills of caring for patients saw planning as paper work to be done when and if there was time. Nurses at workshops have frankly stated that this was their feeling, and Kardexes abound with evidence as the space for nursing care plans has remained blank or reiterated the medical diagnoses and treatment plans.

As the complementarity of nursing's functions to other disciplines becomes clearer, the areas of nursing accountability come into increasingly sharp focus. Professional autonomy is more clearly reasonable and realistic.

REFERENCES

Heusenkveld, Karen. "Cues to Communicating with the Terminal Cancer Patient," *Nursing Forum* 11:105-113, No. 1, 1972.

Kübler-Ross, Elisabeth. "What Is It Like To Be Dying?" "Learning About Death and Dying," *American Journal of Nursing* 71:54-59, January, 1971.

Robinette, Tasker K. "What Is Health Planning?" *Nursing Outlook:* 33–35, January, 1970.

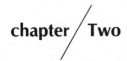

chapter / Two

The Plan:
a *product of process and knowledge*

The nursing plan that is created for any individual or group is only the visible end product of a dynamic, ongoing process. It is as sound as the skills and knowledge that are used by the person constructing it.

The term "nursing process" has been coined to label a concept involving a pattern of observation and logical thinking that is the basis for formulating the nursing care plan. This concept is not peculiar to nursing but is an adaptation from very general usage. The elements are those which maintain the functioning of any open system.[1] The concept has been examined in terms of mechanisms for maintaining homeostasis, for achieving change, for learning, for problem solving, and for decision making, among others. Often the labels used to describe the steps vary with the discipline, but the essential intent remains unchanged.

Since health care planning, and more specifically nursing care planning, is our focus, the labels used will be those of the health professions. The approach will be to divide the process into five general steps: assessment, diagnosis, prescription, implementation and evaluation.

ATTRIBUTES OF THE NURSING PROCESS

The concept of the nursing process has several general properties. This pattern of thinking and behaving:

1. is cyclic and recurring
2. may be carried on with awareness, or almost automatically
3. can be learned in terms of skill and speed
4. may be carried out with varying speed ranging from almost instantaneous thinking to protracted deliberation

[1] An open system is a set of elements in interaction involving exchange of energy, matter or information with the environment. It receives input and releases output to the environment. By a self-regulating feedback mechanism it is able to maintain patterns and organization despite ongoing changes in its environment.

5. integrates priority setting and feedback mechanisms into every step
6. is dependent upon the effective use of a body of knowledge
7. involves verbal symbols (words)

These attributes are an integral part of each of the steps as well as the totality of the concept. Test them as you examine the operational definition of the process that follows.

THE NURSING PROCESS, OPERATIONALLY DEFINED

The five major components of the nursing process can be operationally defined in terms of the behavior needed to achieve them. From these activities the necessary skills can be determined.

Assessment

Assessment is the collection of a data base followed by the formation of impressions of the situation. It is the foundation for the remainder of the process. If the assessment component is weak or inaccurate all that follows will lack validity.

Collection of Subjective Data. The subjective data are concerned with the individual's view of what he is experiencing. *It is the area in which the client is the expert.* It includes the systematic collection of data via the nursing history and the medical history. It also includes the ongoing comments that reflect the individual's perceptions of himself and the world as he sees and experiences it.

Collection of Objective Data. This assessment activity involves the use of any and all sense organs to perceive cues about the status or responses of the client. Done in a systematic fashion it is labelled a physical examination or a functional assessment. Beyond this initial systematic review it is supplemented and updated by continuing observation in contacts with the client, his environment, and persons that are important to him.

Forming Tentative Impressions. Once the data base has been initiated, it is possible to organize the units of information into logical clusters as a basis for formulating initial impressions or possible interpretations. Occasionally the data are pathognomonic (have only one possible meaning). More often there are several possible interpretations and the firm conclusions are delayed until the next step is taken.

Validation of Impressions. Given several possible conclusions, the next step in the assessment process involves the collection of more focusing data from the situation in order to narrow the options to the most specific one that describes it best. This step is comparable to the physician's differential diagnosis.

Ruling Out Problems. The ruling out of problems is as active a process as that of ruling them in. In this step the data are used to confirm that certain problems do not exist for the individual at this time, or that he is coping with them effectively and therefore does not require nursing assistance with them at present.

Diagnosis

Precise Statement of the Situation. For the nurse, as for the physician, this step involves translating the data into words that precisely communicate the client's situation. For the physician it is often a term accepted as meaning a certain syndrome or a particular form of pathology, i.e., uremia, hypothyroidism, cholelithiasis. For the nurse the diagnosis is usually a statement of the impact of a functional deficit on the lifestyle, and as yet we have not compacted these syndromes into single words. Thus the nurse's statement of diagnosis is likely to be a statement rather than a word, i.e., Sev. dyspnea → inability for any ADL or, Dyspnea → rest periods between usual ADL. Perhaps nursing will move toward one-word labels for cue syndromes within its field of knowledge, or perhaps (as in psychiatry) one-word stereotyping labels will come only to be seen as counter-productive for planning therapy.

Predicting Outcomes and Goals. The data base and the resulting diagnosis make it possible to discern the direction the disability or functional deficit is likely to take. From this the practitioner can develop statements of the client's and the nurse's potential/desired outcomes or goals.

Prescription

Prescription is the creation of specifications that certain forms of activity or therapy will be undertaken. First, there is a consideration of the options for action that will enable the client to achieve the desired outcome within present circumstances. From these options, a selection is made of actions which are predicted to most effectively achieve this result. Finally, the prescriptions are put into the specific terms necessary to have them accurately interpreted as a directive for action.

Implementation

Implementation involves the carrying out of the prescribed therapy, by the one who did the prescribing, or by another. When the activity is delegated, implementation involves effective communication of prescriptions to the persons to whom it is delegated and assurance that it has been therapeutically accomplished. This activity could be compared to the physician's writing his medical orders for delegated functions, and then checking back on his next visit to determine the manner in which the activities were carried out.

Evaluation

Evaluation is concerned with the setting of criteria for observing/measuring client response as a basis for judging the effectiveness of any part of the process. The physician uses such criteria as a return to normal ranges of laboratory values, x rays, and vital signs, as well as reported and visible increase in well-being. The nurse may establish criterion measures involving increased competence, greater endurance or strength, less pain, more involvement, more reported satisfaction, evidence of initiative, and so forth.

The Next Step

The next step (there seems to be no final one) is a return to the data collection step in order to obtain data within the evaluative criterion measures. Thus one continues in the cycle.

OUTLINE OF OPERATIONALIZED NURSING PROCESS

Assessment	Collection of subjective and objective data.
	Formation of tentative impressions.
	Validation by collection of focusing data to confirm or revise initial impressions.
	Ruling out problems where there is evidence they do not exist, or where the client is coping effectively.
Diagnosis	Precise statement describing the situation.
Prescription	Prescribing of specific therapeutic behavior.
Implementation	Personally acting in terms of the prescription or delegating the activity to others, with follow-up to assure its accomplishment.
Evaluation	Development of observational criteria and collecting data on the effectiveness of any and all portions of the plan.

ILLUSTRATION OF THE CLINICAL APPLICATION OF THE NURSING PROCESS

A community health nurse is making a follow-up visit to a diabetic client, Mrs. Solvig Sunnerstrom. She rings the doorbell and is greeted by a sturdy, middle-aged man with a weatherbeaten face smoking an equally weatherbeaten pipe. "You must be the nurse," he says, "I'm Hjalmar Sunnerstrom. Come in. My wife will be right down."

As he takes the pipe from his mouth to greet her, the nurse notices a quarter-inch encrusted area on his lower lip.

Assessment

Collection of subjective data.
1. How long has he had the lesion?
2. What is his perception of the cause of the lesion? (fall, cut, bump)
3. How has he attempted to treat it?
4. History of smoking habits?
5. Does the lesion cause difficulties in any activities such as eating and drinking?

Collection of objective data.
Observable cues: He speaks with a decided Scandinavian accent. Complexion—fair. Hair—blond. Sex—male. Age—appears to be in his fifties. Skin—appears leathery and weatherbeaten. Pipesmoker. Small encrusted area on right outer third of lower lip where his pipe was resting.

Impressions.
An encrusted lesion on the lower lip could be the result of a herpes simplex virus, trauma or neoplasm.

Factors weighting impression of neoplasm—Predisposing factors of male, older age group, fair complexion, Scandinavian origin, exposure to the weather, pipe smoking over time. Evidence of non-tenderness since the pipe rested on the lesion originally and was returned to this position.

Validation

In response to a question Mr. Sunnerstrom tells the nurse, "Oh I've had this little thing on my lip for about two months. It doesn't hurt or bother me. I just leave it alone and it will go away pretty soon. My pipe? Well I've smoked a pipe since I was a young man—I started when I went out on the fishing boats in Sweden."

The nurse notices a photograph on the mantle. It is a much younger version of Mr. and Mrs. Sunnerstrom standing before a moored fishing boat bearing the name, Solvig. "Is that your boat?" The question launches Hjalmar Sunnerstrom into a narrative that takes him from his boyhood days on his father's fishing boat in Sweden through his immigration to the Pacific Northwest and and his career as a fisherman in Alaskan waters over the years. As he talks he smokes his pipe, shifting the stem to several positions without grimacing. Palpation of lymph nodes in the neck gives no evidence of enlargement.

Ruling Out
A cold sore would not last two months and would be tender.
There is no reported history of injury.
The lesion is not painful or tender.
It does not interfere with eating or drinking.

Diagnosis

Based on the subjective and objective data obtained from and about Mr. Sunnerstrom the nurse concluded that the most likely diagnosis was a neoplasm of the lip.

Given the probable direction this lesion would take, it became the nurse's goal to encourage him to seek medical attention as promptly as possible, to confirm the diagnosis and plan for necessary treatment. However it is necessary for the nurse to make further assessments as to Mr. Sunnerstrom's goals and factors that would affect his use of the health care system:

What has been his previous experience with health care?
What are his perceptions regarding needed medical care?
What knowledge does he have of cancer and its predisposing factors that might influence his participation in treatment?
What cultural factors will enter into his decisions?
How long will he be on shore before his next fishing expedition?

Prescription

The nurse learns that Mr. Sunnerstrom is not aware of the potential implications of the little sore on his lip, that he has never had need for a doctor's services in this country, that he sees himself as a virile, healthy, relatively young man in a family known for it longevity and where ailments are a sign of weakness. With this in mind, the options for action seem to fall within the area of building trust and using the ethnic and personal values as factors in assisting him to make the decision to see a physician. The prescription is for exploration and dialogue in these areas, with reinforcement of movement toward seeking medical help.

Implementation

Initially the implementation rests with the nurse. If and when Mr. Sunnerstrom chooses to include his wife, she too may be involved and the nurse will help her to participate as effectively as possible.

Evaluation

Criteria for evaluating the effectiveness of the process:

1. Does Mr. Sunnerstrom make contact with a doctor?
2. Does he express satisfaction with the decision?
3. Was the diagnosis of malignancy confirmed? If so:
4. What evidence is there that he is coping with the knowledge of change in his image of himself generated by the diagnosis?
5. How is he responding to the anticipation of therapy?
6. How are he and his wife coping with the daily stress responses they are both experiencing?

Summary

The situation involving the Sunnerstroms in the health care system is obviously not remaining static. As long as they engage the services of the nurse, the nursing process will be the method by which the plan for their health care is kept in tune with their current situation.

APPLYING BASIC KNOWLEDGE IN THE NURSING PROCESS

Attempting to use the nursing process without a knowledge base would, of course, be impossible. Knowledge shapes the action and direction of each step. Neither the process nor the knowledge can stand alone. We have all seen academic whiz kids who were a total loss in the clinical situation because they were unable to apply the facts they had learned to interpret the patient's situation. We have also seen those who religiously carry out each step of the nursing process but never with any success because their body of knowledge is inadequate to lend meaning to the situation. It is the combination of an adequate knowledge base plus skill in the nursing process that determines the quality of planning that finally emerges.

Because of the importance of this relationship of knowledge and the nursing process, the next pages will be devoted to clinical situations illustrating this relationship. As you read, consider other nursing situations in which knowledge or lack of knowledge became a critical factor in the plan of care.

Knowledge and Assessment

Knowledge is the key to assessment. It is a major determinant of attending to significant cues from the client and his environment. As Bruner wrote, "Discovery, like surprise, favors the well prepared mind."[2]

The concept of normality and the knowledge base to recognize responses that fall within this range form the basis for assessment of deviation from the norms. This knowledge must of necessity encompass norms within physiologic parameters, cultures, psychology, sociology, biophysics, biochemistry, pharmacology, and a host of related disciplines.

On the foundation of the knowledge of normality is built the awareness of deviations from normal. A nurse unfamiliar with normal and abnormal electrocardiographic tracings might well ignore a shift to fibrillation, or become alarmed at an abnormal tracing produced by a shifting in the client's position. To an observer who does not know that most suicidal individuals verbalize their intent before taking action, the remark, "Life isn't worth living anymore" might be seen as a passing comment rather than as an important sign. Many persons who suffer myocardial infarction have prodromal symptoms of fatigue, shortness of breath and intermittent chest pain prior to the acute episode, if any one had bothered to observe or ask. Neck veins that remain distended when the individual is sitting up at an angle of more than 30 degrees represents venous back pressure, again an important consideration. The loss of an earlier arrhythmia following digitalization can indicate digitalis intoxication—not improvement.

The nurse can discontinue the assessment process prematurely unless knowledge of various etiological factors keeps the observation open. One cannot as-

[2] Jerome Bruner, *On Knowing, Essays for the Left Hand* (New York: Atheneum Publishing Co., 1966), p. 82.

sume that the patient's poor appetite reflects anxiety without systematically collecting data about his pattern of eating habits, the significance of food to him, the sociocultural and economic factors that may influence his eating behavior and his food preferences and dislikes. Knowledge about the mechanisms and factors influencing appetite and satiety gives direction to the nurse's assessment in problem areas involving eating.

Knowledge also offers the key to the determination of urgency of attention. If one attends to the disorientation caused by cerebral hypoxia rather than to the respiratory obstruction, the error in priority could lead to disastrous outcomes. Airways must be cleared and circulation restored within a limited period of time if permanent damage is to be avoided. Adequate knowledge of the significance of priorities can become very important in high risk areas of response.

In addition to knowledge needed to distinguish between normal and abnormal and between degrees of urgency and priority, the nurse also needs knowledge of the resources and techniques for acquiring data within the assessment process.

Knowledge and Diagnosis

The role of knowledge in determining a differential diagnosis is obvious. The welter of information we take in is organized and processed into logical groupings on the basis of knowledge. One cannot diagnose a response of anxiety unless the criteria for defining anxiety are known. One cannot make a judgment on whether a person is in a diabetic coma or insulin shock unless the differentiating cues are recognized. And how does one distinguish between the phenomena of unconsciousness related to sleep and coma unless there is knowledge of the criteria for defining each? The accuracy of diagnosis is directly related to the extent of the individual's working knowledge.

Let's look at a situation in which a diagnosis was made that seemed to rest on inadequate knowledge.

> Miss Gertrude Greer, an 82-year-old retired school teacher, entered the waiting room of a free nursing clinic in her retirement residence. The nurse noticed that she walked slowly, did not smile, looked unhappy. Her posture and demeanor seemed to droop. She was not as well-groomed as she had been on previous visits.
>
> She is coming to the clinic to have her blood pressure taken as a check on her response to the reserpine her doctor has prescribed for her. She missed her doctor's appointment last month in order to attend the funeral of her closest friend.
>
> As she sits down at the table the nurse asks, "How have things been going, Miss Greer?" There's a pause, then she responds, "Just terrible. I'm no good for anything. I haven't felt like eating for weeks. I don't feel like doing anything anymore. I'm tired all of the time, even when I get up in the morning."
>
> Suppose the nurse had arrived at a diagnosis of depression: certainly

there were data to document this. However, she might well have overlooked other causative factors in Miss Greer's obvious state of depression: manifestations of normal grieving, nutritionally based iron deficiency anemia, or possible toxic effects of the reserpine. Each of these diagnoses would ·necessitate differing forms of therapy, so the accuracy of the diagnosis becomes crucial.

As nurses assume greater responsibility for expanded and extended functions in high risk areas, in more remote localities, and at times when physician backup is less available, the importance of accurate diagnosis on the part of both nurse and physician is increasing. Furthermore, regardless of physician backup, professional nurses are going to be expected to make valid nursing diagnoses in all settings.

Knowledge and Prescribing

It is only as one understands the underlying mechanisms involved in a particular phenomenon or situation that one can prescribe actions with any degree of security about the outcome. This is as true for nursing activities as it is for the physician who knows which antibiotic will predictably halt the growth of a known organism.

Consider the following nursing situations:

If the panic of anxiety is a response to the mechanism of sensory overload and "jamming," then the nurse will deliberately refrain from introducing additional stimulation. She won't touch. Her verbal communication will be short. She will not speak loudly. She will not introduce more visual input than is necessary.

If a high level of anxiety is a deterrent to learning and a stressful, anxiety-producing situation is rapidly approaching, the nurse will not choose this time to introduce new learning. She may even anticipate that the client will forget previously learned material and show some lack of coordination.

If a person with gonorrhea comes from a cultural group that does not include the germ theory in its belief system, an approach other than a discussion of gram-negative diplococci will be needed.

If deep breathing is known to produce coughing whenever there are secretions in the bronchial tree, why prescribe deliberate attempts at coughing?

If self-feeding is shown not to produce ischemic tracings on electrocardiograms of persons with cardiac damage, why prescribe routine feeding?

If effective learning occurs more readily with active involvement, why prescribe "telling" as the predominant form of health care teaching? Why not seek more participant action?

Knowledge is the basis for decisions as to what is prescribed, when the prescription is carried out, its duration and frequency, as well as the degree of client involvement.

Knowledge and Implementation

Beyond prescribing, knowledge is needed for implementation as well, whether one carries out the prescribed activities personally or delegates them. If the prescribed activity involves suctioning a tracheostomy, the nurse must have knowledge regarding proper suctioning techniques in order to remove the secretions without traumatizing the mucosa. Or in another example, the nurse cannot safely change the position of a quadriplegic patient unless there is knowledge of body alignment and prevention of deformities and contractures.

In addition to being personally knowledgeable and competent in the techniques involved in carrying out the prescribed behavior, the nurse needs some additional knowledge when the care is delegated. Here the knowledge base concerns not only techniques and rationale, but also the process of delegation, motivation, dynamics of group process, leadership and organization, learning and a host of other areas. Consider the knowledge that is needed in order to delegate client care to the following colleagues if you know that:

> Ella Brown, LPN, has difficulty relating to authority figures.
> Jean Gregory, RN, had a radical mastectomy six months ago and the client who needs care has a diagnosis of metastatic cancer of the breast.
> Etta Spaulding, 72-year-old single lady, refused to sign the operative permit until she could see and hold her cat. The hospital policy prohibits pets in the hospital.
> The home health aide dislikes caring for elderly women, but the needs at present are those of women in the retirement residences.
> The head nurse believes that good nursing care is epitomized by efficient service in which clients are bathed by 11 a.m., yet Mrs. Sutter has been awake much of the night and needs to sleep. Also she prefers to take her shower in the evening.

Implementation on the current nursing scene necessitates the creative use of knowledge from a wide variety of disciplines.

Knowledge and Evaluation

In a similar fashion, development of criteria by which to judge the efficacy of prescribed therapy must be based on knowledge of what constitutes valid indicators of response within a given goal or to a particular intervention. For example, an increase in body weight is a positive indicator where increase in body size is the goal, but a negative indicator when fluid retention is the problem. Many nursing criteria are much less direct, more elusive, more complex in their relationship to both goals are interventions.

Medicine, as well, is struggling with indicators of effective medical practice, particularly with the ambulatory chronically ill where physiologic change is minimal or slowly ebbing toward the negative. However, knowledge creatively applied can help the nurse develop accurate, observable indicators of client response.

SUMMARY

Nurses use the same pattern of inquiry and thinking as other science-based practitioners as they seek to plan nursing care that is valid for a particular individual's needs. The nurse requires the same rigor in use of a knowledge base. And in the end, the skill which the practitioner applies in inquiry and critical thinking as she blends the data on the specific situation with the knowledge needed to interpret, prescribe, and evaluate will be a major factor in the quality of care the client receives.

chapter / Three

Values That Affect Nursing Care Planning

Having made a case for the quality of care planning being based on the level of skill in the use of the nursing process and a firm theoretical framework. It may now seem incongruous to suggest that the most scientifically sound plan can break apart on the hidden shoals of consumer values. Yet examples of this abound:

> The hospital facilities for delivering babies are as safe and convenient as current hospital architecture and technology can make them, the staff prepared to offer competent service. Still, hundreds of women are having their babies in their homes or in communes. Why?

> Clinics are being set up in shabby rooms with cast-off furnishings and equipment and part-time volunteer workers, despite the presence nearby of large, established outpatient departments with the latest in equipment and supplies. Why?

> Boards of consumers of health services who are organizing to develop community-based health care services are excluding available, well-prepared health professionals from their membership. Why?

If the planned and delivered services were consonant with the consumers' values and expectations, there would be little need to go outside the system for desired health care. What are consumers experiencing that leads them to believe that the system and the actions of its practitioners are inimical to their best interests as clients? Let's listen to reports of their experience with the health care system and the beliefs these seem to generate. Perhaps there will be some answers to our questions.

> "When I came to the clinic with my little girl, I needed help. Right now! But they seemed to feel they couldn't do anything for us until they took care of the paperwork."

> **Belief: The system sets priorities of paper over people.**

> "Even when you got an appointment you wait and wait and wait. I had an appointment at 2:00 and I didn't get in until 4:30. And I wasn't as bad off

22

as the man next to me in a wheelchair. He kept sliding down till he was lying on the middle of his back. And someone would come along and yank him back up again. But they didn't take him any sooner."

Belief: They just don't care about people.

"There is this credibility gap. They don't seem to believe what you tell them. And you don't know whether to believe what they tell you. Either that or you get the runaround. They think you park your brains with your valuables when you are admitted."

Belief: They think they know what is best for you. You can't trust them. They don't trust you.

"If you're not an interesting clinical phenomenon, they aren't much interested in you. And if you have something wrong with you that is unusual, you're so interesting that everyone has to prod and question you. They make rounds and talk over you, around you, but not to you."

Belief: Pathology is more interesting than the person who has it.

"We were told we needed to have a community health nurse come and check my husband after his operation. Well, I needed someone to help me bathe him, so I figured this would be a good service. The nurse came and asked if we understood the medications—I didn't know the names, but I knew what they were for and when he had to take them. She said, 'That's good. You seem to be doing fine.' Then she gave us a bill for $13.50. Later I learned you have to get a home health aide if you want help with care."

Belief: Nurses talk and cost more. Home health aides do and cost less.

"There was this sign in a doctor's clinic—right next to the reception desk, 'Welfare cases not accepted.' I guess the payments aren't enough to take care of the paper work. You feel that you're not wanted when you need help."

Belief: Government supported service may mean no service or less service from the system.

"I had this lump in the upper outer quadrant of my breast. I told the surgeon, 'If the frozen section shows malignancy, just sew it up. No radical mastectomy for me with the odds this location has!' I had to argue, shout, and finally threaten to go to another surgeon before he would agree to my choice of options."

Belief: You lose your right to choose once you enter the health care system.

These examples have focused on some beliefs that come from disillusioned consumers in their use of the health care system. No doubt, as many examples could be cited of people who have had positive experiences. But the point is that even though lives are being saved and therapy is sounder and more pre-

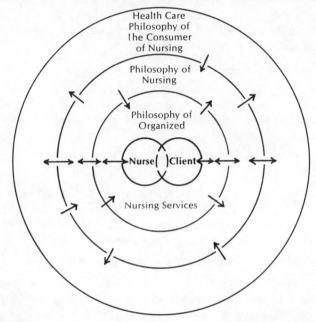

Health Care
Philosophy of
the Consumer
of Nursing

Philosophy of
Nursing

Philosophy of
Organized

Nurse Client

Nursing Services

A MODEL OF INTERACTION OF VALUES INFLUENCING HEALTH CARE PLAN-
NING. Many values of both individuals and groups influence the health care planning at all levels. The relationship may be likened to this group of concentric circles, with forces of influence flowing in both directions—from larger circles to
those within and from the smaller circles to those without.

dictably effective than ever before, still there is this strong undercurrent of dissatisfaction. And, while there are more and better prepared health care workers,
there are widely held beliefs that the health care personnel and the system are
more self-serving than they are concerned with meeting the expressed needs of
the consumers.

What then is the point of considering the widespread negative opinions consumers hold about health care personnel and the system? What has this to do
with health care planning? Each of us as individuals and members of groups,
whether we are providers of health care services or consumers, perceive, interpret, function, make choices and react in terms of the values we hold, even
though we may not be aware of them. It is the *interaction* of these values, and
the behavior that results, which becomes a crucial part of any planning for health
care. Within the health care system, and nursing in particular, there are several
groups whose values are particularly significant in their interaction—consumer
groups, nursing professionals, organized nursing services and the individual client
and nurse. These values and beliefs and their interaction are interwoven throughout the entire planning process.

THE CONSUMERS' PHILOSOPHY OF HEALTH CARE

A philosophy that affects health care is that of the public. Health, illness and the treatment of illness are important segments of the value system of every culture from the most primitive to the most advanced.

Consumers' Expectations for Health Care Services

There has been a growing acceptance of the idea that consumers today believe health care services are a basic right, not just a privilege. This is held to be true regardless of race, age, sex, religion, socioeconomic status, geographic locale, moral values or lifestyle.

Expectations Regarding Rights as Individual Consumers. Beyond the basic belief that it is their right to have health and health care, consumers have expectations as to their rights when they as individuals purchase health care services. They expect:

to be treated as a person rather than as a disease entity, a set of symptoms, a thing, a number or a member of some particular group.

to be given the opportunity to participate knowledgeably in decisions regarding the care being offered.

to be kept as comfortable as modern science permits and they desire.

to be accepted in a state of dependency when this seems necessary to them.

to be helped to understand the status of health, illness, and the therapy being experienced.

to experience acceptance of their lifestyle and cultural values together with the coping behavior these generate, but to understand the relationship between lifestyle and the health care options.

to decline and die in the manner they choose for themselves.

to feel cared about as well as cared for during the experiences of illness and dying.

to be evaluated in terms of personal well-being as well as objective response to treatment.

to have access to a health care advocate as a guardian of their rights, particularly when illness renders the individual or his family unable or unknowing.

Consumers' Beliefs About the Characteristics of the Health Care System. In addition to the beliefs consumers hold about their rights as individuals, they have expectations regarding the nature of the system and characteristics of the services. They believe the service should be organized in such a way as to make them:

Available: obtainable in reality as well as in theory, to all segments of society. "If I'm poor, can I obtain health care?" "If I can't afford insurance premiums, is health care available?" "Do I have to live in a city to have medical care?"

25

Individualized: facilitative of individual assessment and participation rather than stereotyped and routine. "Why do I go to bed in a hospital at 10:00 P.M. when I normally do so at 1:00 A.M.?" "Why can't I be given information about myself on which to base decisions?

Socially relevant: offered where the consumers need the services within the context of the social systems of which they are members. "Why is it so difficult to get a home delivery?" "Why are my culture-based health beliefs and practices not respected and used?"

Accessible: located and scheduled so that, for emergency or ongoing care, consumers are able to reach them with reasonable effort and expense. "Why are settings for care of the mentally ill, the retarded and often the aged so far away from people centers?" "Why is it so dangerous to become ill on a weekend?"

Coordinated: harnessing modern technology in communication to reduce gaps, duplications and fragmentation of data gathering and therapy currently being experienced by both the consumer and health care practitioners. "Why are tests and histories repeated at every entry point to any part of the system?" "Why are they not communicated and revised as I change?" "Why is care so fragmented?"

Comprehensive: effective reinforcement (with status and rewards) of prevention, rehabilitation, and maintenance care as effectively as emergency, lifesaving, and cure have been. "Why is the emphasis on curing my acute illness?" "Why is there so little status in maintaining me at my highest level of functioning when I have chronic illness or a declining state of health?" "Why is there so little financial support for maintenance?" "Why does maintenance equal custodial and custodial equal a negative word?" "Must I be a negatively viewed 'custodial case' just because I can't get better?"

These values and others collected from health care consumers associated with the service and care of the individual can provide insight and guidelines for planning and implementation of health care at any level.

COMPONENTS OF A PHILOSOPHY OF NURSING

Nursing at its core concerns: (a) human beings who take on or who are placed in reciprocal roles of nurse and client, and (b) the interaction and relationship between them when they are in these roles. Thus, a nurse's philosophy must include beliefs about man, about the reciprocal roles of client and nurse, and about the transaction between them which is labeled nursing.

Beliefs about Human Beings

Since human beings occupy both the roles of nurse and client, they have much in common that affects them as they assume differing roles. Obviously, beliefs and values about the nature, the rights and responsibilities of human beings precede thinking about specific roles a person might occupy.

Here are some "building blocks" you may consider as you build your philosophy.

As human beings we:

Vary in our ability to cope successfully with the stress of illness physically and psychologically, on the basis of both genetic endowment, experience, and environmental influences.

Are equipped with mechanisms to maintain a relatively stable internal state provided the magnitude and/or duration of the stressors do not exceed our immediate capacity and reserves.

React totally to the stress of illness: physiologically, emotionally, and intellectually.

Have individual worth.

Have the right to continued autonomy during health care or illness.

Have the right and the responsibility to participate in our health care in illness as in health.

Have the capacity to change our behavior (to learn).

Are not separable from our culture.

Are goal-directed in our behavior.

Experience anxiety when exposed to the unknown.

May mature as a result of learning successful adaptive behavior in or with experiences of illness and disability.

Are not isolated, but belong to some constellation of fellow human beings, family, friends, and others important to us.

Tend to interpret and to respond to a current situation on the basis of past experiences.

Experience needs in a hierarchy wherein survival and safety assume priority over needs for love, esteem, growth, and self-actualization.

Obviously these 14 statements do not exhaust the beliefs and values one may incorporate into a philosophy of man, but they may serve as stimulants to consider others or may evoke variations more compatible with your beliefs.

Beliefs about the Client Role

Who is a Patient or Client? Under what circumstances does a person become a patient or a client of health professionals? When does he assume this particular role in his life? One belief might be:

When a person acknowledges, or by circumstances beyond his control is forced to admit, that he does not have the resources, skills, or knowledge to effectively deal with a health problem and its effect on his daily living, he tends to accept or be placed in the role of client in the health care system.

In addition, relatives or those close to a person seeking or receiving health care services also may become a nurse's clients.

This belief covers clientele in the usual sense of those who seek services of the health care system on their own. But it also would accommodate the preventive concept of case finding. A person identified as having a potential or current health problem may take one of three options:

1. He may choose to seek help and therefore accept the client role.
2. He may, in the case of certain diseases or behavior, be forced into the role, i.e., commitment for mental illness or restriction because of communicability of diseases.
3. He may choose not to accept the health care services at this time and thus reject the role.

Beliefs about Responsibilities Expected in the Client Role

The next belief area that would seem relevant to a philosophy of nursing would be that of changes in lifestyle associated with shifting from being a non-client to client. What is different about being a client in the health care system? What are the responsibilities associated with the role? More importantly, what do *you* expect of a person in the client role?

Do you believe he should:

cooperate readily with the plan of care as it is carried out, since health workers are educated to know what is best for him, and participate in the decision;
or
make his decision after being apprised of the options and probable outcomes whenever he is able?

accommodate to the routines of the health care system;
or
seek accommodation of the system to his ways and needs?

divulge any data the health care workers ask of him in terms of history, feelings, and the functioning of his body;
or
require and retain privacy in areas he selects?

communicate only those messages that will be safe and comfortable to the staff;
or
communicate openly and genuinely what he is experiencing at the risk of making others uncomfortable at times?

assume the ways of the culture of the people in the health care system in areas where he recognizes it and can do so;
or
continue in his own culture-based behavior without attempt at modification?

This is a sample of a few possible opposing alternatives of expectations held for people who become consumers of nursing. As you build your philosophy in this area and test it in real-life situations, you will find many others. It is helpful to consider the most extreme contrary possibilities before deciding where your own values fall within the continuum.

Again, illustrations may be in order to show how these beliefs about the consumer affect the nature of the nursing care offered. A Nursing Clinic was offered to the residents of low income housing for the elderly. When it was established, one basic belief about the clientele seemed to become a guiding force in almost every decision. The nurses believed that these women and men should maintain the highest level of independence possible in all areas of their lives, since remaining in these valued apartments required functional independence. The case that follows demonstrates the application of this belief:

> Mrs. Brant, a 78-year-old widow, dropped into the hobby room that served as a clinic to report that she was to have cataract surgery on her right eye in two weeks. The nurse realized that she would have the eye patched and shielded for a week to ten days. This would pose a problem since Mrs. Brant's other eye was virtually visionless due to long-standing glaucoma. Since Mrs. Brant wished to return to her apartment, the two of them set about planning practice sessions and techniques to enable her, with the help of other residents, to cope with daily living during these days. Mrs. Brant patched the right eye, then practiced bathing and dressing herself without stooping over. She practiced moving from room to room, locating furniture and necessary articles by touch. The three rooms were organized for safety. At the market she stocked up on convenience foods to make meal preparation easy. Other residents offered to help with meal preparation and shopping. By the time she went to the hospital she felt secure about managing her living in the face of a temporary visual deficit.

Or, take a hospital-based situation, suppose you are a nurse with the functional assignment of passing medications. What you believe about clients, their right to knowledge about therapy and their role in maintaining or regaining their health will influence your behavior in carrying out this function. If you believe that clients should not know about what they take into their bodies and need not prepare for self-medication, you can, with technical correctness and using all your knowledge of the disease and the drugs effectively, administer the drugs with minimal client involvement. Should you believe that the person needs to be an active participant in his care and learn effective drug taking technique for future self care, you will add to the above by giving more information as you see the knowledge becoming useful to the individual and helping him to plan for his own management in the future. Your choice of approach will be determined by what you believe and value.

Conflicts in Beliefs about Rights and Responsibilities. The opposite side of the coin of expectations and responsibilities is client rights. You may have noted, one alternative offered for expected behavior is the recognition of client rights. There is a hazard in setting up a separate section on clients' rights: they may not incorporate reality. And rights without reality are no rights at all! For example, on a busy hospital unit a client has a right to have his needs met, *provided* the immediate needs of others are not seen as being greater. A client may need relief from severe pain, *but* if another person is choking on his secretions, the first client's needs will wait. Also, a client's right to comfort may depend on whether his definition of comfort coincides with that of the doctor and the nurses. He may be more comfortable lying still, not coughing, but may be asked to move and cough despite the increased pain. He may expect to have no pain following treatment; the health care workers may expect him to tolerate pain within a particular time period before giving another dose of narcotic.

The most honest, realistic philosophies emerge when rights are stated in conjunction with expectations. Clients have a right to:

> free speech *if* they don't mind the flak or withdrawal that ensues should it make the staff uncomfortable.
>
> die with dignity, *but* perhaps not in a manner or at a time they choose, particularly if they choose a manner or a time the staff do not believe is appropriate.
>
> make decisions about their own care *if* they don't disrupt things too much or *if* they have the courage to buck the system when their decision does not coincide with those of the "experts."

Keep your beliefs about clients rights realistic. Should you wish to change the "ifs," the "buts," the "provides" and the "whethers," you'll need to be able to identify them and acknowledge their presence. Then you can determine whether the people involved, the system, and the environment can be modified.

Priorities of Beliefs. One may hold a body of beliefs about clients in general; however the priorities given to particular beliefs, whether they be rights or expectations may vary with differing groups of clientele. For example, the nurses in the recovery room and the intensive care unit quite appropriately give priority to values related to survival and supporting physiological defense mechanisms over autonomy and sometimes privacy; in this the nurse is using Maslow's hierarchy of Needs (Maslow, 1962). The nurse in the public health agency on the other hand may be primarily concerned with values of autonomy, of responsibility for participation, of the capacity to learn, and with the enhancement of feelings of self worth. She too, as a therapeutic agent, needs to give appropriate attention to the mechanisms by which the elderly gentleman in mild congestive failure maintains his fluid and electrolyte balance. However, when he is maintaining a reasonably steady state, these values may assume importance secondary to his learning to live in a satisfying way with chronic illness and the problems of aging.

Beliefs about the Nature of Nursing

The nature of the interaction between nurses and their clients is different from that associated with other health professionals—physicians, pharmacists, dietitians, physical therapists, social workers and others, even though occasional functions overlap. What then do nurses do that constitutes nursing?

The mere fact that nurses carry out activities does not seem to be a particularly sound basis for developing a philosophical definition of nursing interaction. A nurse may draw date lines on a chart, copy information from one source to another, order supplies, answer the telephone, chaperone a client or do a variety of other tasks—yes, these may not be nursing. A better foundation for beliefs about the nature of nursing interaction would seem to derive from an examination of the primary orientation of nursing, the purpose or focus that generates the direction and goals that nurses and nursing take.

Obviously, in reading this book you are aware of the authors' philosophical bent toward a definition of nursing that is complementary to medicine, not competing for territory. In fact there would be no point in planning nursing care if physicians were already doing it. Nor does there seem to be much merit in merely reiterating medical plans and labeling them nursing care plans, although this has been done frequently, according to Ciuca's survey (Ciuca, 1972).

The belief that will be implemented throughout this book is that:

the primary orientation of nursing is to facilitate effective living by the client and his family even as they experience current or potential health problems.

To expand this philosophical statement let us operationalize each of the critical concepts—"facilitate," "effective living," and "current or potential health problems."

Facilitate means "to make easier." To us, it implies assessment of strengths, resources, and deficits and then acting in such a way as to make it easier for the clients to function. There is a continuum to the behavior in terms of amount and type of activity. It may range at one end from doing nothing so that clients can exercise their own capacities, to taking over the activity entirely, such as managing the fluid balance, with intravenous fluids and an indwelling catheter or dialysis machine, or providing a means of breathing for him with a respirator. Between these extremes may be the provision of an environment within which it is safe for the client to practice activities such as crutch walking or being angry or saying no or measuring insulin. The nurse may provide a cheering section to encourage his efforts, or supply knowledge or resources. But the entire thrust is to use what the client has and only to add those dimensions that are assessed as being needed.

Effective living can be defined by both the client and the nurse, and often these definitions will differ. Essentially we tend to believe that it is the client's right to define effective living for himself, but it is the nurse's responsibility to enable him to perceive the options and gain enough insight to make a responsible choice.

Current or potential health problems constitute deficits in well-being as documented by the client and/or the nurse. In the case of a *current problem* the nurse collects enough data to enable her to outline an area where health has been diminished or the client reports this to be the case. *Potential health* problems exist when there is a diagnosis of high risk based on data of history, present client status and environment or predictable future conditions. Cheraskin and Ringsdorf, in their series, *Predictive Medicine,* present some interesting concepts that apply equally well to nursing (Cheraskin and Ringsdorf, 1973). For definitions of health, we suggest reading Milio's Prologue to *9226 Kercheval, The Storefront that Did Not Burn* and Wu's chapter, "The Concept of Wellness" (Milio, 1970; Wu, 1972).

You will see our beliefs about the nature of nursing implemented in each step of the nursing process from assessment through to evaluation. You will also see it in the discussion of nursing's emerging role expansion. In a similar fashion, the belief *you* hold about the entity known as nursing gives direction to your lifestyle as a nurse and to the choices you make. It is important to understand the force that influences such a large part, not only of one's own life, but also, the lives of clients and colleagues as well.

Summary

The beliefs that form a nursing philosophy serve as guidelines to whatever individual or group its values represent. From them emerge objectives, options for action, and criteria for evaluation. In succeeding sections you will see a variety of philosophies, first of departments of nursing service, and then of units within these departments, and finally, of the vital core—the relationship of individual nurse and client philosophies.

RELATIONSHIPS OF PHILOSOPHY OF NURSING TO NURSING'S OBJECTIVES

A philosophy is a statement of beliefs; an objective is a statement of goals. A philosophy is abstract; an objective is concrete. A philosophy can only be reported; achievement of an objective can be measured. Objectives are always the superstructure of a philosophical foundation.

In the pages that follow, you will see examples of philosophies of nursing subscribed to by departments of nursing service. Also included are adaptations of these for wards and individual clients. If there are objectives for which no explicit statement of beliefs is included, try to put into your words the belief that you think supports that objective.

You will notice some common components in the philosophies. They include beliefs about:

the nature of the clientele
the nature of nursing
the roles of the nursing staff
the organizational characteristics
the relationships to the community and
the nature of commitment to staff development.

PHILOSOPHIES OF DEPARTMENTS OF NURSING SERVICE

Both the American Nurses' Association and the National League for Nursing acknowledge the importance of a philosophy for nursing service. The League cites as its first criterion for evaluating a hospital department of nursing service, "The department of nursing service has definitive statements of philosophy and objectives."[1] Similarly, the first standard the ANA sets for assessing nursing service is, "The nursing department has stated beliefs and stated objective which reflect the purposes of the health care facility and give direction to the nursing care program."[2]

In the philosophies of nursing service that are in use in agencies, the influence of the clientele can be seen. As an inner circle, nursing service maintains the characteristics of its governing authority, but it also seems to absorb the characteristics of the circles within it, including the innermost circle—the client.

County Owned Hospital

The first sample philosophy was that of a county owned hospital in a metropolitan area. It was tax-supported and responsive to the local government and to the public. It had had long affiliation with the schools of nursing and medicine at the nearby state university. The philosophy and objectives developed by the department of nursing service were as follows:

Philosophy of King County Hospital Department of Nursing[3]

Our philosophy of nursing is based upon respect for the dignity and worth of the individual. We believe that each patient has the basic right to receive effective nursing care which is a personal service based on his needs as they relate to him as an individual and to his clinical disease or condition.

Recognizing the obligation of nursing to help restore the patient to the best possible state of physical, mental and emotional health and to main-

---

[1] Criteria for Evaluating a Hospital Department of Nursing Service, p. 4. New York, National League for Nursing, Department of Hospital Nursing, 1965.

[2] Standards for Organized Nursing Services in Hospitals, Public Health Agencies, Nursing Homes, Industries and Clinics, p. 8. New York, American Nurses' Association, 1965.

[3] This institution has since changed to a medical center with a philosophy modified in keeping with the changed governing body and service.

tain his sense of spiritual and social well-being, we pledge intelligent cooperation in coordinating nursing service with that of the medical and allied professional practitioners.

Understanding the importance of research and teaching for the improvement of patient care, the nursing department will support, promote and participate in these activities.

Objectives of Nursing Service

To develop recognition of the patient's need for independence, his right for privacy and his desire for self-awareness in relationship to this illness.

To provide effective patient care relative to his needs insofar as the hospital and community facilities permit.

To encourage interaction with the patient in order to assist him in his acceptance of and adjustment to his condition.

To carry out the therapeutic measures ordered by the doctors with intelligent application to the individual needs of the patient.

To create an atmosphere conducive to favorable patient and employee morale and to personnel growth.

To appreciate and acknowledge the contribution and worth of all personnel in assuring improved patient care.

To continually evaluate the competency and attitude of all employees in the nursing department.

To provide an inservice program for orientation of new employees and for the continued education of all personnel in the nursing department.

To develop an awareness and understanding of the legal responsibilities in nursing.

To study and evaluate the quality of nursing care and implement improvements.

To interpret, implement and uphold hospital policy.

To support the financial plan of the hospital.

To support and participate in research and educational programs.

To cooperate with all departments within the hospital in furthering the purposes of the institution.

To foster and maintain good public relations.

This philosophy places first its belief that "nursing is based upon respect for the dignity and worth of the individual." Some persons who enter the doors of a county institution may seem to have lost their own sense of dignity and worth. Nursing service administrators have expectations that nurses who work in this setting will not accept these individuals' current estimate of themselves, but will accord service based on the foregoing ideal. Restoration to the best possible health and sense of well-being are natural outgrowths of this belief.

Belief in educational obligations is reflected in both the philosophy and its objectives. The goals of creating high employee morale, of continued opportunities for growth, and acknowledgment and appreciation of achievement, indicate that educational goals are pervasive and do not relate only to students in the setting.

Objectives related to organizational, financial, and public relations goals undoubtedly tie in with those of the governing authority and the hospital's connections with the surrounding community.

Psychiatric Institution

The philosophy of the Illinois State Psychiatric Institute (George, 1967) differs from those previously cited in both format and content. The current statement of philosophy is a revision of the original, which was written in 1961 (Norris, 1962). The introduction to the present philosophy indicates that it reflects a shift in the nature of therapy. In addition to the philosophy, a preface describes: the physical setting of the Institute and its nursing units, the administrative hierarchy, interdepartmental relationships and nursing functions. The philosophy itself is stated as a series of concepts followed by the subconcepts that contribute to the concept as well as the relevance to nursing functions.

The twelve major concepts incorporated in this philosophy are:

Concept   I: Man is an integrated biological, emotional, intellectual, and social being. All of man's life experiences become part of his total being.

Concept   II: Man goes through various sequential phases of growth and development in striving for maturity and personal integration. Opportunities for growth continue throughout the life of the individual.

Concept   III: Man cannot live alone. What he is endowed with at birth is developed by his contacts with others. Man becomes much of what he is through his life experiences.

Concept   IV: Man cannot be understood apart from his culture.

Concept   V: Man has an innate desire to experience life as meaningfully and as fully as he has the potential to do so.

Concept   VI: All human beings have a need to experience relationships with others which lead to self-fulfillment.

Concept   VII: Each person is a separate and unique being who is ultimately responsible for himself. Because we are part of mankind, we are also responsible to each other.

Concept VIII: All human beings have potential for change.

Concept   IX: Behavior is meaningful and can be understood.

Concept   X: Anxiety, which is common to all people, can be a motivating or an inhibiting force.

Concept   XI: Readiness for learning must be present before learning can occur.

Concept   XII: Communication occurs on several levels simultaneously, and can be understood through consideration of both its content and the relationship between the individuals involved (George, 1967).

An illustration of one of the concepts and the expansion of subconcepts and nursing implications give a further idea of how this philosophy was developed.

Concept   IX: Behavior is meaningful and can be understood.

Behavior has motivation and is purposeful. It is a response to stimuli from within and without, and it in turn has effects or consequences. All behavior is a function of the person's perception and represents both a conscious and unconscious reaction to past living experiences, present relationships, and the anticipated future. A particular behavior might be understood in a number of ways and a variety of thoughts or feelings may be expressed in the same way behaviorally. To understand behavior one must examine it in the context in which it occurs.

In order to develop skill in understanding the behavior of another, the nurse must understand that her own behavior conveys different meanings and, therefore, she must consciously examine the effects her behavior has on others. Through the development of a relationship, she can help the client to understand and validate others' perceptions of his behavior. She can examine with him his reasons for his behavior and help him to consider alternatives (George, 1967).

The expansion of ideas under each concept demonstrates the way in which this philosophy of nursing service is used to guide the preceptions, interpretation of interaction, and the actions nursing personnel undertake with clients in this particular setting.

Institutions for Mental Retardates.   Institutions devoted to the care of retarded members of our society have problems that are different from those of other institutions, and, as one might expect, this factor is incorporated into their philosophy. The following philosophy is that of a nursing service department in a center for retardates:

1. The mentally retarded differ in degree, and not in kind, from other human beings.
2. No one should enter an institution who can be cared for in the community; no one should remain who can adjust to the outside.
3. Education and training of the retarded should prepare them to adjust to as many current demands and responsibilities of society as they are able.
4. An institution caring for the mentally retarded should create an "inside" society which differs from the "outside" society only when institutional demands require it.
5. The institution should enlighten the community about the problems of mental retardation and continue to cooperate, coordinate, and even merge with community agencies (Ebbeson, 1967).

This philosophy may be very helpful in setting guidelines and priorities for nurses who function in this setting. For example, the item related to the belief that their "education and training should prepare them to adjust to as many current demands and responsibilities of society as they are able" forms the framework for many of the learning experiences provided. Society demands that its members be dressed and groomed to certain standards, that they be able to eat comfortably with others, and that they be able to handle the currency of the land. It also demands that its members contribute to its productivity whenever possible. Thus, trainable retardates are taught to dress, to set some standards for grooming, to acquire acceptable manners as they eat, and to relate to each other in group settings. They are also provided with situations in which they may learn to handle money. Those who have the potential are also placed in employment situations within the institution and thus may learn to be employable. Some of them learn to care for other residents, some are able to work in the kitchen or in the cafeteria, in the laundry, or on the grounds.

Then too, while the beliefs about education and society are being accomplished through care of the individual and modifications of the environment, the retardate is also being acquainted with his role in the "outside" society and is being readied to move into the outside world.

Nursing Home. Finally let us look at a philosophy for a nursing home. This is a care setting in which the values and beliefs of nursing service are of paramount importance. In contrast to the doctor-oriented climate of the general hospital, the nursing home tends to rely much more heavily upon independent nursing decisions and judgment.

The following philosophy is not that of a specific nursing home; rather, it is one extrapolated from literature devoted to the nursing care of persons in long-term care facilities:

1. The chronically ill person who is hospitalized for long periods has physical, emotional, and social deficits that must be compensated for.
2. Every client, no matter how disabled physically and emotionally, has some strengths that can be used in his rehabilitation.
3. Relationships within families of chronically ill undergo prolonged stress and disruption.
4. The older chronically ill person experiences family separation, the loss of his contemporaries, and the narrowirng egocentric world of the aging. The institution becomes the social world, the day-to-day family, and "important others" in his life. Room selection, roommates, socializing situations, and planned interactions assume an important priority in the objectives of care for them.
5. Diminution of sensory acuity and cerebral changes of aging make subjective reports of condition an unreliable sole source of data upon which to judge current status.
6. The client has a right to expect that hostile, agitated, depressed behavior will be understood and effectively handled by personnel.
7. Clients can be helped to adjust to physical, intellectual, and emotional

limitations and still find satisfactions in daily living.

8. Clients have a right to independence and autonomy in areas in which this is possible.

9. Clients have the right to experience social and intellectual stimulation on an ongoing basis.

10. Clients who are becoming increasingly ill, or who are dying, have the right to support, understanding, and companionship, as well as physical care.

11. Chronically ill or aging persons have a right to individualized nursing care that encourages their participation, yet serves them with dignity and graciousness in the areas in which they have deficits. When they can no longer create a world in which they belong, a world in which they can experience a genuine sense of belonging should be created for them.

Nurses who work in long-term care institutions:

1. Need to be helped to find personal satisfaction and pride of accomplishment in making days pleasant and comfortable for clients who will not get better, as well as in the small advancements they can accomplish among those who are stable or improving.

2. Need a work environment that stimulates flexibility, experimentation with new ideas, and creativity in approach.

3. Need regular communication with nurses and workers in other institutions through workshops and continuing education programs as a source of new ideas that may be employed in the care of their clientele.

4. Have an obligation to contribute to the body of nursing knowledge through their experience and research by presenting their knowledge and findings in publications and in professional meetings, both locally and nationally.

This philosophy takes cognizance not only of the nature of the clientele in this setting and the particular problems, but also of the particular needs of the nurses if they are to give satisfactory and satisfying care, which grows and develops rather than becoming stagnant and stereotyped.

Summary. The examples of nursing philosophies included have been those of institutions. However, nursing service departments in other agencies, such as public schools, business and industry, group-practice office nurses, and public health agencies, can derive like benefits from compiling a consensual statement of beliefs and objectives of their nursing service.

To recapitulate, the philosophies of nursing service departments incorporate the beliefs of the larger governing body. They make general statements of beliefs about the nature of the clientele they serve, their obligations to the nursing personnel in their department, their expectations of them, and their responsibilities to affiliating agencies and to the nursing profession.

Changes in Philosophies of Nursing Service

The following statement of the philosophy of a teaching and research hospital was included in the first edition of this book.

Teaching and Research Hospital. The nursing service philosophy in a teaching and research hospital that is part of a university community conveys slightly different emphases.

The Philosophy of the Nursing Services, University Hospital, University of Washington

The Nursing Services Department of the University Hospital recognizes and accepts the overall philosophy of the University of Washington and the University Hospital. As an integral part of these organizations, the Nursing Department will support and facilitate the teaching and research program of the University. We further acknowledge that the primary responsibility of Nursing Services is to assist the patient with meeting his needs of daily living.

We will strive to maintain and promote a democratic environment within Nursing Services so that each member of the department recognizes and respects the patient's human dignity and human rights.

In a Teaching and Research Hospital the patient is participating in experiences that will uniquely influence his activities of daily living. Nursing Services has a responsibility to help interpret these experiences and to provide support for the patient.

In order to achieve a patient-centered department, we will work closely with other professions and services within the hospital and the university.

Nursing Services accepts the responsibility of providing students with an example of high quality nursing care so that they may acquire attitudes, values and behavior patterns which will serve as a guide for development of excellent patient care.

Nursing Services recognizes the need to maintain an environment in which staff development and learning geared to improved patient care can take place.

Nursing Services has an obligation to study what constitutes effective nursing care measures, and to exhibit leadership in finding answers to many of nursing's unsolved problems. Nursing Services has the unique advantage of being in close proximity to clinical problems and in being able to assess the results of nursing actions. Nursing Services should be able to make significant contributions to the theory of nursing.[4]

In the interim between 1964 and the present the Department of Nursing Service, using a committee of volunteers who represented every category of worker in the department, developed an updated philosophy. It was rough-

[4] The Philosophy of Nursing Services, Objectives of Nursing Services. Seattle, University Hospital, University of Washington, May, 1964.

39

drafted then sent out to all the units for discussion and exploration about means of implementation. This is the new version of their philosophy:

> The Nursing Services Department of the University Hospital recognizes and accepts the overall philosophy of the University of Washington and the University Hospital. As an integral part of these organizations, the Nursing Department supports and facilitates the teaching and research programs of the University. We acknowledge, however, that the primary responsibility of Nursing Services is to the patient. We believe that this is fulfilled by meeting his needs of daily living in order to help restore him to his optimum state of health or support him toward a dignified, peaceful death.
>
> In a Teaching and Research Hospital, the patient participates in experiences that will uniquely influence his physical and emotional state of being. Nursing Services, as the patient's advocate, has the responsibility to help interpret daily experiences and to provide emotional, physical and spiritual support for the patient as well as helping him to maintain his family and community role. Since we believe that each person is a unique individual possessing human dignity and worth, his rights regardless of race, creed, color, sex or age must be preserved and protected. The patient has the right to make decisions regarding his care.
>
> We believe that the patient can best be served by collaboration with other professions and services within the hospital and the University. A democratic environment is necessary within Nursing Services to help each member of the department recognize and respect the human dignity and human rights of patients, families, and personnel alike.
>
> Nursing Services recognizes the need to maintain a milieu conducive to staff development and learning, focused on improved patient care. It is our belief that nursing personnel are unique, self-actuating individuals. A democratic environment is basic to individual growth and development because such an environment encourages self-realization and opportunities for self-expression.
>
> Nursing Services accepts the responsibility to act as role models in providing exemplary nursing care and attitudes, values and behavior patterns which may serve as a guide for the development of excellence in patient care.
>
> Nursing Services has an obligation to study what constitutes effective nursing care measures, to exhibit leadership in finding answers to many of nursing's unsolved problems and to be responsive to changes in patient care. Nursing Services has the unique advantage of being in proximity to clinical problems and in being able to assess the results of nursing actions. It is our belief that Nursing Services can and should make significant contributions to the theory of nursing both in practice and in publication.

We suggest you compare them. Note: (1) the broader approaches to the purpose of nursing and the purposes of experiences provided for clients; (2) the spelling-out of kinds of nursing support offered; (3) the inclusion of families; (4) the making mandatory of protection of client rights; (5) the specification of a collaborative relationship between nurses and other professions; (6) the specification for a democratic environment together with the rationale for it; (7) the broader use of role models; and (8), the commitment to (a) application of theory to practice and (b) publication of clinical knowledge.

Beyond maintaining a currently updated philosophy that reflects the beliefs of the members of the Nursing Service Department, they also utilize the philosophy to develop two sets of objectives. One set is involved with overall long-term objectives of the department.

Objectives of Nursing Services

1. Assist the patient to meet his needs of daily living.
2. Develop productive interdepartmental and interprofesional working relationships.
3. Contribute to student education by practicing quality nursing care.
4. Provide nursing personnel with opportunities for individual growth and development in the practice of nursing.
5. Include the patient and his family in decisions regarding his care.
6. Promote an atmosphere within the nursing services where creative ideas may be expressed.
7. Continually evaluate methods of nursing practice for areas of improvement.
8. Use results of nursing evaluation to effect change in nursing practice.

In addition annual goals are derived from these objectives. These are objectives evolved each year again using the volunteer approach from categories of workers. An annual evaluation of the effectiveness of nursing service is based on the extent and the nature of the achievement of the yearly goals. The analysis is included in the Annual Report of the Department.

Nursing Service Goals 1972-73

I. DEVELOP SELECTED POST-HOSPITALIZATION FOLLOW UP PROGRAMS FOR PATIENTS AND FAMILIES
   A. Evaluate usefulness of present methods of assisting patients and families to adjust to their post-hospitalization.
   B. Facilitate communication between hospital nursing staff and public health nurses.
   C. Develop selected resource files of pertinent available community resources.

II. DEVELOP MEANS OF COMMUNICATING WITH THE CONSUMER.
   A. Involve the patient and family in health care planning and teaching.

       B.   Revise materials provided to patients and families for general information and orientation.

       C.   Increase the participation of the patient in patient centered teaching, including activities such as rounds, case conferences, and discussions between the nurse, other health professionals & the patient and/or family.

III.   ESTABLISH *PROBLEM ORIENTED CHARTING* FOCUSING ON DEVELOPING THE TOTAL PROCESS.

       A.   Continue to review concepts and process of POC with new staff.

       B.   Refine the process as new insights evolve through ongoing use of POC.

       C.   Perform periodic review of patient records.

IV.   DEVELOP PROGRAMS AND RESOURCES AVAILABLE TO STAFF FOR ORIENTATION AND CONTINUING EDUCATION.

       A.   Establish written procedures, library materials, resource files, and guidelines pertinent to needs of individual units.

       B.   Establish special educational program for nursing staff in collaboration with the Inservice Division.

       C.   Perform periodic assessment of nursing care process and include input from the consumer in this assessment.

V.   DEFINE AND DEVELOP NURSING ROLES.

       A.   Study and implement the concept of Primary Nursing Care on select units.

       B.   Investigate role expansion of the primary nurse coordinator.

       C.   Clarify the roles of LPN, Nurse Practitioner I, II & III.

       D.   Assess the psycho-social situation of patients, and their families and utilize this information in care plans.

VI.   IMPROVE INTERSTAFF COMMUNICATION.

       A.   Provide opportunity for all staff to participate on scheduled meetings.

       B.   Explore peer review as a method of communication.

       C.   Continue to work with clinical and administrative nursing staff.

       D.   Evaluate staff scheduling and assess alternate systems of staffing.

PHILOSOPHIES AND OBJECTIVES OF NURSING UNITS

The next step towards increasing specificity is that of the philosophy and objectives of the nursing unit. In some smaller institutions, such as convalescent homes, small infirmaries, nursing homes and so on, there is sufficient homogeneity of clientele so that the philosophy of the nursing service may also serve as that of the unit or units within it. In most institutions, however, some compartmentalization occurs. The result is that clients on a particular ward or service have common denominators of characteristics that permit more precise application of beliefs and objectives.

Common Factors Affecting Nursing Unit Philosophy and Objectives. Some of the common characteristics that assist the nurse in developing philosophical priorities and more specifically relevant goals include:

1. The nature and degree of illness of the clientele.
2. The age of the population.
3. The usual length of hospitalization.
4. The goal of the medical treatment.
5. The usual prognosis.
6. The goal of the service.
7. The depth and nature of the nursing staffing pattern.

The nature and degree of illness of the clientele is a factor in unit philosophy and goals. Well-child supervision in the ambulatory care unit may require priorities in values and goals that differ from those relevant to the care of the acutely ill child, although ultimate goals are identical. Psychotic clients who are somatically healthy would call for objectives differing from those applicable to the person who is somatically ill but coping psychologically with stress.

Age of the population can be another variable. The objectives most relevant to the nurse caring for a population of neonates can be quite different from those of the nurse caring for a preschool, adolescent, adult, or aged population.

Length of hospitalization is another important factor in selecting the objectives that will have priority. The nurse's expectations regarding her role and the goals she will be able to achieve alter with the duration of the client's hospitalization. The nurse who consistently works with clients for less than 24 hours in the labor and delivery room, with postpartum mothers whose length of stay is two to three days, or with someone undergoing surgery who stays five to eight days cannot meaningfully set out to accomplish goals requiring long-term contact. On the other hand, the nurse who works on the rehabilitation ward or convalescent units would be doing a disservice to the client if she were to deal only with goals attainable within one to eight days.

The goal of treatment, both medical and nursing, is still another influence. Consider the objectives of nursing care that would be germane to treatment goals of: (1) isolation of the person with a communicable disease while his infection is being treated; (2) health teaching and control of disease, as in diabetes mellitus and emphysema; (3) conservation and palliation, as in rheumatoid arthritis; (4) reconstruction and return of function in burns or trauma; (5) palliation and comfort in terminal malignancy; or (6) diagnosis in any of many conditions.

Are there particular segments of the philosophy and goals related to prognosis that come to the foreground? Will the person who is dying benefit from care with goals that are different from those that are set for someone whose disease is self-limiting or responsive to therapy?

The purpose of the unit influences the beliefs and objectives of the nurses who work there. A prime example here is the research unit, in which the primary goal is the acquisition of data and the secondary goal is the treatment of the individual.

Finally, the depth and nature of staffing of the unit with nursing personnel must of necessity influence the philosophy, and, particularly, the objectives of a unit. To claim that the nurse is a major source of social interaction for a particular group of clients, when the workload of technical procedures severely limits her contacts with them, is unrealistic. True, she can use each moment as effectively as possible, but she probably will still not be a major part of their social interaction.

Nor can the goal of personalized care plans for each client be realized unless there are prepared personnel, time to create them, and a place where the distractions and stress associated with the nurses' station do not detract from the necessary thinking processes (Cleland, 1967).

Philosophy of a Research Ward. This research ward is located in the university hospital whose philosophy was quoted earlier. Again, it is possible to see that the values and beliefs of outer philosophical circles have filtered down to this extrapolated ward philosophy, but they are made more specific to the particular clients.

1. Clients volunteer for participation in research conducted on this ward. Nurses and the care they give should support him in his satisfaction with his original decision and in his continuing decision to remain in the study population to the end of the study.
2. There are segments of control which the patient relinquishes in order to participate in the study. It is important that the nurse support his autonomy in those segments of his daily living that are not affected by the research design.
3. Patient understanding of the research commitment and the role expectations held for him are important to his successsful collaboration in the study.
4. Nurses who participate in research projects must have:
   (a) A passion for accuracy in following the procedures and timing of data collection and
   (b) Integrity in reporting any deviations from the prescribed research design.

The support of the client participating in the experience of medical research is reaffirmed in the ward philosophy, as is the belief that nurses should support and implement research.

Philosophy of Cardiac Recovery Unit. Two nurses who worked in the cardiac recovery room at the University of Oregon Medical School Hospital incorporated statements of that unit's philosophy of nursing care in an article—"The Apprehensive Patient." In their view, the person in their recovery room has the right to:

1. Gentleness of touch and voice.
2. Expert nursing care, particularly nursing skill in relation to emergency procedures.
3. Dignity.
4. Clear explanations of procedures, even though he may not fully understand them at the time because he is not completely conscious or is under sedation.
5. Personalized care suited to his needs.
6. The presence of a nurse when he wants one.
7. Honest answers to his questions. (Powers, 1967).

This philosophy emphasizes special needs of clients in a cardiac recovery unit, although it is largely applicable to any unit.

Philosophy and Objectives of a Ward of the Chronically Ill. The residents on this ward were ill with lung diseases with an average hospitalization of about eleven months. They were all men, with a mean age of 46 years. One fourth to one half of the 54 men on the ward were diagnosed alcoholics. Most of them had less than high school education and worked in laboring or service type positions. Their family ties in many instances were very tenuous. Using the above data, and findings from previous studies that had characterized individuals with tuberculosis as tending to be dependent and passive, the following philosophy and objectives were evolved by four psychiatric nurse specialists. These nurses stated that the men on this ward had:

1. Worth.
2. A right to know about their medical condition and treatment as a basis for reasonably intelligent collaboration.
3. A responsibility to participate in their care in the hospital as a preparation for self-care after dismissal.
4. A right to personal autonomy in those areas not restricted by the communicability of their disease.
5. A right to experience meaningful interaction with others within the restricted hospital setting.
6. A right to a maximum sense of well-being during hospitalization.

From this philosophy the following general client objectives emerged and were approved by the nursing service administrative staff and the ward physician:

1. A better understanding of self (behavior, feelings, thoughts).
2. Increased ability to relate to others.
3. Ability to view the present situation (past and future) realistically.
4. Understanding of own medical condition and status (quarantine, modified quarantine—legal restriction on the compound).
5. Factual knowledge about tuberculosis and/or alcoholism and its treatment.
6. Achievement of emotional satisfaction through discovery of new spheres

of interest and development of new creative and emotional outlets.

7. Achievement of greater level of maturity:
   (a) Increased tolerance of frustrations through more constructive ways of dealing with frustrations.
   (b) Taking responsibility for own welfare, actions, etc. (Little, 1965).

From ward philosophies such as these are derived the guidelines and major objectives which are then individualized in terms of each client's observed problems.

ADAPTATION OF THE WARD PHILOSOPHY AND OBJECTIVES TO THE INDIVIDUAL

Moving again toward the center of the philosophical circles, we come to the innermost pair of intertwined circles. In one of these, the nurse filters the nursing service and unit beliefs through her own values and her perceptions of the client to integrate them into her plans for nursing care.

We have shown examples of various applications of the broader, more abstract values at each level—first, the departmental level, and then from departmental to ward level. The same process takes place as the ward objectives become specific client objectives.

The previously cited nurse specialists in their seventh objective (above) wished to encourage the men to take responsibility for their own welfare and actions. Let us look at the way this general goal was actually translated into specific nursing actions that vary from client to client.

Mr. Strand was an elderly blind man, quite content to remain in the safe confines of his room and allow the world to come to him. Actually, the nursing care would have been easier and less time consuming if the nurses had been willing to allow him this degree of dependence and withdrawal. However, they felt that he would benefit from developing a sense of responsibility based on being able to care for himself. With this in mind they fastened a cord to the wall of the corridor from his room to the bathroom, so that he would not get lost. In the beginning, personnel walked with him, but gradually he was able to find his own way. They set his tray in the community eating room with other older men, in order to increase his contacts and to encourage him to socialize with others in his institutional world.

Another man, Mr. Ramirez, had his environment modified in another way to enable him to assume responsibility for his own care. A system of self-medication of antituberculosis drugs had been introduced to the ward. Mr. Ramirez would have had difficulty in adjusting to this because of his inability to speak or read English. With the help of another resident, the instructions, labels, and the record forms on which he was to write were translated into Spanish. Mr. Ramirez was then able to take his own drugs and keep the records on them.

For a third man, the ability to take responsibility for his own actions depended upon his acquisition of knowledge. Mr. Taylor was a young American Indian whose background included a childhood spent on a reservation. In the hospital he was taciturn and withdrawn, albeit friendly, but speaking only when spoken to, making no requests. As he slowly developed a relationship with his nurse, he began to share his perception of tuberculosis, as well as his lack of understanding of what was happening to him therapeutically in this alien hospital environment. A lung hemorrhage had precipitated his admission. When he had been hurt or ill in the past, his grandmother, an effective medicine woman of the tribe, had "sucked out the poison" from his infected cuts and had used herbs and native remedies to treat his ailments. The current pattern of therapy left him bewildered. His nurse began with simple diagrams to show him about the nature of his lungs, and about the respiratory system and its connections with his mouth. She told him how the tuberculosis germs could enter the body and how he could spread them to others. He looked at her and said, "We might've been passing t.b. germs along with that bottle." From this level of understanding about his body and the routes of communicability of his disease, it was not hard to move on to greater understanding and acceptance of staff precautions and to his own active cooperation with them. When he had reached a point of sufficient understanding and health, he began to attend group sessions on the ward; but his nurse always checked with him afterward, to find out if his interpretation of the movie or the discussion was in keeping with reality. Respect for different cultural orientation to health and treatment and a sharing of knowledge were the keys to self-responsibility in one area for this patient.

A fourth man, Mr. Rusk, illustrates the application of the objective when cardiac decompensation necessitated reduction of physical exertion in a very independent person. Mr. Rusk liked to assume responsibility and to take care of himself. His problem was that he wanted to do too much. The nurse had to find ways to permit him to care for himself without placing too many demands on his heart. Obviously, he should not be wheeling the oxygen tank and aerosol equipment out of his room and back to the alcove. Instead of giving him his aerosol treatments in bed, would the doctor permit him to walk slowly to the treatment room—if he showed no ill effects? Were there other activities that could be adjusted so that he could take over—some that would give him the satisfaction of self-care? There were. And so it went from day to day, with nurses and nursing personnel seeking significant aspects of his care that might be adjusted in terms of his potential for self-care. In addition, the staff took pains to note the contributions he was making to his own care and to the well-being of the ward. Here the goal was achieved by making some aspects of self-care possible.

And so it went on this ward, from one to another. The overall goal of trying to gain wider acceptance of responsibility for self in a population accustomed to being cared for was implemented with each one. The individual goal and the supporting nursing approaches, however, were as varied as the men themselves. The fact that all personnel on the ward were aware of the common objective helped them to create a consistent environment in which progress was not only much more possible, but more comfortable for all concerned. The same situation could hold with other ward goals that encompass the care of all persons on the service.

CLIENTS' PHILOSOPHIES

Finally we come to the centermost philosophical circles: nurse and client. Like the nurse and other health workers, the client is a member of the universal group called "the public," and as such he has had the opportunity to assimilate the value system of this group. But as a discrete individual he also has the potential for deviating from it in many respects. He may represent a blend of cultures, as exemplified by Mr. Ramirez and Mr. Taylor, who were discussed earlier in this chapter. Stereotyping of cultural values is dangerously misleading; each person must serve as the source of the information on which you make judgments regardings his beliefs.

In the original diagram the client's and the nurse's philosophies regarding health, illness, and nursing care were pictured as overlapping slightly:

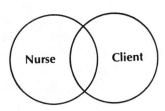

In truth they may overlap extensively—

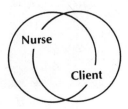

or they may not overlap at all.

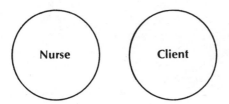

Because the client's objectives also grow out of his values, it is conceivable that objectives could be as disparate as the philosophies. The end result may be that the client and the nurse tend to pull in opposite directions.

Usually both make adaptations and adjustments in terms of one another's value system. There was a time when most nurses—female, Caucasian, and middle-class, as they tended to be in the Western world—functioned on the assumption that their system of values was applicable to everyone. Any discrepancies that emerged placed the client in a position of default, which he was supposed to rectify. Today the nurse as a therapist in the situation is charged with the responsibility of being aware of and showing insight into the nature of the conflicts of values and goals between herself and the clients, and of initiating action that will either assist him in adjusting to goals that are not entirely his own, or modify the situation so that adjustment is minimized.

Sometimes potential clients take the initiative in selecting health services that minimize goal conflict between themselves and health workers. For example, there have always been many diverse beliefs associated with childbirth and infant care. Prospective parents and health workers may disagree on some of these; also, institutions may not have the flexibility to accommodate the varying desires of clients. For this reason many prospective parents have scouted among their friends to find the doctor who not only share their beliefs regarding care during labor and delivery and in the postpartum period, but who also practices in a hospital that has facilities to make this kind of care available. For example, if they believe that they have the right

1. To have a say in the type of anesthesia used.
2. To have the husband present during labor and delivery.
3. To have natural childbirth.
4. To have the infant "room in."
5. To successfully breast feed the baby.

they may select an obstetrician who is in agreement, and who practices in a hospital that has a policy permitting the above.

In pregnancy, with its built-in preparation time, adjustments such as this are often possible. Others may not be so fortunate as to be able to pick and choose either their physician or their surroundings, and serious conflicts that interfere with healing and well-being can arise.

In nursing we believe we are beginning to reach an "age of enlightenment" wherein we accept differences and allow clients' beliefs and goals to vary from ours. It may be just so much lip service unless we maintain an awareness of differences in beliefs and a respect for the rights of others to hold to their beliefs just as we want to hold to ours.

INFLUENCE OF PHILOSOPHIES OF LARGER HEALTH CARE SYSTEMS

Consumer and nursing philosophies of health care as presented here may have been oversimplified. We have alluded to the need for reality, yet have not considered the constraints and influences imposed by beliefs and values espoused by larger health care system components.

In case there is any doubt that the values of far-removed governing bodies influence the health care services right down to the day-to-day contacts of nurse and client, let's have a closer look.

In the United States, Medicare exemplifies a national bureaucracy concerned with providing for health care to a segment of the population—those over sixty-five years of age. One official belief within Medicare that influences the behavior of the individual practitioner and the client is that of the validity of norms in the time required for institution-based therapy. That is, a given ailment responds to treatment within a given period of time and therefore X number of days will be reimbursed. Review committees have been established to make decisions in individual cases within these guidelines, and higher review committees may reconsider or revoke the decision of the original committee. Clients who deviate from the norms by responding to treatment more slowly or by learning to cope with disability less effectively within the given time limit may find their health care services terminated prematurely. Or at least payment for them is terminated—which may amount to the same thing for those with limited resources.

How does this affect nursing care? If, for instance, a nurse is charged with helping a new elderly diabetic learn to cope with a change in his lifestyle, she must either structure the activities during the days of hospitalization in such a way that he can really obtain a working knowledge of living with his diabetes within the reimbursed time span, or she risks sending him home inadequately prepared. (This presumes that the client is competent in physical and mental status to learn as needed.) Many nurses can cite instances where their clients were not adequately prepared to cope on their own and returned to the hospitals with problems created by their lack of understanding, skill, strength or motivation. Thus relationships and content in every contact between a nurse and a client can be influenced by the values of boards or commissions thousands of miles away.

50

Institutional Values and Nursing

In addition to values that define legitimate services to be offered or reimbursed, there are value systems of governing bodies which reflect the purpose of the immediate system within which the nursing department functions. A university system has education as its primary objective. Thus, a teaching hospital within this system would incorporate in its philosophy values that reflect its dual clientele—students and clients. A Veterans Administration Hospital will give priority to treatment of service-connected disabilities and illnesses of veterans of the armed forces. The newly emerging health maintenance organizations (HMOs) give priority in values to keeping their clientele healthy in order to keep costs down. Thus, prevention and maintenance may receive greater budget and priority, and staff will be hired for their interest and expertise in this area. An acute care institution is obviously going to espouse values related to diagnosis and cure. Each system or agency has an official (and unofficial) system of values dictated by its purpose and clientele. Individual nurses as well as nursing departments functioning within these larger systems will have their priorities in values influenced by those of the institution.

Viable institutional values, strongly held, can shape the nature of the facility in many ways. It can modify the architecture, the color scheme, the nature of the staff, and the lifestyle.

A psychiatric unit in a Canadian hospital was architecturally designed to support the belief that fostering openness and interaction with others will facilitate the return to mental health. This unit is shaped as an opened flower. The staff area is an open space in the center where the only physical barriers are some narrow work surfaces, no doors or glass. Records on movable carts fit into a recess in the wall when not in use—so the focus is on people not paper, even in terms of visibility. Around this center and its surrounding space, clusters of client units form petals. Each petal is made up of a sitting room opening onto the center and three individual units set against the outside walls of the petals. There are no doors between the individual unit and the sitting room of each petal, nor between the petal and the center area, only sliding partitions. The quality this communicates is one of unobstructed openness and unimpeded movement toward —not away from. Only two isolation units exist, places obscurely away from the flow patterns. Small, barren, and functional, they are used in extreme crises for short periods. The room in which treatments are given several hours each week is transformed within minutes back to a lively stereo and billiards room by folding the carts and storing them and other equipment in a closet. Treatment is important, but living is more so. Wood, warm colors, shapes and lines that flow upward from the center further communicate the climate of a sharing, people-oriented place.

Even more easily than in wood, stone and paint, a philosophy flows into the reality of job descriptions, patterns of administration, staffing patterns, policies, rewards, dress, and the working lifestyle of practitioners. In fact it would be difficult to find a facet of institutional life that would not be reflective of the institution's beliefs and values.

The advantage of knowing the dimensions and the nature of the institution's philosophy is that it enables those who practice their profession there as well as those who are served to know the expected nature and range of services offered as well as the institutional climate.

THE NURSE IN THE MIDST OF VALUE SYSTEMS

Carl Rogers, in discussing a modern approach to valuing, traces the shift in sources of values from the infant experiencing and valuing what pleases him to the adult who tends to develop values in order to receive affection and approval by pleasing others. He suggests that the mature person needs to once again restore contact with his own inner values, then to see them in relation to the values of those who are seeking to shape him (Rogers, 1969).

A parallel is seen in nurses. Attitudes and values change as students in the health professions are socialized into their professional roles (Mauksch, 1965, Kramer, 1968, 1974). Once they become professionals they find that value systems and priorities must again change when they move from one bureaucracy to another if they are to receive approval from those around them (Corwin, 1964; Kramer, 1970, 1974).

Perhaps it is time to examine our own values and then those of our consumers, our colleagues, and our employers. Perhaps we should become aware of the forces that are being used to reshape our values and the actual reshaping that is being attempted. Only then can we make a mature decision as to whether it is advisable to change our own values and priorities or to strive for an accommodation to them.

SUMMARY

Values are like an ever present current. Sometimes it is visible. More often it flows below the surface. It is a current, however, that strong or weak, modifies direction, decisions, and pace in any interaction. It can be anticipated that these value currents, obvious or subtle, will frequently take differing, sometimes opposing directions among interacting individuals, professions, units, and institutions. Sometimes the current of values that is overt in terms of the stated or written form is quite different from the strong undercurrent that is the real force in the operating value system.

The professional needs to have a high degree of awareness for the impact of value systems held by self, by clients, colleagues, professions and organizations on health care services. The professional needs a high level of consciousness about personal values and the way in which these are shaping his observation, interpretation, decisions and actions—including the ways in which he may be striving to make others conform. The professional needs to deliberately seek data on values involved in presenting situations and to incorporate these data into the planning process.

REFERENCES

Ciuca, Rudy. "Over the Years with the Nursing Care Plan," *Nursing Outlook* 20:706-711, November, 1972.

Cheraskin, E. and W. M. Ringsdorf. *Predictive Medicine, A Study in Strategy.* Mt. View, Calif.: Pacific Press Pub. Assoc., 1973.

Cleland, Virginia. "Effects of Stress on Thinking," *American Journal of Nursing* 67:108-111, January, 1967.

Corwin, Ronald. "The Professional Employee: A Study of Conflict in Nursing Roles," in Skipper and Leonard, *Social Interaction and Patient Care.* Philadelphia: J. B. Lippincott Co., 1965, pp. 341-356.

Ebbeson, M. "Care of the Retarded Spotlighted," *Newsletter,* King County Nurses Association, 20:1, February, 1967.

George, G. R., et al. *"Revised Philosophy of Nursing,"* Chicago, Ill.: State Psychiatric Institute and Associated Facilities, 1967, 10 pp.

Kramer, Marlene. "Role Models, Role Conception and Role Deprivation," *Nursing Research* 17:116, March-April, 1968.

———. Role Conception of Baccalaureate Nurses and Success in Hospital Nursing," *Nursing Research* 19:428-439, September-October, 1970.

———. *Reality Shock.* Saint Louis: Mosby Co., 1974.

Little, Dolores, et al. *Nurse Specialist Effect on Tuberculosis.* Appendix C-4 ff. USPHS Grant, #Nu-0094-01, 1965.

Maslow, Abraham. *Toward a Psychology of Being.* Princeton, N.J.: Nostrand Company, Inc., 1962.

Mauksch, Hans. "Becoming a Nurse: A Selective View," in Skipper and Leonard, *Social Interaction and Patient Care,* pp. 327-340.

Milio, Nancy. *9262 Kercheval, The Storefront that Did Not Burn.* Ann Arbor: The University of Michigan Press, 1970. "Prologue," pp. xiii-xiv.

Norris, C. M. "Administration for Creative Nursing," *Nursing Forum,* 1:88-105 Appendix: Philosophy of Nursing by Louise M. Atty, et al, pp. 106-117, Summer, 1962.

Powers, M. E. and F. Storlie. "The Apprehensive Patient," *American Journal of Nursing* 67:59-60, January, 1967.

Sparer, P. *Personality, Stress and Tuberculosis.* New York: International Universities Press, Inc., 1956, pp. 65-101, 169-170.

Wu, Ruth, *Behavior and Illness.* Englewood Cliffs, N.J.: Prentice Hall, Inc., 1973. "The Concept of Wellness," pp. 75-88.

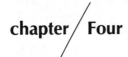

chapter / Four

Cues and Inferences:
foundations of nursing care planning

The skills that are most basic to nursing care planning relate to the perception and accurate identification of information in the environment and the assigning of valid meanings to the situations. The terms that have come to be used to describe this process are cue identification and inferencing. The concepts of cues and inferences and the associated skills will be explored in this chapter as a foundation to their use in the subsequent steps of the planning process.

CUES: WHAT ARE THEY? WHAT ARE THEIR SOURCES?

What Is a Cue?

A cue is a unit of sensory input—a single message that is noticed and usually named. The noticing, unless the cue is very obvious, is an outgrowth of knowledge, both theoretical and experiential. Even small behavioral responses or changes in the environment can assume significance to the skilled and knowledgeable observer. Some examples may add clarity to this idea of cues:

a surname having potential ethnic implications

a home address having economic, environmental or transportation and service implications—the ghetto, the suburb, a remote, rural area

a statement regarding degree of devotion to particular religious practices that influence diet or treatment

the reported concern of a mother regarding the wellbeing of her two preschoolers

the drawing together of eyebrows, quick intake of breath, clenching of teeth, or sudden rigidity of body following a particular stimulus

a sudden cessation of speech

lack of eye contact

a dry hacking cough

a fruity odor to the breath

felt resistance when range of motion is attempted

Cues for the nurse come as data about the status, environment and response of the client and those around him.

Cue noticing is an important part of the nurse's expertise. Once noticed, the naming or description is as objective and precise—quantitatively and qualitatively as the observer's skill and vocabulary permit. For example a report of "thready regular pulse of 140" is more precise than, "rapid pulse." This naming may not be written or even spoken, but it is thought. The precision of description applied to cues in *thinking* obviously precedes and influences any subsequent verbal communication to others as well as any decision making. This is where the discipline and expertise begin.

It is also important to keep in mind that the cue is *not* the phenomenon itself. Just as a photograph or a painting are only representations of reality, never the reality itself, so our perceptions are only our personal imagery of the actuality. Photographs can record accurately or they can distort, foreshorten and de-pattern. So too, we internalize accurate or inaccurate versions of our environment. What then becomes fact or reality for us may or may not match the situation that generated the input.

All this prefaces the idea that, because the environment outside ourselves is so elusive and changing, nurses as humanists and science-based professionals must take all possible pains to insure that they capture and internalize precise and accurate labels or representations of reality. After all, once the fleeting stimuli are no longer present, our representations, whether they be words or nonverbal impressions, are all that remain for us to use.

What Are Cue Sources?

Cues in the nurse's world can come from a variety of sources, internal and external. They may be verbal or nonverbal.

External Sources.   One of the most important sources of cues for the nurse is, of course, the client. He is the *primary* source of data and *the expert* on what he has been or is experiencing. Persons around him and records about him are *secondary* sources. These represent their own reality and perceptions of the person. Cues are also available in the environment of both the client and the nurse. Cues emerge from conditions, events, people and records about people.

Internal Sources.   In addition to cues in the external environment of an individual, it is also possible to identify cues within oneself. These are known as subjective phenomena. Examples of these might be: feeling unable to keep your eyes open in that one o'clock class, the stiffness in a joint when you try to move it after it has been immobilized for some time, a dream, hunger pangs. . . . When these experiences are verbalized to someone else they become cues to the other individual as well.

Later sections of this chapter will explore in more depth the important sources of cues for persons in the nursing role.

Developing a Working Definition of Cues

Since recognizing cues is a skill that must be applied in an unending variety of situations, merely recalling the words of the definition is not enough. There is a need to be able to use it effectively. So before continuing further, try using your knowledge of the characteristics of cues:

> a single unit of noticed information
> received through any of the senses—sight, hearing, smell, touch, taste and
> and proprioceptors
> described as objectively, accurately and precisely as possible.

Set yourself to receive cues from another person, verbal and nonverbal, for about 15 seconds. Write them down. How many did you notice? What sense organs did you use? Could you have gotten more by using others? Ask yourself, "Would another person in this setting be able to identify the same cues? Would he be likely to label as I did?"

Now read the following description

> A 40 year old clean-shaven male, lying on his left side. The fingers on his left hand are flexed slightly. There is a little resistance when I straighten them. He rubs his forehead with his right hand. His lips have a bluish cast. His respirations are rattling on inspiration. The skin feels moist and cool. His gown is damp. He does not speak. Both eyes are open, pupils are dilated and even. The room is light. There is an odor of cigarette smoke about him.

What sense organs were used in this cue recognition? If you were in this situation, could you receive comparable sensory input and supply similar labels to describe the cues received?

Skill in cue identification is very much in keeping with the admonition to "Tell it like it is!" to yourself and others.

WHAT ARE INFERENCES?

If cues are units of sensory input representing reality, what then are inferences? Inferences are *subjective*, personal meanings assigned to a situation by an individual based on input, usually a *group* of cues. Inferences are made behind the eyeballs of the beholder.

Inferencing is a giant step away from the original reality in that it depends on information that has first, been *screened* by sense organs, which may or may not be transmitting accurate signals and second, *processed* by a brain where the input can be modified by attention, previous experience, knowledge, and the language available for description, to say nothing of being modified by the beholder's value system as well.

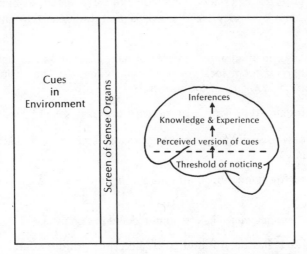

Cues from the environment pass through or are picked up by the sense organs and may be sent on in an accurate or distorted version. If noticed in the central nervous system, they are combined with previous related experience, available knowledge and usually vocabulary to arrive at inferences or assigned meanings.

Just as there are words associated with cues, so there is an inference-oriented vocabulary that appropriately describes cue syndromes or impressions/conclusions drawn from these clusters of related cues. Words such as angry, worried, happy, sleeping, comatose, immobilized, elderly, rich, intelligent, incompetent describe judgments that have been made as a result of combining multiple cues. You can undoubtedly think of many others in your own vocabulary. One of the skills in assessment comes in being aware of the cue-oriented vocabulary and its distinctness from inference-oriented words.

Nurses are paid to infer. In nursing as in other sciences, basic and applied, observation is not an end in itself but is done with the purpose of understanding relationships within a situation and making decisions regarding subsequent actions. However, given the multiple factors that can and do influence the assignment of meaning—inferencing—there ought to be room for recurrent healthy skepticism when inferences are made. They are highly subjective!

THE PROBLEM OF BLURRING CUE IDENTIFICATION AND INFERENCING

There would seem to be an easily recognizable difference between identifying cues in a situation and assigning meaning to them or drawing conclusions from them. Yet often these behaviors are used interchangeably, without awareness. Keeping them separate is not as simple as it would first seem. After all, in each instance, whether describing cue input or making a judgment, one tends to use words. In order to experience the challenge for yourself, examine the following admission note and identify the words that indicate that inferences have been made:

> Elderly, obese, man admitted per wheelchair. Discouraged at being readmitted. Angry at room location. Very demanding. Will not help himself. Lies on his back. Glares at the nurses.

How many inference-type words or phrases did you select? Did they include:

> elderly, obese, discouraged, angry, very demanding, will not and glares at the nurses?

Now go back to the admission note and see if you can find five cues. Did they include:

> man, admitted, per wheelchair, readmitted and lies on his back?

One technique that has been found to be helpful in differentiating between cue identification and inferencing is to ask yourself, "How did I *KNOW* that?" If you can identify units of information (cues) that led you to the conclusion that a certain status or situation existed, you have made an inference. The units of information that you were able to identify as enabling you to *KNOW* were the cues. For example, the inference was made that the man was elderly. How could one draw this inference? What cues contributed to it?

> The dome of his head was bald and the remaining rim of hair, his eyebrows, and mustache were white.
> His face was creased with deep wrinkles.
> His back curved forward, his shoulders rounded.
> The knuckles of his hands were enlarged and twisted, the gutters on the back of his hands between the bones and tendons were deep.
> There was a palsy type of tremor in his hands.
> He was without observable teeth, his lips and cheeks were sunken.
> He wore thick-lensed glasses, bifocals. His irises were ringed with a light edge.
> His voice quavered.
> He cupped his hand behind his right ear when people were talking.

Each cue taken alone would not permit the observer to conclude that this individual was "elderly" (although some carry more weight than others in creating the impression). Taken together, they reinforce each other and suggest the conclusion that was drawn.

In order to experiment with this further, take another one of the inferences made about this client. Then determine what cues in his appearance or response would enable you to derive the inference that was recorded. Notice how easy it is to slip into including other inferences. Did you find yourself using general terms such as "facial expression?" That could mean a host of responses. Try for precision so that another person who did not have this experience could share in it vividly.

If you are a pragmatic person, by this time you are saying that such a tedious review of cues to arrive at an evident conclusion is belaboring the obvious. Or, on the other hand, you might suggest that the other extreme is equally possible —that almost anything is an inference and that one could be endlessly caught up in minutiae (Wilson, 1963, 18). Even so obvious a characteristic as being male is an inference based on cues of anatomical features, body shape, hair distribution, and voice, as well as clothes and mannerisms associated with the male role in our culture. In either case, the point is well taken. Still, if we as nurses are to be accurate and objective in our assessments, we need to walk a middle road in which we decide what cues constitute any given inference and then read the cues in each situation accurately before making inferences. Recent nursing literature has begun to call a group of cues that often or always makes up a given inference a *cue syndrome*. Medicine has been doing this for some time, including a few cues that are pathonomonic of particular diagnoses (inferences).

WHY IS IT IMPORTANT TO DISTINGUISH BETWEEN CUES AND INFERENCES?

What difference does it really make whether a nurse uses cues and inferences interchangeably? Obviously a nurse must infer at some point. The difficulty arises when the nurse's judgment *about* a situation is used as if it *were* the actual situation.

Take an extreme hypothetical example from a related field. Suppose you had an abrasion on your lip. On a visit to the doctor for a routine physical examination you hear the doctor say, "We're going to have to do something about that lesion on your lip. We'll schedule you for a radical excision tomorrow, or as soon as we can get you in. And you better plan your life around a postoperative course of x-ray therapy." The doctor would have taken a cue, the lesion on your lip, and translated it into a judgment—malignancy, then acted as if the inference were fact. "No doctor behaves that way," you say. Admittedly, the example is far-fetched, but there are everyday nursing situations much closer to home where nurses use judgments as facts.

A film used to test nurses' identification of cues showed a man who was given a tray of food, but did not eat. Some of the nurses who viewed the film said that the man could not feed himself, others, that he would not feed himself. Actually, what they saw was that he did not feed himself (Verhonick, 1968). When this example has been used in workshops and classes, many nurses have

59

indicated that they treat patients who "can't" differently from those who "won't" —particularly when things get busy (Crowell, 1968; Pearson, 1968).

Or take another example. An elderly man was hospitalized because of inability to manage the activities of living as a result of advanced organic brain syndrome. In occupational therapy a specially adapted eating utensil was developed and he learned how to feed himself. There had been visual cues that he was able to feed himself. Yet at mealtime he would eat only a few bites before saying, "I can't do it." The nursing staff "knew" he could. At each meal an, "I can't!" "You can!" verbal tug of war ensued until the man would begin to cry and a member of the staff would feed him grudgingly. Eventually an additional cue was noted. He stopped feeding himself and said he "couldn't" when he spilled on himself for the first time each meal. When he was given a clean start, he could again feed himself. With this additional information the nurses' inference became, "Feels unable to feed himself when he is aware he has spilled." The verbal can-can't struggle was replaced by a nursing action of using protective covering that could be replaced or wiped off. Staff and client were happier.

Frequently the inference is made that a client has reached a level of unconsciousness that renders him unable to hear. Discussions take place over and around him that weren't intended for his knowledge or he is treated as an object of attention, not a person, and never spoken to. The memories these individuals report upon recovery of ability to speak make our nursing and medical care seem inhuman.

There are also situations in which an inference is made that the person in the client role hasn't the capacity to understand or utilize honest information and he is given evasive or simplistic answers.

Can you think of other situations, nursing or non-nursing, where treating an inference as if it were fact led to ineffective behavior?

TECHNIQUES FOR INCREASING AWARENESS OF CUES AND INFERENCES IN DAILY LIFE

After offering many workshops in which distinguishing between cues and inferences was stressed as a part of the program and activities, we have learned that merely talking or reading about this behavior does not make much of a change. The skill seems to require follow-up of day-to-day effort. And certainly the ability to differentiate data-gathering from making judgments about the data must precede subsequent assessment skills.

In order to assure yourself that you are ready to move on to the next assessment skills, try some of these activities in clinical or nonclinical settings.

Listen to others describing clients, situations or coworkers. In your own mind *separate* the cues from inferences.

Try to separate cues from inferences in what you read, or what you hear and see on television or in the movies.

Listen to yourself! Become aware of the times when you are using cues, not only in your speaking but also in thinking. How often do you hear yourself BSS-ing (making *B*road *S*weeping *S*tatements with little supporting evidence)? Have you heard others BSS-ing?

When you find yourself making inferences, ask yourself, "Now how did I *KNOW* that?"

In order to overcome the blind spots in this behavior that each of us has, why not ask a friend to listen to you in terms of the cues that you use and the inferences you make?

When you are satisfied that you are pretty consistently aware of the uses you make of cues and judgments, when you notice the differences in the reporting of others, when you separate cue vocabulary from inference-oriented words, you are ready to move on.

FORCES THAT INFLUENCE CUE RECOGNITION AND IDENTIFICATION

Scholars have devoted years to the study of perception and factors that influence what we notice. At the risk of oversimplifying a very complex concept, it still seems important to examine some of the forces that influence nurses' cue recognition and identification.

It comes as no surprise that we tend to notice in our environment that which we:

desire to see

expect to see

have been trained to notice

have been led to believe will be present or

are able to encompass with our vocabulary.

In a walk along an ocean shore: a rockhound *desires* to see agates, jasper and jade; a driftwood collector *expects* to see water-battered branches and roots; a marine biologist has been *trained to notice* and *identify* marine plants and animals; while the clam digger may have been *led to believe* that the little holes in the sand mean the presence of the clams he is seeking. Each of these individuals can encompass his area of interest within his *available vocabulary* but may not be able to identify with that of one of the other beach-walkers. The clam digger may not have the vocabulary of the rock hound regarding semiprecious stones and neither may have the marine biologist's terminology. In the health field too there are desires, expectations, trained observations and vocabulary associated with the discipline as well as input from others that can modify what is noticed in the environment and the manner in which it is identified.

Preset Expectations

Diagnosis. Many newspapers carried a story of eight persons who, wishing to investigate conditions in mental hospitals, feigned insanity. The diagnoses that resulted in their commitment was, for most of them, schizophrenia. Once committed they reverted to their usual behavior, behavior that had been seen as normal in the community. The cues spun off by this usual behavior were duly noticed and recorded by the staff to validate abnormality. Schizophrenic behavior was what they expected to see in a person so labeled, and that was what they did see. Their fellow inmates, on the other hand, presumably did not have the label and the associated knowledge to modify their observation. They saw the cues as representative of nonpsychotic behavior and wondered what the game of the phoney psychotics was in getting themselves locked up. Even the psychologist who initiated and reported the project indicated that he was aware that he tended to see what he had anticipated, despite his honest desire to be objective (Rosenhan, 1973). Knowledge of a diagnosis can color our perceptions —it can be a help in locating cues that might otherwise be missed, but it can also cause us to stereotype where it is not appropriate (Scheff, 1965).

How often do you tell the cues what they are to say to you, instead of letting them speak for themselves first?

Context of Cues. The context within which cues are seen tends to influence whether we notice them and what labels we use to describe them. A worn paperback book on the library shelf is a library book; that same dogeared book in the garbage dump might be seen as refuse. In the hospital persistent attempts at self-care by the post-myocardial infarction client in the coronary care unit is labelled as noncooperative behavior, while the same behavior on the rehabilitation unit is recorded as evidence of motivation and cooperation with treatment goals. Desire for client response results in different labeling and differing value judgments being applied to similar behavior.

Clientele. For the nurse, a variation on the idea of context relates to the nature of the particular clientele and the priorities certain cures have in their diagnosis and care. Sometimes age-related behavior is a dominant feature, as in the very young and the very old. On some units, cues related to responses to treatment get first attention. In the oncology unit, where chemotherapy for malignancy has a high risk of toxicity, there is importance attached to symptoms indicating the degree of expected responses and indications of dangerous intolerance. On the rehabilitation units or intractable pain clinics where operant conditioning is being used as the treatment approach, the responses related to complying with the treatment plan become important. Occasionally, it is the response to pathology or progression of a normal phenomenon that is deemed important, as in congestive heart failure, obstruction of a body lumen (airway, intestine, or blood vessel), or progression of labor and delivery. The very act of focusing on one particular set of cues may tend to blur or render unnoticed other significant cues unless the client makes it impossible for us to ignore them.

Client Perception of Nurse Interest

The expectations which health professionals hold about the cues they want to or should notice tend to be communicated in some way to the client. In turn, this can and does affect the cues that clients make available. Ambulatory care nurses in clinics with medical specialists often are given data seen as too trivial or of no interest to the doctor. A spry 90-year-old told the nurse, "My heart and pacemaker are working fine. It's the rheumatism in my knees that keeps me from getting around." Or, another client in this same cardiac clinic whose postoperative status was very good told the nurse she didn't know how to go about getting the metatarsal arch supports she needed. In each of these instances the noncardiac data were made available to the nurse, not the cardiac specialist whose interest and priority were data on the heart status and related responses. Health professionals, both doctors and nurses, can, intentionally or not, influence the cues that clients share.

Colleagues' Attitudes

In a similar fashion the comments and attitudes of our coworkers toward particular clients or groups of clients has the power to influence our behavior toward cue recognition, identification and inferencing. Both verbal and nonverbal communication can modify the noticing of cues, as well as our neutrality or lack of it. The nurse can influence or be influenced toward alert openness and objectivity or to premature narrowing, prejudgment, and stereotyping that restricts and colors both reception and assignment of meaning.

Pretend for a moment that you are coming on duty in the morning. The night nurse reports that Mrs. Eaton, a 38-year-old woman with long-standing asthma, has had a most uncomfortable night. She's been wheezing and short of breath, has slept very little and been quite anxious and miserable. After report you walk down the hall to Mrs. Eaton's room to check on her. She says, "Oh, Miss Reader, would you mind rubbing my back? I've had a terrible night—hardly slept at all." What thoughts go through your mind in response to this request?

Now let's replay the scene. You are back listening to the night nurse's change of shift report. She says, "In 139 you've got a real problem. Mrs. Eaton is a middle-aged chronic asthmatic who sure seems to enjoy ill health. She's using her condition to manipulate her husband, her children, her parents *and us!*" After report you go down to see this client. As you enter the room she says, "Oh Miss Reader, would you mind rubbing my back? I've had a terrible night—hardly slept at all." What thoughts go through your mind in response to the same request this time?

Testing Biasing Influences.   A fresh personal experience has more impact than either vicarious experience through reading or even recall of an earlier experience where your own receptiveness to stimuli was modified by the attitudes or words of others. To test this personally, enter into a situation (clinical or not) with the goal of allowing others to influence your receptiveness to cues and the labels you would assign to them. Any individual or communication media can be used. After you have experienced it yourself then try another experiment. Deliberately seek to influence and color the cue-noticing behavior of others. Then find out where you, by your words and manner, were a force upon the way another person viewed events and subsequently interpreted and responded to them. Listen to change of shift reports or assignment conferences for influences that may shape subsequent observations of the participants. Then look at your responsibilities for maintaining a climate where data can be neutrally, objectively perceived and validly interpreted.

Awareness of the Observational Climate. It would seem wise for the nurse who is identifying cues in a particular situation to stand back occasionally and try to examine forces that may be working in this situation to cause her to narrow her focus, modify the response of the client or color her perceptions. Prior knowledge and experience in cue recognition are invaluable to the nurse, but like so many virtues they can be a vice as well, as they tend to shape perceptions toward conformity with that which has occurred before. The skilled practitioner will maintain a balance between using her expertise to locate and identify cues and continuing openness to data and meaning. Give the data opportunity to reach you in its own form, then use your knowledge to organize it for making inferences that are valid *for this occasion.*

Vocabulary as an Influence

There is another potential force in cue recognition and identification—vocabulary. While there is some disagreement about the role that a person's vocabulary plays in the attention given to cues in the environment, some authorities do believe that the words one has available and the knowledge they represent affect not only *how* one describes what is noticed, but more particularly, *what* one is prepared to notice (Postman and Weingartner, 1969, 99-101). Suppose, for example, a very young nursing student with a limited vocabulary related to the respiratory system and its dynamics was asked to check the patient's breathing. She might well come back and report, "He's breathing." Once her vocabulary and concomitant knowledge include the relevant descriptive terms and phrases she would *be prepared to notice* many additional cues other than the rise and fall of clothing or bedding covering the chest. The vocabulary usually includes terms such as: rate, shallow, deep, equality of chest expansion, accessory muscles, flaring nares, duration of inspiratory and expiratory phases, wheeze, rattle, sighing, pursed lips on expiration, depression of the sternal notch on inspiration, paradoxical breathing, rales, flail chest, and so forth.

Level of Precision. By the same token, it would seem that a general or precise type of vocabulary might well influence the detail of data gathering. Pretend for a moment that your descriptive vocabulary for identifying the nature of client response is limited to a few general qualifying terms: good, fair, poor, well, some, normal, moderate. Now describe some familiar client responses. Did you find yourself using such phrases as: tolerated well, looks good, respirations poor, fair evening, usual day, moderately active, some pain? Do these phrases sound familiar?

If, indeed, vocabulary is a force in determining *what* we are able notice in the environment, then as nurses our competence in assessment must include attention to a vocabulary that permits us to "see" what is available and to retain its word picture with appropriate precision.

Being Multilingual

While we are considering vocabulary and cue identification it may be the time to note the importance of a nurse's being multilingual. Often we think of multilingual as referring to languages other than our native tongue. There is, however, another aspect of being multilingual—*within* one's own language (Engle, 1969, 354). For the nurse, this means having a working knowledge of the jargon of the related health care disciplines with which she regularly works and that of groups of clientele she regularly contacts.

The physician group will be most comprehending if data are offered to them in medically oriented terminology, sometimes even within the vocabulary of a subspecialty. A skin lesion, for instance, can be described in lay terms, but it can also be translated into the dermatologists terminology to him to communicate precisely the nature of the observation. A brown spot could be described as a nevus, a reddened area may be erythema, hemangioma, macular or papular rash, or a combination of both, and it may be dry or weeping. Each term conveys a particular precise meaning to the dermatologist.

By the same token, if we wish to be understood and to understand the data clients offer, we obviously need to know the words and meanings of their day-to-day vocabularies. A student once reported a situation where a physician was both concerned and angry when a client was readmitted with a flare up of his peptic ulcer, reportedly due to a heavy bout of drinking. He decided to try to frighten the client out of repeating this pattern by showing him the relationship between the drinking and the symptoms. The doctor, accompanied by the nurse, went in and in a loud, obviously negative tone of voice, pointed out the relationship between methyl alcohol and hemorrhaging or perforating ulcers. When the client seemed properly cowed the tirade ended and the doctor stalked out. The client then turned to the nurse and said, "He sure was mad. What was it all about?" It then became the nurse's role to translate medical terms to lay terms so that the content as well as the feeling tone was understood. As nurses, we can't collect subjective data unless we can use the client's language in our questions and understand his meaning in his responses.

It is tremendously important for the nurse to be multilingual within the English language, at least in terms of health care disciplines and clientele, in order to collect cues and to communicate them.

THE NEXT STEP

Two basic component skills have been discussed so far—first, making the differentiation in your own thinking between cues (objective data on reality) and the subjective inferences drawn from them; second, awareness of forces that influence cue identification. Beyond these foundational skills are others related to knowledge of cue sources and identification of cues in verbal and nonverbal forms using the various sensory receptors.

SOURCES AND SKILLS IN IDENTIFYING VERBAL CUES

The most tangible cues, if not necessarily the most valid ones, are verbal—words, written and spoken. Here the skills are related to capturing verbal messages as they are heard in spoken cues and in knowing where and what to look for in records or other written sources of cues.

Cues in Written Form

Cues in written form have the advantage of being stable and available for reexamination. They tend to be about the client rather than from the primary data source except for the relatively rare situation where the client or people important to him have put material into writing. The major source of written data is records *about* the clients that are maintained in some form in almost every health service. Records tend to be kept on:

> data collected—subjective and objective, inferences made, services performed,
> client response to activity, therapy or pathology.

Any practitioner can survey the forms and records available in a given health care setting and determine the range of accessible data. Of course, *when* the data become available, and *which* information actually will be collected seem to be less predictable in most settings. But even here the nurse can look for patterns as a basis for use of the materials.

Admission or intake records often accompany the client to the unit or agency. A referral form may precede a contact. Even the least formal of the nonestablishment clinics probably make some notation of an initial contact. One discovers that medical histories and physical examinations or nursing assessments are taken and written up within hours of admission or in X number of days. The physician and all other disciplines who make contacts tend to make notations on progress or consultation forms. Routine laboratory work includes specific items in each particular clinical service or type of setting and becomes available after so many hours or days. Some records are kept in the immediate area, some farther away. But in each health care setting, formal or informal, establishment or nonestablishment, there evolve some record system and some norms of expectations for kinds of written data and the times when they become available. The nurse learns record resources, locations and norms of availability as a basis for skillfully using the cues in recorded data.

Beyond learning the system, the nurse decides, in any given client situation, what it is essential to know and the range of desirable data. Then she uses the system skillfully to obtain those data which it can predictably provide.

Cues in the Admission Sheet. The admission sheet is an example of a regularly available data source on an institutionalized client. It is so readily available that it is often overlooked as a source of important, useful cues. To test this out, scan the admission form of Lois Graham. See what you know about her when you finish reading it.

Use the data on this sheet, including the addresses and cities as if they were real, whether you the reader live in Montana, another state, or another country.

How many cues did you find? There should have been more than twenty.

Our Local Hospital

ADMISSION RECORD

Name: Graham, Lois Eileen   Date: 8/6/76   Time: 10:20 A.M.
Patient number: 1-2-345-67
Usual address: 408 West 2nd Street, Kalispell, Montana
Age: 46   Sex: Fe   Birthdate: 1/7/30
Birthplace: Montana   Marital: M   Religious Preference: Assembly of God
Social Security Number: 517-26-1799   Phone—Home: 756-4321
Employer: Grant's Hardware Store   Address: 360 West 3rd
                                                    Kalispell, Montana
Length of employment: 6 years   Occupation: Stock clerk
Legal next of kin: John Graham   Relationship: Husband
Address: 408 West 2nd Street, Kalispell, Montana
Person to notify: John Graham   Relationship: Husband
Address: (current) Evergreen Motel   (in reader's city) Phone: 321-6500
Admitting Diagnosis: Low Back and Right Leg Pain—acute exacerbation
                    Chronic Disc Syndrome
Attending Physician: Dr. Oliver Parker
Admitting Service: Neurology

You, without seeing Lois Graham know a great deal about her already. You have data that say she is a 46-year-old woman, admitted on an August morning with low back pain and pain in her right leg. She has had it before and has been diagnosed by someone as having chronic disc syndrome. Her legal next of kin is her husband John who is with her in town, staying at a motel in your area. They share the same home address in Kalispell, Montana. John is to be notified if any need arises. Despite her previous back problems, Mrs. Graham has for six years worked as a stock clerk in Grant's Hardware Store in the town where she lives, probably a couple of blocks from her home. Grant's Hardware Store is her current employer so she may have responsibility for a return date. She has a social security number. They have a phone in their home. She lists a fundamentalist church organization as her religious preference rather than a more general category such as Protestant. Dr. Oliver Parker is her physician on this occasion. She has been admitted to the neurology unit.

When you add your knowledge of: (1) your town or city, (2) Dr. Parker's philosophy of medicine and treatment of low back pain in particular, (3) the nature of the neurology unit (substitute an appropriate clinical unit if your setting does not include a neurology unit), (4) the presence or lack of a Church of God or related denomination in your area, (5) the distance of your location from Kalispell, Montana, and (6) the resources in your town available to visitors —you've pulled together quite a host of working data in a short time. And this hasn't begun to bring in your knowledge of the pathophysiology and other scientific bases. If you were experienced in using an admission sheet in this way, the identification of cues and tying them in with your related knowledge took only the time needed to scan the admission sheet. The looking and the thinking can be very rapid processes. In addition to giving you: (1) an immediate block of background information about the client, (2) stimulating consideration of these cues in relationship to your knowledge of the current environment and the resources it offers and the underlying pathophysiology of the presenting complaint, these data serve another purpose. This review of the written cues also suggests other areas of nursing implications. (See Uses of Single Cues, pp. 76-79) and a need for additional data. It results then in the creation of an *observational shopping list* of items to be explored in the upcoming client-nurse contact as a basis for arriving quickly at an accurate current assessment of the client's status and nursing needs.

Cues in Other Sections of the Clinical Record. Obviously you could perform this same activity with laboratory sheets, order sheets, nursing assessments, nursing care plans, physical examination sheets, or any other form on which data about a client are recorded. To check your own growth in using data on forms for cues you might:

1. keep track of the time it takes you to use a particular data source; it should get shorter as you gain skill and speed.
2. notice whether you are making use of more cues in your planning and subsequent assessment of the client

3. notice if you have developed different combinations of sources of information with changing clientele, data needs, and situations.

To compare your perceptions in screening records to those of others, ask another nurse on your unit or in your class to screen the same record independently. Then compare the cues you noticed and your reasons for selecting them. When you have differences, look to the logic of your choices. This activity can also be used profitably as a mini-team or ward conference on a regular basis. **Written Material: Primary and Secondary Source Material.** Occasionally, in some settings the client will write about himself or produce some written material that can be used as data. But for the most part written cues are about, not from, the client. This means that they constitute some other person's recorded perceptions or the report of a machine's measurement of the client. They are an invaluable resource, and, being written, they stay put. Stability however should not be equated with validity. Written data are only a point of departure for the next contact with the client—that constantly changing person.

Cues in Spoken Form

More transient than words written on paper, but often closer to the sender at that point in time are the words that are spoken. In speech, too, one often experiences more spontaneity. Still, there is the added difficulty of catching the words and their intended meaning on the fly. They're here and gone so quickly! The skill comes in capturing and storing these verbal cues in an accurate form for later retrieval and use.

The sources of spoken data can be either primary (a person revealing himself in words), or secondary (a person other than the client talking about the client). Of course, the person who talks about the client also is a primary source since his words reveal himself, his perceptions of the client and the relationship as he sees it. These too can be valuable cues to the nurse.

The nursing and medical histories are examples of deliberate, systematic search for primary verbal cues. These interview guides seek to elicit the client's description of what he is experiencing and what he has experienced. His report on what has happened to him is *his area of expertise*. In addition to the history, which is seen as a one time interaction in any entry to a health care system, there are the day to day contacts between health care personnel and the client during which verbal cues are offered on what he is experiencing or, perhaps more accurately, what he wishes you to know about that he is experiencing. It can include symptoms, thoughts, dreams, ideas, interests, feelings, goals, and any other perceptions.

Some examples of spoken cues from secondary sources include conversations or reports from family members and acquaintances. It would also include reports from any others involved in care or services, both professional and nonprofessional.

IDENTIFYING NONVERBAL CUES

Verbal cues represent sensory input that someone has already noticed and named. As such these cues have a certain concreteness and identity. But, as individuals, we also receive sensory input from our external and internal environment that is nonverbal and which we ourselves notice and name in order to use it purposefully and communicate it effectively to ourselves or others. We take over the function of translating nonverbal cues to a verbal form.

It has been said that 90 percent of interpersonal communication is nonverbal. Yet nurses, in common with their fellowmen, experience the greatest difficulty in delineating cues in nonverbal areas. The most blurring between cues and inferences occurs in this nonverbal dimension. We tend to be less observant, and more vague and nonspecific. To validate this for yourself, try the following activity. Observe another person as you interact with him. Note the cues being sent in facial expression, position, distance, body movement, voice pitch, rate of speech and speech patterns (not content). What is being communicated? Are you finding, like the rest of us, that inferences roll in almost unbidden? Did the elusive cues seem to slip away before you could catch them to be quickly replaced by equally fleeting new ones?

Subliminal Amplitude in Cues

As teachers we've often been aware that a class is just not with it on a particular day without noticing how we have gotten this impression. Once the situation is recognized it is sometimes possible to identify the usually nonverbal cues that transmitted the message in the first place. Sometimes we resort to a perception check to validate the impression by asking the students—What's happening? Have we lost you? What's operating? In the same way some nurses seem to tune in, without being really aware, to subliminal input of cues. They know a client is taking a turn for the worse even before it becomes obvious. Again subliminal cues—cues of insufficient amplitude to be noticed and identified are coming in. At least some kind of input has generated the impression. This is not unusual in nursing or outside of it. There are innumerable occasions when you "just know," but can't quite identify the critical cues in the situation that enabled you to "know." As important as intuition and hunches are, for nurses they are primarily an antecedent to the search for the input to validate the impression.

Skills in Identifying Nonverbal Cues

The skills in making nonverbal cues useable are related to increasing sensitivity to the input and having the available language to identify, usually with words, that which is noticed. Skills in cue identification, like any others, are achieved by *appropriate* practice, not merely reading about the associated ideas. The nurse who is interested in gaining skill will not only read, but will practice: (1) wider and more intensive use of sense organs to take in cues in the environment, and (2) development of language to translate the cues into precise, useable, retrievable units of information.

Visual Cues

The complexity of the visual world around us has forced us to resort to selective inattention, screening out some stimuli so that we do not become overloaded and uncomfortable. But, unless one checks out occasionally what is being ignored, there is a risk of depriving one's self of richness of visual input that may be available. Periodically it is wise to reverse the direction from screening out stimuli to opening ourselves to the fullness of the visual environment, just to be sure we are not excluding necessary or desirable cues. It may also demonstrate that the capacity for noticing and using cues is in fact greater than had been suspected.

Receiving Visual Cues. Sometimes it is necessary to go outside the usual sphere of activities to renew personal skills. A place to start sharpening vision may not be in the clinical situation, but in another environment, one with a nonnursing orientation. An art appreciation class can offer dimensions of seeing color, shapes, and relationships that may foster fresh eyes and words for these stimuli. This then can be brought back to offer greater precision in the clinical situation. Some nurses have told us that a beginning drama class sharpened their vision for noticing cues of body language and related areas. An anthropology class was found to enable the nurse to interpret cues of territorial preferences and body language in terms of differing ethnic meanings. Sensitivity workshops, which focus on cues, meaning, and response and exclude so many extraneous demands and constraints, enable participants to experience input of cues with greater intensity in the visual field as well as in other sensory dimensions.

Each of these ventures away from nursing suggests new vistas so that on returning to the clinical field, the practitioner can view the client, the environment, and self with a different perspective—a readiness to see with fresh eyes.

Sending Visual Cues. Beyond the seeing of visually available cues there is another area of concern to nurses. That is the nature of visual cues or messages which the nurse is sending to others knowingly or unknowingly.

To test the visual cues you send, set up a role-playing experience with one other person.

> Ask that individual to assume the role of a client who has turned on his signal light to request some small personal service which he can't do for himself. Then assume the role of a nurse answering this light. Behave as if you were working on a very busy unit and answering the light of a client about ready to go home. This particular client has been "sitting on his light" all shift long. This final little request is the last straw. Do not permit yourself to communicate any of your frustration and impatience verbally. Be verbally polite and do what is asked. However in visible, audible nonverbal

behavior try to communicate the idea that his behavior in making this request is highly unacceptable and has made you very upset. Discontinue the role-playing as soon as you have completed the requested service. Then ask your "client" what he experienced.

In workshops and classes where this learning experience has been used, within seconds the "clients" reported receiving messages of hostility, anger, "she didn't want to do it," "she couldn't wait to get out of the room" and similar feelings of rejection.

Ask your client what there was in your behavior that enabled him to "know" that you were upset since you were being verbally professional and actually carrying out the requested task. Compare the cues your partner recognized with those you intended to send.

In the groups where this experience has been used one often sees: distance being maintained between nurse and client except while the service is performed, rapid movements, and the setting down of objects with vigor. The posture of the nurse, if the client talked at any length, tended to be that of placing the weight on one foot rather than on both, hands behind the back or in some cases on the hip and movement was away from rather than toward the patient. "Clients" also reported lack of smiling and eye contact as well as short responses.

In a few seconds the service has been given, the nurse has been professional and the client has received a message that his request was disturbing to the nurse.

From earliest student days nurses are taught about verbal communication. The visual cues that are sent, though insidious, can drown out our well chosen words. Obviously we can't establish a continuous awareness and control of the visual cues we send, but as health professionals we can't ignore the reality of our cue-sending behavior either. We can strive for growing awareness and skill in sending cues that effectively and authentically communicate clear messages. At the least we may shed the delusion that we can conceal our real feelings from our clients.

Vocabulary in Visual Cue Identification. Increasing the range and precision of vocabulary available to retain visual stimuli will be directed toward adding words which depict several dimensions. Words and quantifying symbols related to color, gradation, shape, size, relationships in space, location, movement, speed and distance are needed.

Activities to develop your vocabulary in this area can be undertaken with very little disruption of your day. To test this take a minute to try to think of all the words you could use to indicate the particular shades and values of a color, such as red. Or try this activity with a partner: Alternate naming a shade of the color until one of you is unable to continue. With just a few minutes spent regularly in this type of activity your immediately retrievable working vocabulary related to visual cues in each dimension can be expanded. This in turn can affect *what* you are prepared to see.

Nonverbal Auditory Cues

It is paradoxical that in a time of increasing noise pollution where "tuning out" is almost essential in some parts of our lives, the nurse must try to "tune in" effectively to a variety of subtle auditory stimuli in her contacts with clients. Deliberately introduced activities may be needed to prevent the tuning out which the nurse may do in the nonclinical segment of her life from creeping into the clinical portion where astute focused listening is an essential professional skill. Words represent only part of the auditorily received cues that are available and needed. Reading and participant activities can be undertaken to sensitize or resensitize the student, practitioner or team member to the art of listening, beyond or in addition to the words—listening to people and nonpeople oriented sounds.

Receiving Nonverbal Auditory Cues. Activities to increase nonverbal auditory receptivity are primarily oriented to the nurse role; however exercising the listening-cue labelling behavior in a variety of settings involving many sources of nonverbal auditory input can add acuity in a wide range of situations. The goal is to develop sensitivity to nonword cues—changes in pitch and volume of sounds, including the voice, noticing *when* sounds occur or fail to occur in a situation, attending to the rate of flow of words in speech, the duration of utterances—any dimension of sound that does not deal with the content of the words.

Try to separate sight from sounds by listening while looking away from the speaker or the source of the sound. Turn off the video portion of the TV or movie film. Listen to tapes, to the radio. Make tapes and listen to yourself.

Listen to another person without looking at him. Try to extract cues about the sounds and speech patterns from what you hear.

Areas in which cue collection may be possible include: rate of speech (words per minutes if you wish to quantify), voice inflections, pitch of the voice, length of utterances, interrupting or overriding of the speech of others, sentences shortened or interrupted by breathing activities, sighing, grunting, groaning, sobbing, giggling, wheezing, rattling, quavering, silences. . . .

Listen to a change of shift report. Are there any messages conveyed by the voice rather than the words? Identify them. What changes in voice or speech patterns led you to notice them? By changing your speech patterns could you communicate a similar mood or message?

Listen to the sounds in the client's hospital environment as if you were not a nurse and therefore did not know their meaning. What do you hear? Listen from various parts of the unit. Does the sound of the environment vary? Listen at different hours of the shift, different shifts. What do you hear? Do these sounds which project cues to the client have any implications for your nursing care? Try setting a tape recorder in various parts of the unit at differing hours of the day. The sounds may astound you.

Check with the client as to the sounds he hears and what they as cues communicate to him.

Again the goal is to listen with a fresh approach. With or without a tape recorder it is possible to set oneself to listen more widely—to allow sounds to be noticed which have been tuned out before. In the end the decision may be that it is efficient to tune them out once more, but it will be a decision based on a recent experience, not on routine or habit.

Sending Auditory Nonverbal Cues. As with visual cues, nurses send nonverbal auditory cues. The tape recorder can enable an individual to hear himself and gain some insight into what he communicates unknowingly. Encounter groups serve this purpose too, as do some communication classes. There are many resources for gaining insight into nonverbal auditory behavior. Learning to know ourselves in this dimension can add insight to our nursing skill if the initial discomfort of hearing oneself when it does not sound as we might have expected or wished can be tolerated.

To test how different moods might change the sound of the same words try using the following sentence,

Sally Burton asked me to trade days with her, so I'll have tomorrow off.

to communicate: delight, disgust, anger, neutrality, disappointment. If you have a tape recorder available, record the performance and listen for identifiable differences. Try to describe them. Or ask a friend to listen and tell you what sounds different.

Begin to listen to yourself more attentively. Is the tone of your voice sending the same messages as the words?

Vocabulary in Auditory Cues. Vocabulary in auditory cues will seek to communicate accurately the nature of the sound, volume, pitch, tone of voice, rate of speed of sounds, monotony or variability, patterns, frequency of sounds. It can also be used to indicate relationships to antecedent or current events.

Tactile Cues

Tactile cues are used to communicate data about both current status and response. One has only to contrast the tactile exploration by the infant of his world with the lack of use of this sense by most adults in their assessment of the environment (excluding the blind of course), to realize how diminished our use of tactile cues has become. True, in the clinical area touch is used to rule out and rule in certain pathology—the heat and hardness of a potential inflammatory response, the size, shape, firmness, and texture of a mass, the smoothness or roughness, dryness or moistness, of a skin lesion, the crepitus of bone fragments or friction in a joint.

Beyond these, touch also communicates units of information about response, mood, territory and sometimes custom (Plackhan, 1968). Here, cues on speed, force, impact, area of contact, degree of firmness, or absence of touch are dimensions that communicate important data. Contrast the messages of response via the tactile cues of: lips touching lips, a hand having vigorous impact on a face, the stroking of hands on a back, the contact of a hand firmly grasping a limp, flaccid one and quickly withdrawing.

Receiving and Sending Tactile Cues. The receiving and sending of cues by touch has implications for nursing care (Durr, 1971). Avenues may be available that have not been fully used. Learning experiences in sensitizing, exploratory thinking, and testing are appropriate in increasing the nursing fitness of the tactile sensory input system. Look for situations in which tactile cues are: (1) available and (2) significant in nursing care situations. Seek the experience of receiving tactile input from animate and inanimate objects to refresh yourself in the receiving of these cues and to heighten the discrimination of differences you may discern. Experiment with interpersonal cue sending and receiving through the sense of touch.

> To increase awareness of tactile input, deliberately seek out and identify tactile cues that you have recently experienced without noticing—the nap of fabric, the slippery coldness of condensation on the outside of a glass of ice water, the satin feel of hand-rubbed wood, the slivery sensation of rough-cut cedar siding, the fragile softness of a flower petal. Don't neglect the sense organs on other parts of your body—your feet, your back. Experience the texture of the chair, the bed, the cement sidewalk, the "give" of the padded rug, the gravel road. Experience anew the tactile input you have tuned out, not used.

> If a group activity is desired, bring in a number of objects representing variety in tactile stimulation. Ask group members to experience the objects through their fingers and hands—without looking at them. Then describe the tactile cues they received. Compare descriptions.

> Try to "see" another person's face through the touch of your hands and fingers as the unsighted might. Close your eyes. Touch and trace the person's face. Note the features, planes, movement, temperature, textures, tension of musculature. Verbalize the cues as you experience them. If this is done as a group activity, each participant should have the opportunity to "see" and to be "seen."

Vocabulary in Tactile Cues. Vocabulary to retain descriptive, precise impressions of touch can include words expressing variants in location, texture in depth or surface, consistency, pressure, outline of shapes, smoothness or friction between moving parts, degree of dryness or moisture, force, impact, and temperature.

Other Senses

While sight, hearing, and touch are undoubtedly the most frequently used sensory receptors, the remaining senses—taste, smell, and proprioceptors (body sense) cannot be omitted if the fullest range of input is to be experienced. Having read and participated in the activities of the previous sections on nonverbal sensory input, try to create your own activities and vocabulary for your own learning and that of a group, if you have responsibility for staff development. Highlight experiences using taste buds, the sense of smell, and the widely distributed proprioceptive organs that contribute to self knowledge on position and body image (MacRae, 1969, 659).

CUE IDENTIFICATION—SUMMARY

Cues, individual bits of sensory input, constitute an individual's images of reality. They form the building blocks for structuring subsequent inferences, decisions, and actions or attitudes. This is true whether one is aware of the nature of the input or not. As health professionals we owe our clientele and ourselves real competence in the several dimensions of cue identification:

knowledge that heightens noticing of significant cues

openness and sensitivity to cues that are available, even when their significance is not immediately apparent

working knowledge of cue sources in the clinical setting

a vocabulary adequate to: permit receiving communication from clientele in data gathering; describe objectively and precisely the input being noticed and communicate data to other disciplines

curiosity enough to search for identifiable cues when intuition or hunches suggest that a particular situation is occurring

a growing awareness of the cues one is sending as well as those being received

an awareness of forces that shape noticeability and identification of cues in any situation.

CUES, THE BUILDING BLOCKS IN INFERENCING

For the health professionals the collection of cues is an active, deliberate process carried out for a purpose that goes beyond the mere accumulation of information. Yet the planning process has tended to break down at the point of using collected cues effectively to formulate valid inferences. Again, this is a skill that can be isolated and practiced for greater effectiveness.

Skills Related to the Use of Single Cues

Cues may be likened to bricks. Given a single brick, you could conceive of many uses, the ceiling being the limits on your experience and imagination. Stop reading for a minute and in that time write down all of the uses you could make of a brick.

How many were you able to think of?

Did you consider using a brick for:

a paperweight

a weight for pressing flowers or glued materials until they dry

a book end

a weapon

a hammer

a nutcracker

an elevation or prop for an object or some part of it

an obstacle to prevent movement of a car wheel

a foot warmer

a weight for traction or muscle building

a counterweight in a pulley system

an art object (a surface for painting)

a decorative object for texture or shape

a base for a vase or flower pot

a planter

a water saver when placed in the toilet water tank

a weight to facilitate rooting in plant propagation by layering

a door stop

a stool for standing on to reach a high object

a support for a book shelf

a fulcrum in a lever system or small teeter totter

a dam for a mud puddle

ground cover or drainage (crushed up)

a scraper for removing mud and dirt from shoes

This does not begin to suggest the things you could start to build with one brick.

Such an activity results in *divergent* thinking—a consideration of all available options or implications. This type of thinking in turn tends to minimize premature closure, narrow, ritualistic thinking, and invalid stereotyping.

To apply the same type of creative divergent thinking to nursing that was attempted with the brick as the object, take a single cue and consider the widest range of *nursing* implications. Try this out using the cue:

human—five days old

Allow yourself a few minutes to write down all of the normal attributes related to this cue and the resultant parallel nursing implications that come to mind. Then check the chart on the following page and compare ideas.

With both the brick and the five-day-old cue activities, unless you had attempted them earlier, the range of ideas probably was narrower and emerged more slowly than they would on repetition. When this type of activity has been used in workshops, no one ever has reported having all of the items proposed by

Client Status Cue—Five Days Old

NORMS	NURSING IMPLICATIONS
Inefficient temperature regulating mechanisms	Control body coverings and temperature of environment, food, and fluids.
Small capacity and inexperienced digestive tract. Sucking capacity but unpredictable	Small, easily digested formula or breast milk offered at signs of hunger. Control size of opening of nipple if bottle feeding. Sucking and swallowing compatible with ability.
Multiple sleep cycles throughout the 24 hour period	Short periods available for feeding, cleaning, sensory input around the clock when awake. Implications for sleep and rest of mother/father.
Fragile skin	Need to check and protect airway. Support head moisture/irritants. Use of protective films—oil, powder. Avoiding strong chemicals.
No control of elimination	Need system for absorbing and catching wastes and removing them. Easy opportunity to evaluate normalcy of urine and stool.
Low resistance to certain pathogens	Minimize exposure via respiratory, gastrointestinal tracts and skin. Regular observation for any signs of infection.
Inability to lift head or turn self	Need to check and protect airway. Support head and spinal column.
Open fontanelles	Avoid pressure or impact on unprotected brain area.
No verbal communication	Interpret needs via voice sounds and patterns plus body movements.
Minimal ability to provide own sensory stimulation within the narrow desirable range	Consider norms of recent intrauterine life and offer sound and visual input in amplitude and duration compatible with recent shift. Offer holding and motion to maintain intrauterine norms.

pooling the contributions of all members of the group. And all participants agree that in a second go round, time, not lack of ideas, would be the major factor limiting productivity, at least up to a point.

This same approach then can be used for staff development for the individual or group. Cues that are significant to the clientele being served could be the focus for short staff development activities.

Identify the cue to be used.

Ask each member of the group to write down the nursing implications it brings to mind within a minute or two at the most.

Pool the resources by writing the contributions on a chalk board if there is one in the room or a large piece of newsprint or easel paper hung on the wall.

Leave it there for the rest of the day.

As other ideas occur, they can be added if you leave the chalk or marking pen handy.

One person might volunteer to check a book or journal article for additional ideas.

An expert in the field may also be consulted for input.

This activity serves two purposes for the staff. It fosters divergent thinking in all members—a set to look for options to be validated rather than immediate answers and closure. Second, it brings together for more effective storage and more rapid retrieval the ideas that should be triggered in noticing the cue.

Within each work setting or each category of clientele, no doubt priorities of cue importance and commonality occur. These clinical or client-oriented priorities tend to dictate the cues for which immediately retrievable nursing implications are important. In the coronary care unit cues related to the ECG tracings, types of pain, heart sounds, lung sounds and particular symptoms become urgent. Concomitant cues related to coping responses and resources of the individual, his relatives, or important others also assume significance. On the other hand, in the labor and delivery room, emergency room, hypertension clinic, oncology unit, mental health clinic, or nursing home, other cues suggest the need for immediate response. Thus the frequency of significant cues in one's work setting may order the sequence of staff development conference topics in the cue and nursing implication exercise.

Once the significant/urgent cues common among a given clientele have been brought up to date in the practitioner's repertoire, other cues can be refurbished, reexamined, and reorganized. Eventually, it would seem productive to reach out for cues that might be overlooked in the situation. The goal is to achieve openness, not only to the implications of obviously significant cues but to all cues that the client or his environment may offer which affect his health care and related life-style management.

Use of Multiple Cues

To return to the bricks. When you were asked to imagine or to recall all the uses you could make of a brick, you reached out for ideas or memories. On the other hand, when you see many bricks combined in a certain arrangement, the direction of thinking as to its meaning or identity is convergent—a focusing-in. The arrangement of the bricks suggests a walk, a wall, a barbecue pit, a house, an office building, a street, a border, an oven, a kiln, and so forth. The organization of the individual bricks and their relationship to each other permit assignment of a specific identity.

The same phenomenon holds true with cues. Individual cues combined in particular arrangements or relationships suggest more specific meanings or inferences. Often there are still options of meanings, but the range narrows. In some situations where clusters of cues have a predictable meaning, they are called cue syndromes. The cues are the operational definition of the label. Take the following examples:

Presenting Cues

History of current bed rest

Change in body position from horizontal to upright without an interval in the sitting position.

Complaint of dizziness and feeling of faintness

"Everything's getting black"

Observable pallor

Loss of consciousness, slumping or falling

Increase in pulse rate

Blood pressure lower than previous readings.

LABEL: Orthostatic Hypotension

Presenting Cues

Symptoms being experienced by the individual on a regular basis.

Doctor has informed the person in language he understands and on several occasions of the findings on diagnostic studies, the diagnosis or meaning of the findings and the probable outcome.

Individual deviates regularly from prescribed regimen of medications, diet and activity schedule.

Individual reports feeling better or decrease in symptoms when objective data and observation of his responses indicate continuation or progression of pathophysiology.

LABEL: Denial of disease

Nursing's body of knowledge will achieve increments as cue syndromes related to *its* definition and primary focus in health care are identified and tested for scientific soundness and predictability. The nurse's expertise, as the physician's, will lie at least in part in being able to detect the subjective and objective cues in the client's situation and then arrive at an accurate nursing diagnosis as a basis for productive health care management.

SUMMARY

Skills in extracting information from the environment, retaining an accurate representation of it, assigning valid meanings and being able to communicate these precisely to others are basic to the care planning process. These skills will be integral and essential components of subsequent chapters as we move into the steps of care planning.

REFERENCES

Crowell, Carolyn. "A Study to Determine What Cues are Utilized by Selected Senior Students in Nursing When Making an Inference About the Condition of the Patient," Unpublished Master's Thesis, University of Washington, 1967, 117 pp.

Durr, Carol. "Hands that Help . . . but How?" *Nursing Forum* 10:392-400, 4, 1971.

Eisman, Roberta. "Criteria Registered Nurses Reportedly Use in Making Decisions Regarding the Observation of Respiratory Behavior of Patients," Unpublished Master's Thesis, University of Washington, 1970, 65 pp.

Engle, George E. "On the Care and Feeding of Faculty," *The New England Journal of Medicine* 28:351-355, August 14, 1969.

Gibson, Eleanor. *Principles of Perceptual Learning and Development.* New York: Appleton-Century-Crofts, 1969, Chapter I.

Gore, William J. *Administrative Decision Making: a Heuristic Model.* New York: John Wiley and Sons, 1964.

Kaplan, Abraham. *The Conduct of Inquiry.* San Francisco: Chandler Publishing Co., 1964, pp. 126-138.

Lombard, George F. "Self Awareness and Scientific Method," *Science* 112:289-293, Sept. 5, 1950.

MacRae, J. H. "Speculation, A General Theory of Perception," *Developmental Medicine and Child Neurology,* 11:654-662, 1969.

McDonald, Florence. "Inquiry," in *Behavioral Concepts and Nursing and Intervention,* Carolyn Carlson, ed. Philadelphia: J. B. Lippincott Co., 1970, pp. 269-280.

Moore, Larry. "Problem Recognition in Nursing Service Administration,"*Nursing Forum* 8:94-102, No. 1, 1969.

Parnes, Sidney. *Creative Behavior Guide Book.* New York: Charles Scribner's Sons, 1967, pp. 3-41.

Pearson, Betty. "A Study of Cues Which Staff Nurses Reported They Utilized in Making an Inference of a Patient State," Unpublished Master's Thesis, University of Washington, 1968, 68 pp.

Pluckhan, Margaret. "Space the Silent Language . . ." *Nursing Forum* 7:386-397, 4, 1968.

Postman, Neil and Charles Weingartner. *Teaching As a Subjective Activity.* New York: Delacorte Press, 1969. "Meaning Making," pp. 82-97; "Languaging," pp. 48-132.

Rosenhan, D. L. "On Being Sane in Insane Places," *Science* 179:250-258, January 19, 1973.

Scheff, Thomas J. "Typification in the Diagnostic Practices of Rehabilitation Agencies," in Marvin B. Sussman, *Sociology and Rehabilitation.* Am. Soc. Assoc., 1965, pp. 139-147.

Trabasso, Tom and Gordon H. Bower. *Attention in Learning: Theory and Research.* New York: John Wiley and Sons, 1968, pp. 1-43.

Verhonick, Phyllis, et al. "I Came I Saw I Responded: Nursing Observation and Action Survey," *Nursing Research* 17:38-44, January-February, 1968.

Wilson, John. *Thinking With Concepts.* Cambridge, England: Cambridge University Press, 1963.

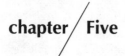

chapter Five

The Role of Knowledge in the Assessment– Diagnostic Process

How does assessment differ from the cue and inference activities discussed in the previous chapter? It does and it doesn't. Actually, the cue and inference activity is the basic unit of the assessment process. Assessment, however, seems to go well beyond these basic skills to a complex, systematic investigation in which a body of knowledge is used to test combinations of the cues and inferences made against a variety of diagnostic concepts to arrive at valid productive explanations—nursing diagnoses. This is true whether the assessment is a comprehensive one involving many areas or a presenting problem approach.

For example, suppose the nurse entering a room in a nursing home sees an elderly woman sitting hunched over a wheelchair in the corner. Her gnarled, thin hands lie motionless in her lap. She is in stocking feet. Her thin gray hair is wispy and looks uncombed. She doesn't move, look up, or respond verbally when you speak to her. You could combine these few cues into several possible diagnostic possibilities: aging, deafness, depression, disengagement, immobilization, preoccupation, sensory deprivation—to name a few.

The assessment process is a continuous flow between data sources and the observer's body of knowledge, drawing on one and then on the other. The data serve to generate the possible explanatory concepts that need to be drawn to awareness in the person's bank of knowledge. The knowledge in turn generates criteria that must be met by the data if a given diagnostic explanation is to be an appropriate fit. The process continues until the assessor is satisfied that, for the moment, the data and the explanation have a good fit. Physicians do this in arriving at medical diagnoses, detectives in solving a crime, and nurses in arriving at nursing diagnoses.

A critical factor in this assessment process is knowledge, particular kinds of knowledge from a variety of disciplines. This knowledge must be organized and stored in such a way as to make it effectively retrievable in the assessment–diagnostic process.

Unless a doctor knows what signs and symptoms, and what etiology are involved in a given diagnosis, unless he understands what the mechanisms of the pathology are in a given diagnosis as well as the host response, unless he has some idea what external interventions are effective in reducing the pathologic effects and supporting the host's defense mechanisms, and unless he knows what cues indicate progress or regression in the course of the given diagnosis he is not functioning very effectively. Dr. Foley wrote of the logic of medical diagnosis proceeding from:

> identification of symptoms and signs (phenomenologic diagnosis)
> specifying the disturbed physiology (physiologic diagnosis)
> localizing the anatomic area of disturbed function (anatomic diagnosis)
> determining the underlying pathologic process (pathologic diagnosis).

He further suggested that whenever this protocol is abandoned in favor of a short cut or intuition, the patient is not well served (Foley, 1973, 26).

The same discipline holds true for nurses, whether they assist in making a medical diagnosis or are involved in arriving at nursing diagnoses. They too must seek data on the desired client and nursing goals, on the barriers to achievement of these goals, on the coping resources the client has available and the skill to use, on deficits in coping resources, and on the underlying mechanisms in a given situation as a basis for arriving at a statement of the nursing diagnosis. For nurses as surely as for doctors, any short cuts or purely intuitive approaches do not serve their clients effectively either. Obviously, this complex, disciplined type of critical thinking requires a body of working knowledge stored and used in a skilled fashion.

As nurses, for the most part, we have rather taken for granted the process by which we combine data and knowledge in the critical thinking skill we call assessment–diagnosis. In this chapter we will attempt to make more explicit three ways in which knowledge is used in this process:

1. to determine significance of cues in the presenting situation
2. to suggest the range of alternatives of explanations/diagnoses for the presenting cues
3. to guide the branching logic involved in searching the situation for additional cues to validate and sharpen the precision of the explanation (diagnosis).

KNOWLEDGE AND ASSIGNING SIGNIFICANCE TO CUES

How do nurses know, among the welter of cues in the environment, which ones to notice and which to ignore? How do they recognize that certain data signal the need for immediate action? The answers lie of course in the knowledge of what mechanisms these cues represent and the danger or discomfort they indicate for the individual. In fact, much of the education of both nurses and doctors is devoted to learning to identify cues—to differentiate and assign weight to them in terms of diagnosis and urgency of response.

Let's take some examples. Since, in the hierarchy of needs, physiologic changes pose the most immediate threat to life, we will use these as our examples,

CUE	SIGNIFICANCE
Rhythmic spurting of bright blood from a wound.	Urgent! Arterial bleeding.

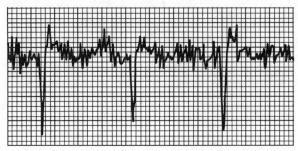

MCL[1]	Not significant—artifact of movement about in bed.
	Significant! Asystole leading to ventricular fibrillation.

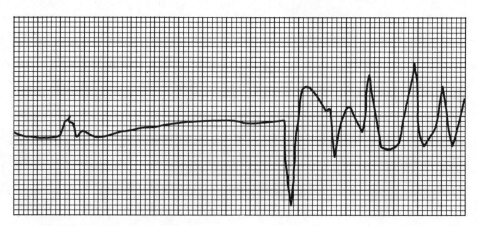

No. ECG 100[1]

Euphoric confusion in an individual with history of chronic obstructive pulmonary disease whose current medical diagnosis is pneumonia.	Significant! Symptoms of cerebral hypoxia.
Urinary output of less than 30 cc per hour.	Important! More than 30 cc of output are needed each hour to maintain renal function.

[1] Tapes and interpretation courtesy of Sandra Underhill, Coronary Care Nurse.

with the acknowledgment that psychosocial crises also can be urgent. In each of these situations knowledge was necessary to cause the nurse to notice the critical cues amid all the others and then to alert the observer to the significance and the relative urgency of the symptoms (Ledley and Lusted, 1959, 9).

This has implications for the way knowledge is stored. When a nurse is acquiring knowledge from any source—about physiology, psychology, anthropology, sociology, microbiology, pharmacology, pathophysiology, law—the deliberate storage pattern should include highlighting the pattern of critical cues associated with each particular nursing diagnostic concept. This in turn should ensure more effective recognition of important cues in the presenting situation and accurate assignment of significance and urgency to them.

KNOWLEDGE AND MOVEMENT TOWARD A DIAGNOSIS

A second use of knowledge in the assessment process is related to the steps involved in arriving at an accurate diagnosis. A definitive diagnosis of a situation is rarely reached in one giant leap. Rather, it emerges as a type of chain reaction in which the cues noticed in the environment trigger ideas within the pool of available related knowledge; this in turn sets off a search for more related data. Wortman, in describing this thinking-searching process, called it a "serial generating and testing process" (Wortman, 1970, 334).

Diagnostic Criteria and Good Fit

Any diagnostic concept includes the criteria that must be met in order for it to fit the situation and offer appropriate explanations of the dynamics involved. The more closely the presenting data and the diagnostic criteria fit, the more accurate and useful the diagnosis will be. Let's look at an example of diagnostic criteria associated with the diagnosis of rubeola (red measles):

> Prodromal fever, conjunctivitis, coryza, bronchitis, Koplik's spots (bluish white pinpoint spots opposite the first molar on the buccal mucosa), exposure to someone having measles from 8 to 13 days earlier (usually 10). By the third or fourth day a dusky-red blotchy rash appears beginning on the face and becoming generalized, lasting 4 to 6 days. Leukopenia.

Prior to the advent of the measles vaccine, and today among those who are not immunized, persons regularly are called upon to recognize this combination of signs, symptoms, and etiology to associate them with the measles diagnosis or consult health personnel to do this.

Now let's take more of a nursing diagnosis and examine how a similar matching of criteria and data occurs. For the diagnosis of *frustration* to be applicable there must be data present in the situation showing that there exists:

1. a desired goal

2. a barrier to achievement of that goal which the individual did not surmount or avoid
3. an uncomfortable feeling ranging from uneasiness to strong disappointment and/or sense of defeat related failure to achieve the desired goal. The intensity of the feeling will tend to be related to the importance of the goal to the individual.

As an example—a nurse sees a baby sitting in a highchair playing with a rubber duck. The duck falls to the floor. The child twists and squirms trying to get out of the chair, strains and reaches toward the floor for the toy, makes increasing noises during the retrieval attempts. When the baby is not successful in reaching, climbing out of the chair, or getting attention by verbal calls, his face flushes, his movements become more vigorous, and he begins to cry. In this classical situation each of the criteria of frustration are met—there is the desired goal of reaching the toy, the barrier of the chair, and the failure of someone to respond to his calls and then his crying. The diagnosis of frustration could be said to be appropriate in explaining the dynamics of the situation.

Let's take another diagnosis common to nursing—*dependency*. If this diagnosis is to be used to explain the presenting situation, data must be present which meet the diagnostic criteria of:

1. a desired goal
2. barrier(s) that prevent the individual from achieving the goal himself
3. availability of resources (other than one's self) that would, if used, enable the achievement of the goal.

To illustrate how the dependency criteria and data can fit, look at the following situations:

an individual with renal failure (barrier) wishes to continue to live (desired goal) and a home dialysis unit plus training, health personnel, and funding are available (external resources to enable achievement, if used);

an elderly Italian lady was deprived of schooling during her childhood so she never learned to read or write (barrier), but she wishes to maintain communication with distant friends (desired goal). Long distance phone calls are prohibitive on her pension (barrier). She has neighbors, visitors, and relatives who can read her mail and write for her (resources) if she chooses to accept their offers or request their help.

Obviously, with either medical or nursing diagnoses, the concepts must be created to include the clearest criterion statements that are available and appropriate (see pp. 300–301). Knowledge stored in this way can help the nurse to check the fit between the presenting data and the criteria. On the other hand, fuzzy, ambiguous, incorrect, or incomplete criteria can make the assessment/diagnostic process both difficult and inaccurate.

The Pool of Working Diagnostic Concepts as an Influence

In nursing as in other disciplines, the quality of assessment–diagnosis is also closely related to the number of well-developed, usable diagnostic concepts the individual possesses. The hallmark of brilliant medical diagnosticians is their ability to scan the greatest number of relevant diagnostic possibilities and their skill in recalling the cue syndromes against which the data must be matched. Obviously, the depth and breadth of the knowledge base as well as proficiency in making connections in novel situations are important. Ledley and Lusted suggested that the errors involved in failure to consider a possible diagnosis are much more common than any other sources of diagnostic mistakes (Ledley and Lusted, 1959, 9). In other fields, too, the ability to scan multiple options before making a judgment is seen as the most creative and effective approach to decision making (Parnes, 1967, 87).

The poor diagnostician, by contrast, may be characterized as having a pool of diagnostic concepts that are inadequate in number and variety. We have seen new students acquire a new diagnostic concept such as immobilization or anxiety and use it to explain a large number of situations where other concepts would be more productive. The poor diagnostician may have an adequate number and variety of concepts but construct them so ambiguously or inaccurately as to make them dangerous. The chances that the diagnostician with few concepts or poorly constructed concepts will move efficiently toward valid, productive diagnoses are markedly reduced because of the caliber of his knowledge base.

There is an old joke about a man who was returning in the wee hours of the morning from a party where he had taken on a considerable amount of alcohol. As he stood on his darkened front porch fishing awkwardly for his keys and trying to fit one into the elusive keyhole, he dropped them. He looked about for a moment or two, shrugged and staggered down to the sidewalk where he began to search about under the street light. A neighbor came along and asked what he was looking for. "I'm trying to find my keys. I dropped them trying to get them into that lock." The neighbor asked why he was looking so far from where he had apparently dropped them. The party goer's response was, "Well, it's light out here. You don't expect me to be able to see in the dark, do you?"

Knowledge is like light, and like the man who lost the key, we as health professionals tend to try to solve problems within the area lighted by our available knowledge. Clients are lucky if their problems are to be found there—and unlucky if they lie outside our range of knowledge. Nor are nurses alone in looking for problems where the light of knowledge is. Balint suggested that doctors may seek to proselytize clients into having the kinds of diseases that they think are feasible, given the focus of their knowledge (Balint, 1957). For example:

A nurse practitioner was assuming ongoing health management responsibility for a 45-year-old man with essential hypertension, among other diagnoses. His blood pressure had been well controlled with guanethidine for several years. A cardiologist had noted earlier on the progress record (shortly after the guanethidine therapy was begun) that the man reported changes in his sex life. The client was referred to a urologist for a consultation. The urologist recorded that there was no organic problem and referred the client for a psychiatric consultation. No further note was made on the problem.

The nurse practitioner's working knowledge included awareness that some drugs regulating hypertension had potential for producing side effects of reduced sexual ability, aldomet and guanethidine being the worst offenders. The man and his wife had lived with the problem for about three years before learning that he was not losing his virility in either an organic or psychological respect, nor was she at fault. The change in their sexual relationship was the price they were paying for pharmacologic control of his blood pressure. Given this knowledge, he could make choices. He and his wife could deal with the problem on a valid foundation just as he was dealing quite knowledgeably with other aspects of his cardiovascular problems and the therapy regimen.

Here was a situation where the light of working knowledge of several health practitioners had not extended to include the side-effects of antihypertensive drugs.

But there are many situations closer to nursing too. Suppose you were given the information that a client you were about to see had a "poor diet." Think of all the explanatory options you might need to consider and on which you would be collecting criterion-related data as you participated in the assessment interaction before you could settle on a definitive nursing diagnosis. Now, see how your list compares with the ideas listed below.

Did you think of these possible explanations?

Is it a *lifetime pattern,* as in the case of the man who never learned to eat fruits and vegetables and now at 75 is not about to change?

Is it *religiously based choice* as in some vegetarian or macrobiotic diets?

Is it *finances,* not enough money in the check, the social security or the welfare payment?

Is it impaired *personal mobility* or lack of transportation to the store?

Is it *lack of knowledge* about what constitutes a balanced diet or a therapeutic diet?

Is it lack of translating that knowledge into *shopping skill?*

Is it *enjoyment of a particular food style,* as in a young mother with liver disease whose total personal diet consisted of cokes and candy bars, though she gave her children a balanced diet?

Is it *lack of skill in cooking* as in the case of the widower whose late wife was a marvelous cook while he never learned how to boil water?

Is it *lack of cooking facilities* so that there is no place in the room to prepare food? (And no availability of Food Stamps for the same reason?) Or more recently lack of anyone to go and get the stamps in person?

Is it *lack of interest due to* preoccupation with other things to the neglect of eating?

Is it *loneliness* at mealtimes as in the case of the widow who had always fixed meals for and eaten with others and is alone at meals for the first time in her life?

Is it *lack of appetite?* Any signs of stress or pathophysiology associated with anorexia?

Is it *poor dentition* (sore teeth, loose teeth, missing teeth, or lack of dentures)?

Is there *preoccupation with food* leading to overeating because of boredom and lack of other interests?

Obviously, this does not complete the list of possibilities. However, it does incorporate some major areas of possibilities. And each conjecture leads to a variety of explanations of the general diagnosis, "poor diet." In turn, each different choice of explanation would generate a direction of search in the assessment process and subsequent decisions regarding ways of acting to help the client manage his nutrition more effectively.

The alternatives of diagnosis become crucial to subsequent data gathering and decisions for action. It is essential that nurses have:

1. enough working concepts to encompass at least the commonly occurring coping deficits so that alternative explanations can be considered as the assessment is going on, and
2. facility in scanning concepts to include all potential nursing diagnoses from which an eventual differential diagnosis will be made.

KNOWLEDGE AND BRANCHING LOGIC

The term branching logic in medicine is used to suggest the economy of "going where the money is" (Yarnall et al, 1971, 11). It is the testing portion of Wortman's "generating and testing" process. Thus, it grows out of and is dependent upon working knowledge. The presenting data available in the situation leave a cue trail to be both *followed and predicted* for more rapid arrival at a diagnostic destination.

Given certain groups of cues there are usually a limited number of directions that logical explanations can take. One collects cues related to the criteria, then matches them against the diagnostic criteria to see if they fit, much as a woman goes to a particular size rack for clothes, then tries them on for suitability. If she is a junior petite, she will not go to the Tall Shop or the Half Sizes. And, within the junior petite sizes, she will not go to the size 7-P if she wears an 11-P. Once she has found the dresses in the 11-P section of the rack there may be some that look and fit better—this is where the trying on is done for *precise* goodness of fit.

In the same way, for efficiency in nursing assessment, general relevant explanatory areas are selected for the initial search, then data are matched against them until the appropriate level and area of precision in explanation are reached—the fit looks good.

The pattern of branching logic might be diagrammed to look something like this.

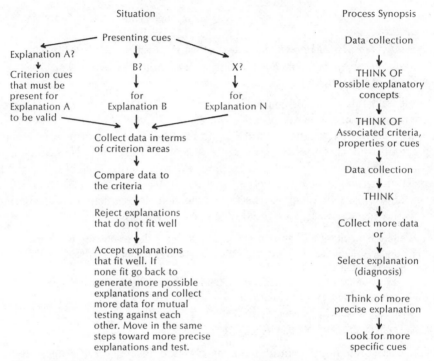

Let's' try this sequence:

Mr. French is a 68-year-old man from northern Alaska who has recently had an above the knee amputation for peripheral vascular insufficiency. He is a former alcoholic who for the past ten years has headed an Alcoholics Anonymous unit in his home town. He has smoked two packs of cigarettes per day for about 50 years. His doctor has explained the importance of his giving up cigarettes in order to get the maximum blood supply to his other leg and his stump, citing the research that shows a relationship between smoking and vasoconstriction. Mr. French still smokes whenever he can obtain cigarettes from someone—despite both pleasant and unpleasant confrontations with the medical and nursing staff and urging by his wife.

In the case of Mr. French, the nurses learned that the explanation for his continued smoking was predominantly addiction, with an element of violation of his normal independence. They heard him saying, "I quit drinking and I'm a

Example of branching logic related to Mr. French's case:

POSSIBLE DIAGNOSTIC CONCEPTS	CRITERIA	DATA COLLECTION
Addiction.	Substance being used by client is known to produce physiologic or psychological dependency (addiction).	Studies show smoking produces physiologic dependency with identified withdrawal symptoms.
	Exposure to the substance long enough to develop physiologic or psychological dependency.	History of heavy smoking (2 packs/day for 50 years).
	Reports of continuing desire for substance and/or withdrawal symptoms/signs associated with lack of intake of the substance.	What kinds of symptoms does he experience when he cuts down or quits? Are there observable differences in behavior when he does not smoke?
		What did he substitute for his drinking behavior?
		How did he manage to quite drinking? (coping with previous addiction)
		How would he see managing to quit smoking if he should decide to do so? (perceived coping resources)
Lack of willpower. (courage)	Reports desire to quit, but says he can't do it; or tries but has obvious difficulty and so engages in the behavior again.	Does he report wanting to quit? What behavior indicates he is trying to quit? Does he return to smoking after cutting back or stopping for any period of time?
Ignorance of consequences. (ignorance)	Reports that he doesn't remember having heard of a relationship.	What does he report understanding of what the health personnel have told him on the subject?
	Reports he does not understand relationship between smoking and circulation.	Is he aware of the research relating smoking to vasconstriction?
Denial of relationship between smoking and vasoconstriction.	Reports having heard about this or having read this information.	What does he think of the studies done in this area—e.g., the Surgeon General's Reports?
	Reports he doesn't believe the research or statements of health personnel.	What does he think of health personnel's expertise in such matters?
	Cites opposing findings.	
Independence.	Reports or behaves as if he does not like having people tell him what to do.	How does he feel about having people tell him what to do?

POSSIBLE DIAGNOSTIC CONCEPTS	CRITERIA	DATA COLLECTION
	Takes initiative in activities.	Does he usually make up his own mind on matters?
	Has history of "doing his own thing."	
Apathy regarding physical well-being.	Says he doesn't care what happens.	Does he speak of wishing he were dead?
	Behaves in other ways to endanger his well-being.	Does he ignore his appearance when he did not do this before?
		Has his attitude toward himself changed in a negative direction since surgery? Does he indicate he is worth less now?
		Does he ignore normal safety precautions?

leader in my town helping other alcoholics. If I can lick alcoholism, I can quit smoking too. I know it's something I must do. But it doesn't help much having you people nag at me all the time, or try to shame me in front of others. I'm no child! What do you know about the craving for that cigarette with your morning coffee while you're reading the paper? I've done it all my adult life. It's going to be easier to manage this when I don't have so much time on my hands with nothing to do and so much pain. When I get back to Alaska I can keep busy, then I'll quit. In the meantime I *am* cutting down, so just get off my back!"

In this example, the presenting situation of an individual who did not stop smoking despite having a good health-based reason for doing so, first caused nurses to consider the possible nursing diagnoses that could be an accurate explanatory framework for the client's difficulty with the treatment regimen. They then recalled the criteria of cues which must be present if a particular diagnosis were to fit, searched the situation for cues that matched and, using the data, narrowed the probable explanations. This is branching logic applied to a nursing management problem.

There is one other way in which branching logic with its inherent knowledge base can be used to lend precision to assessment; it can be used in determining the stage of response in which the individual is functioning. A parallel in medicine would be a situation in which the doctor has made a diagnosis of malignancy and is trying to determine the stage of advancement of the disease—in situ, local spread, distant metastasis. In nursing, too, assessment is often refined to the point of finding a stage in the sequence of responses.

For example, nurses are often concerned with the management of coping problems associated with significant losses in the lives of their clients—loss of a close relative or friend, loss of a way of life as in an undesired or premature retirement from work, loss of freedom to act without having to count the energy cost, loss of function of a part, loss of beauty. Kübler-Ross's concept of the stages in coping with dying (loss of life) is applicable to a variety of significant losses—denial, anger, bargaining, depression, acceptance. The observational criteria offered for each stage permit a nurse to determine the stages at which an individual is functioning in the management of grieving. The branching logic in assessment here would get to the level of precision of: searching for data on the coping mechanisms being used, identifying the stages in the sequence where the individual is functioning and noting its impact on effective management of daily living and personal well-being (Heusinkveld, 1972; Kübler-Ross, 1969, 1971).

MEASUREMENT OF EFFECTIVENESS IN USE OF KNOWLEDGE IN ASSESSMENT

With expertise in nursing assessment becoming mandatory as an explicit skill in our discipline, tests are being evolved to measure the use of knowledge and data in the assessment process using clinical simulations. This has been done for the medical profession (McGuire and Solomon, 1971). Nurses are also developing clinical simulation tests which measure both proficiency in use of knowledge and efficiency in combining the use of knowledge and that of data (De Tornyay, 1968, McIntyre et al, 1972).

SUMMARY

By now it is obvious that assessment and a knowledge base are inseparable. Both elements are involved—a knowledge base and the ability to perceive the cues in the situation and relate them to the diagnostic concepts. The need to use knowledge in this way should influence the way a nurse learns, organizes her knowledge, and masters the skill of knowledge retrieval in the face of cues. There is no such thing as a *routine* assessment. *System* should be strived for, yes, in that the person or the situation are scanned in terms of a planned set of categories to avoid gaps, but routine, never! In each instance a new combination of cues are presented that must be organized according to the most accurate and productive nursing diagnosis. Novelty is the name of the game and knowledge is the substance that holds it together.

REFERENCES

Balint, Michael. *The Doctor His Patient and the Illness.* New York: International Universities Press, 1957.

Butler, Robert and Myrna Lewis. *Aging and Mental Health, Positive Psychosocial Approaches.* New York: Mosby Co., 1973.

Carnevali, Doris. "Conceptualizing, A Nursing Skill," in Pamela Mitchell, *Concepts Basic to Nursing*. New York: McGraw-Hill, 1973.

Chamberlin, T. C. "The Method of Multiple Working Hypotheses," *Science* 148:754-759, May, 1965. Reprint from *Science* 15:92, 1890.

DeTornyay, Rheba. "Measuring Problem Solving Skills by Means of the Simulated Clinical Nursing Problem Test," *The Journal of Nursing Education* 7:34-35, August, 1968.

Foley, Joseph. "Pinpointing Organic Mental Disorders," *Medical World News Geriatrics* 1973, pp. 26-27.

Heusinkveld, Karen. "Cues to Communication with the Terminal Cancer Patient," *Nursing Forum* 11:105-113, #1, 197.

Kübler-Ross, Elisabeth. *On Death and Dying*. New York: Macmillan Co., 1969. "On Learning from the Dying," *American Journal of Nursing* 71:54-62, January, 1971.

Ledley, R. S. and L. B. Lusted. "Reasoning Foundations of Medical Diagnosis," *Science* 130:9-21, July 3, 1959.

Levine, Marvin. "Mediating Process in Humans at the Outset of Discrimination Learning," *Psychologic Review* 70:254-273, 1963.

———. "Hypothesis Set During Discrimination," *Psychologic Review* 74:428-430, 1967.

Lufts, Joseph. *Of Human Interaction*. Palo Alto, Calif.: National Press Book, 1969, pp. 13-15.

McGuire, Christine and Lawrence Solomon, eds. *Clinical Simulations—Selected Problems in Patient Management* and *Atlas of Illustrations*. New York: Appleton-Century-Crofts, 1971.

McIntyre, Hattie, et al. "A Simulated Clinical Nursing Test," *Nursing Research* 21:429-435, September-October, 1972.

Parnes, Sidney. *Creative Behavior Guidebook*. New York: Charles Scribner's Sons, 1967.

Scheff, T. J. "Decision Rules, Types of Error and their Consequences in Medical Diagnosis," *Behavior Science* 8:97-107, 1963.

Wortman, Paul. "Utilization of Probabilistic Cues," *Behavioral Science* 15:329-336, 1970.

———. "Medical Diagnosis: An Information Processing Approach," *Computers and Biomedical Research* 5:315-328, August, 1972.

Yarnall, Stephen and A. Libke. *An Introduction to the Medical History and the Medical Record*. Ed. 2. Seattle: University of Washington Medical School, 1971. Mimeographed, 22 pp.

chapter Six

The Client, The Nurse, and the Nursing Assessment Transaction

The development of a valid, adequate nursing data base is a mutual concern of both the client and the nurse. Each has a vested interest in its accuracy and adequacy. The initial assessment contact is the point where these concerns first intersect. Within the available time period—short or long—client and nurse will participate in sharing themselves in ways that will influence their subsequent interaction as they try to cope with the effective management of health problems and the impact these problems have on daily living.

THE NURSING ASSESSMENT TRANSACTION—
WHAT IT IS AND WHAT IT IS NOT

Over the years the Nursing Assessment,[1] or Nursing History as it was originally called, has emerged in practice as many things—a modified admission procedure comparable to checking clothing and valuables, an orientation to a new environment, a form handed out impersonally to be completed by the client and then collected and filed, a ritualistic question and answer session assigned to the low man on the nursing staff, an extensive systematic review of the client's reported and observable status, a compact collection of high priority subjective and objective information on the presenting situations—it has been all of these. It has been carried out ritualistically or creatively. It has been seen as drudgery or as a stimulating experience. The data base has been used; or it has been filed, unused. It has been made a legitimate part of the client's permanent record; it has also been seen only as a nurses' work sheet.

[1] It is acknowledged that nurses assess clients in almost every contact in some way. Thus we feel a need to distinguish between the ongoing nursing observation and the initial planned systematic collection and recording of the subjective and objective nursing data base (comparable to the physician's history and physical examination). To emphasize this difference, we have used capitalization, so that *Nursing Assessment* is meant to signify the formal protocol of initial data collection.

We see the nursing assessment transaction as a time-limited, focused inter-action in which high priority subjective and objective data regarding the client's presenting situation and his resources and deficits in coping are elicited, observed, and recorded in both physiologic and psychosocial[2] dimensions. The data gleaned become the foundation for plans of nursing care, unwritten or written, involving modification of nursing behavior immediately as well as over the duration of the involvement.

THE CLIENT ASSESSES TOO

Although this aspect of the nursing assessment transaction is less often recognized, the procedure serves as an information gathering situation for the client as well as the nurse. The client may well have an avid need for data, and he may be expected to form important impressions based on this first encounter:

> What information are these people interested in?
> Why does a nurse need information from me?
> Who will use it? What will they do with it?
> Does this person seem to care about me, or is she just filling out another piece of paper?
> Will they be interested in my family or those I value?
> What accommodations will I have to make? Will they make any accommodations to my needs and to me?
> What's the pace of care in this setting?
> Do I feel like trusting them based on this one-person sampling?
> What is it like here?
> Do they listen to me? Do they believe me? Will they help me if I need them?
> Do they seem competent?

Often nurses are not aware of the mutual nature of the information gathering that goes on. They know much of the information *they* have collected, but are less aware of the other side of the coin—the extent and the nature of the data that clients have collected from and about them. And, just as nurses will use the nursing data base for subsequent perceptions and actions, so too the client will modify expectations and responses on the basis of his data base about the nursing staff.

To learn what kinds of information and impressions clients could be collecting from you during the assessment process, try some of the following activities:

1. Tape record an assessment interaction. Don't listen to it immediately, but allow it to "cool" for a few days. Then listen to it *as if you were the client*, not the nurse.

---

[2] "Psychosocial" is intended to include cultural aspects as well.

An alternative would be to ask someone else to listen to it as if he were the client and to give you feedback on the impressions gained from your patterns of verbal communication.

2. Role-play the assessment interaction with a colleague or an acquaintance. Ask the person playing the client role to give you feedback on the messages he received about the nurse and the health care he would predict from your behavior. Then, find out what cues you sent by way of position, movement, voice, choice of words, pace, sequence, and so forth, that allowed him to gain the impressions he did.

   Try different techniques with different partners after the initial experience to see what behavior changes the impressions gained.

3. If video taping equipment with instant replay is available, this offers more evidence of the nonverbal cues as well as verbal ones; it can be invaluable.

   You might develop a videotape in which the nurse's focus during a Nursing Assessment is on anything but the client—on the form, the questions, the equipment, the time, the phone, the visitor . . . . Preface the viewing by asking the nursing audience to assume the place of the client. (This can be facilitated by having the nurse on the tape talking to the camera as if it were the client.) The feelings which the tape generates in them as clients would be an interesting point of departure; initially, cues that generated the impressions could be reported and, finally, recommendations for changes in approach could be discussed.

   Another tape, a client-centered one (the nurse focusing solely on the client) could be used to permit the audience to contrast the differences in cues sent and in techniques used by the nurse-assessor.

Activities such as these can sharpen nurses' awareness of the "information" being intentionally or unintentionally communicated to the client during the assessment interaction. These experiences can also be used to examine values being implemented in the assessment interaction by the nurse and the client and their relationship to each other.

To summarize our definition of the Nursing Assessment: it is a compact information seeking and giving transaction between two or more people involving subjective and objective data, usually in predetermined categories relevant to nursing care. It is, at least on the part of the nurse, a skilled activity requiring thinking and observing as well as interpersonal activity (verbal and nonverbal) in which the direction of observation and the nature of responses are modified on an ongoing basis in accordance with the data being received. At the same time, the Nursing Assessment requires the nurse to behave toward the client in a manner which successfully initiates the relationship needed to deal effectively with the problems of health and illness.

No small order this! And no wonder we recommend that the most skilled personnel, rather than the newest or least prepared, undertake this aspect of nursing care. No wonder we stress that these skills need to be thoroughly taught in educational programs and regularly upgraded in staff development or continuing education programs.

THE RELATIONSHIP WAGON

Human relationships have been likened to a vehicle by Cummings. Some wagons, he noted, carry very little weight before they break down, while others are so sturdy that they can carry much more than their rated capacity (Cummings, 1970, 76). It's the same way with people. Each of us can recall relationships that we take care not to burden with many demands; they wouldn't stand up under them. But we can also think of others that not only hold up but seem to grow stronger under the burden of additional stresses—at least up to a point.

Clients entering a health care system are most often carrying an additional stress load. Sometimes it is relatively light, easily borne alone. At other times the load of stress is heavy, but of short duration. And then there are occasions when the client faces a long heavy haul—uphill all the way.

As nurses, one of our functions is to build the needed professional relationship wagons with our clients in keeping with the assessed weight of stress, so that clients can be helped to handle their burden of health–illness problems to their best advantage.

The initial assessment interaction is the point where the mutual building of this particular relationship is begun, in whatever form it will take. One, both, or perhaps neither party may be fully aware of the nature of the stress load the relationship is going to have to carry, but the initial impressions of demands and contributions each one can bring will begin to emerge in this encounter. So, while the primary focus of the Nursing Assessment is indeed on the collection of data, a concommitant function (and one that grows out of the data gathering), is the initiation of a relationship that will prove useable to the client as he deals with the health-related issues in his life.

It is entirely possible to collect the necessary subjective and objective data for the nursing data base with a minimum amount of relationship building. There are techniques that communicate, "We don't expect to build any strong ties here. You carry your own load." Some of these nonproductive approaches are:

> introducing the Nursing Assessment with a comment such as, "We've got this form we have to fill out on every patient."

> using the editorial "we" so the client knows he is talking to no one person, but to an impersonal and unknown group. "We're interested in. . . ."

> following the sequence of questions on the assessment form from top to bottom each time, regardless of the clients' presenting problems or desires.

> reading the questions from the form exactly as they are written every time, particularly if it is done in a monotone.

> avoiding eye contact throughout.

keeping busy with other activities while you ask the necessary questions.

rushing through, treating any additional contributions of the client or any questions as deviations from the sequence and therefore unwanted interruptions.

behaving as if what the client tells you is suspect, or as if he could not possibly understand what is going on within him.

standing during the assessment interaction, shifting your weight from foot to foot, looking at your watch while the client is talking, and edging toward the door as you get to the bottom of the sheet.

While any one of these techniques will help, combined they are almost sure to result in a rickety relationship at best and at worst a determination by the client not to try to count on the staff in this setting for much in the way of support in carrying his stress load. Surely none of these responses are the accepted goal of professional nurses.

On the other hand, often without taking any more time, it is possible to gather the subjective and objective data for the nursing data base and to initiate a beginning relationship that will be mutually productive. The techniques for creating a sound "wagon building" climate during the assessment interaction will be incorporated throughout the chapter. Watch for them.

ON WHOM ARE ASSESSMENTS MADE?

For all the talk of comprehensive or total care, the truth of the matter is that, in most nursing situations, we give high priority care, and often need luck or exceptional skill to do even that. In setting the priorities for time and attention, many nurses have suggested to us that, if you must be selective about assessments, the ones to eliminate are the short-term clients—those who will have the shortest current contact with the health care system.

Actually, this seems like a rather inadequate criterion for doing or not doing an assessment. Obviously, the duration of the contact dictates how much or what kind of data the nurse will be able to use, but it is not the best guide for deciding on whether to assess or not.

Perhaps a more useful guide would be to predict the stress related to the contact or the health risks associated with the characteristics of the client. A chest cold and a visit to the doctor's office may be nothing to a young adult with no history of respiratory deficits, but it may be a prelude to dying for the emphysematous older person. A trip to the emergency room with an injury to the tip of the left index finger may be incidental to the right handed lawyer, yet a disaster to the violinist in the midst of the "season." A diagnostic D and C, a breast biopsy —simple, relatively painless in and out procedures, until you think of coping with the stress of antecedent knowledge like the positive pap smear or the mother and grandmother who died of breast cancer. Tonsillectomies are often major traumas in the life of youngsters, as well as in those who are not so young.

As experienced nurses we tend to place a different value on what constitutes a coping challenge. Placed against the major surgeries, the massive traumas, and the dramatic lifesaving emergencies, many health problems seem to pose no challenge to coping resources. Still it is the client, not the nurse who must cope and manage the moments and days of living, given *his* version of reality. So it would seem to be wise to make an assessment that at the least will determine what challenges *the client sees* in the presenting situation and whether or not he seems to be meeting them and proceed from there.

We would suggest then that each client deserves *some* systematic nursing assessment by the professional nurse. The extent of the assessment would be determined by the presenting situation from the nurse's *and* the client's perception of their abilities to manage—with or without help from the nursing staff.

TIMING OF THE NURSING ASSESSMENT

Nursing care can't be *planned* in any dimensions until there are data of some sort on the nature of the client and his presenting situation. Thus, logically, the Nursing Assessment should occur at the earliest stage of the client's encounter with the health care system. But, as with all ideals, there are frequently intervening factors that modify their implementation.

Client-Based Intervening Factors

At times the client is in no physical condition to participate in the assessment interaction except on a physiologic, nonverbal basis. He may be in dire straits— in need of an airway, fluids, sleep, prevention of blood loss, treatment of shock, control of pain, or dozens of other high priority physiologic needs. He may be in such a psychological crisis that verbal data gathering must be minimized. Medical diagnostic tests and treatment may have priority. Confused, elderly persons are sometimes transferred to nursing homes without accompanying relatives or friends. Young children may be flown from remote areas without accompanying parents. Or perhaps the client has been subjected to three or four prior data gathering experiences before the nurse arrives on the scene and he's fed up to the teeth with giving information about himself.

On the other hand, Nursing Assessments may have priority over other data gathering sessions. The mere fact that a physician or medical student arrives on the scene when the nurse is in the midst of a Nursing Assessment does not signify that the activity should be immediately terminated in favor of another discipline. The collection of the nursing data base is just as important as others—medical, pharmaceutical, and social; at times it may be more so.

Obviously where the immediate needs of the client have higher priority than the nursing assessment protocol, the nurse will reserve until later the more structured assessment. On the other hand, the nurses in a nursing home who were receiving unaccompanied confused clients decided to make prior contacts with relatives. They found that these relatives were reassured when the nurses who were going to care for their parent showed enough concern to find out about the individual before he came to them. It became good public relations as well as good nursing.

Thus, accommodation to client-based intervening factors may dictate that the Nursing Assessment be moved ahead in anticipation of a client's arrival. Or, it may be delayed until the client can participate effectively and at no expense to his survival.

Nurse-Based Intervening Factors

Staffing. On the nurses' side there are also intervening forces. At times other clients have such overriding needs that they must be attended to before Nursing Assessments can be done. Emergencies can cause unexpected staffing shortages. When these conditions occur the Nursing Assessment, although done, must of necessity be an abbreviated one; obviously, nurses must meet the priorities of their case loads.

However, if this is occurring so regularly that nurses can legitimately say that there is never time to do planned Nursing Assessments on each new client, then something is very wrong! Administration in institutions or agencies may be giving only lip service to the necessity of planned nursing care (and there are some who tool up just in time for accreditation). Often administration has not acknowledged that assessment by nurses, as by physicians, does take time. It is flattering to be seen as being capable of doing all things in less time than it takes anyone else and able to do many things at once, but unfortunately it is not true. Time must be allotted realistically if assessments are to be made. Staffing must be planned which treats Nursing Assessments as a legitimate unit of care per client in just the same way that baths, treatments, or any other aspects of client care are scheduled.

Nurses' interest and skill. One might also find that inadequate staffing is used as an excuse for not doing Nursing Assessments. If a nurse does not care to do Nursing Assessments, or is unskilled in performing this procedure, it is not hard to find other activities to occupy the time. We have found over the years that well-prepared, skilled nurses enjoy the nursing assessment encounters and tend to find time to do them; while those who are not skilled tend to downgrade their importance and find "more pressing" tasks to occupy their time. So, if there is enough staff and assessments are not being done, it might be wise to take a closer look at the skills and the values of the staff.

Summary. In any case, when there is never enough time to do Nursing Assessments regularly on clients—regardless of the client setting, it is time to take stock of what is going on. We should be honest about the working goals of the nursing department, the clinic, the office, and the school health care system. We should examine skills, values, and the level of professional nursing care of the nursing staff. Without systematic assessment, the nursing care can be inept, ritualistic and inappropriate to client needs.

THE NURSING ASSESSMENT: PRESENTING PROBLEM VERSUS COMPREHENSIVE APPROACH

Once nurses have accepted the notion that it is necessary for them to make Nursing Assessments, they, like physicians, face the conundrum of whether to use a comprehensive or presenting complaint approach (Markle, 1971). Some of the same factors pertain, but in nursing there are additional influences.

Factors Influencing Extent of Nursing Assessment

There are multiple factors influencing the extensiveness of the data base in the Nursing Assessment. Some of them are related to the client, some to the nurse, some to the agency and some to government or third party payors.

Client-based factors. Clients influence the approach taken in the Nursing Assessment in two obvious ways. As with the timing of the assessment, both their condition and their desires shape the interaction.

The urgency of their current physical problems is the most obvious influence. In acute emergency conditions, the data gathering is related to diagnosing and dealing with the most immediate physical and psychological crisis type data as a basis for making an accurate rapid treatment plan. Sammy swallowed a whistle; he needs an airway, not talk. Mr. Cutler, suffering the chest pain and anxiety of the onset of an M.I. doesn't benefit by telling his life history and food preferences. Neither Karen, who is moving rapidly into advanced stages of labor, nor the pale nervous young man in the background want to talk until they know things are under control. Jerry, in an acute psychic crisis, is in no position to deal with anything but surviving the throes of his emotional distress. And elderly Mrs. Munson is worried about those stomach pains and her insomnia; she will need to deal with these first. Obviously, a presenting problem approach is the only logical one in these cases. At the other end of the scale, a sliver in the finger doesn't warrant a complete Nursing Assessment.

The ability of the client to participate in the assessment process will also be a factor. Nonverbal, confused persons and young children—unless there are other sources of information—will not be able to yield much subjective data and the focus will then become a search for objective data to determine problems of nursing management. Again, this is not a comprehensive approach.

Client availability for subsequent contacts is another consideration. In many walk-in clinics contacts are often a onetime only affair. Collection of a broad data base would, in most instances, not be a cost effective use of nurse or client time. Likewise in hospitals, with short stays after surgery or delivery, and in the new walk-in, walk-out surgery units, the time available for using data becomes a factor in deciding the amount to be collected. At the opposite extreme is the situation where clientele fall into the health maintenance category. Here, either the presenting problem approach or the comprehensive approach work equally well. In the presenting problem approach there are continued contacts for filling in data gaps; however, there is also justification for collecting the data in one visit and having it immediately available. In the long-term care clinics where the authors tried both approaches, either one seemed to be effective. With this type of clientele there is obvious benefit to the client's health care in having a very adequate recorded data base, whatever method is used. As the nursing data base becomes part of the permanent client record, subject to updating just as the medical record currently is, the comprehensive approach will undoubtedly become more common and essential.

Client desires, overt or covert, are still another influence. If the client is viewed as a consumer of health services, then he presumably has the option to purchase or to use the type of health care he prefers and can afford, within the available services. The private client with ample funds can probably do this with a fair degree of ease; even some low income clients manage to make the system comply to their desires.

Some colleagues of ours work in both volunteer and supported clinics where the clients are predominately male transients and usually, they tell us, suspicious of and alienated from the establishment. The men use a presenting problem approach exclusively with the staff. Any attempt to go beyond the health problem *they* wish to have treated is not acceptable. Trust is built slowly, if at all. Many are one-visit clients. The reputation of the clinics and their growing usefulness in helping this segment of the population to deal with their multiple health problems came about because the grapevine spread the message that the client was accepted on his own terms. This same client-initiated approach was used by the authors in Nursing Assessments at clinics for the independent elderly where reservations about sharing information were not the major consumer hangup, but where this approach to assessment was a reinforcement of their desire for continued independence in all areas of decision making (Little and Carnevali, 1974).

Client-based factors influencing choice of comprehensive versus presenting problem approaches include the urgency of the presenting problem, the ability of the client or his representative to participate in the subjective portion of the assessment, the usefulness of a broad data base for subsequent contacts, and the desire of the client for particular kinds of health care services.

Agency-based factors. In addition to client influences on the extensiveness of initial data collection, and perhaps often overriding them, are factors introduced by the agency. The reality of staffing levels, space available for interacting with clients and examining them, and numbers of clients to be accommodated within a particular time period all place constraints on the amount of time available and the nature of data that can be collected or that will be usable. It is difficult, to say the least, to do a comprehensive assessment when the only space allocated for Nursing Assessments is a chair in the waiting room or corridor while the clients are waiting to see the doctor. This is the arrangement in many crowded clinics and outpatient departments or offices. Nor is a comprehensive Nursing Assessment possible when it must be completed in 5 to 10 minutes—whether it is on a new admission to a busy hospital unit or to a walk-in clinic. Space, time and opportunity for use of the data are some of the agency-based factors that influence the presenting complaint versus comprehensive approach to nursing assessment.

Legislation and third party payors. Increasingly, financial factors are shaped by decisions far from the agency, as the government and third party payors exert control over the nature of health care that will be reimbursed. With the primary interest in health care still focused on the medical model and cure, nursing care and maintenance are not in very influential positions at present. These regulations in turn affect the nature of the data that is collected and subsequently used.

Nurse-based factors. Finally there is the nurse's own belief system about the comparative merits of the comprehensive data base and the presenting problem one. The nurse's attitudes will influence what data are collected and the structure given to the assessment interaction.

Implications of Choices

There are advantages and risks related to a choice of either approach. These must be considered and compensated for when choices are made. As with so many other decisions, it is probably wiser to hang loose, maintaining a continuum of options regarding approaches to the Nursing Assessment. Take a presenting problem approach when this appears to be called for, but continue to exercise the comprehensive option when this is profitable. Seek conditions in the work setting that will permit the comprehensive option to be exercised as needed. With either option the nurse will try to compensate for the disadvantages that are recognized.

RECORDING THE NURSING ASSESSMENT DATA

Should the nurse write in the presence of the client? It is admittedly more difficult to maintain eye contact and the flow of the interaction when one is writing as well, but even more basic is an obvious underlying reluctance among many nurses to write in the client's presence.

Some nurses have assumed that it makes the client uncomfortable to have the nurse make notes during the assessment. Yet, when we have role-played the situation time after time in workshops where each person takes the roles of client and then reverses to the role of nurse in paired assessment interactions, they found that they experienced discomfort in the role of nurse, not of client. This experience is helpful in placing the feelings where they really do exist as an appropriate basis for dealing with them.

Some techniques for writing in front of clients that the authors have found helpful (through both role-playing and actual clinical experience) may prove usable to the reader. We, for example, found it more comfortable in both the client and nursing roles when the person in the nursing role sat where the client could see what was being written—that is, they both faced the same direction. It increased the sense of working together in the management of health problems and reduced the sense of the secrecy of health records. The client didn't worry about what the nurse was writing; it was visible. Where the physical arrangement did not permit shared visibility of the writing, we found that commenting aloud on what was being noted decreased the feeling of exclusion. For example, we might say as we make a note of it, "You get up four to five times a night to go to the bathroom after you've taken the diuretic and you're taking the pill on even numbered days at present." (Obviously the recording is an abbreviated note of this commentary.)

Other role-playing experiences yielded additional insights which we have subsequently validated with our clientele. The climate of trust was felt to increase when the person in the nurse role said, "I'd like to make some notes on what you tell me so I won't forget the important points, but if you want to talk about things that are to be 'off the record' just say so and you can be sure I will keep them in confidence." It offered the rationale for writing but gave a way out for discussing materials that were not to be shared. Again, nurses, particularly from smaller towns, have indicated that they need to be careful of what they record and share. The health care workers are also neighbors, not professional strangers.

The problems related to writing as one makes the Nursing Assessment also caused us to revise our estimate of the number of pages needed for the assessment tool, as well as the spacing and arrangement of headings. Multiple pages kept us flipping papers trying to find the right slot for the material being shared, and again our focus shifted from the client to the papers. As a result we now favor headings on the side of the form in a column, with the remainder of the page a blank space for writing. The headings can be underlined in the recording context where the notes are being made. There is no problem of wasted space nor crowding, and no hunting for the right space on the page. For example:

Sleep: Orthopneic. Has PND c̄ time he falls off his 3 pillows → panic for him ē wife. Other nights sleeps 11p – 7³⁰ā s̄ interruption. Occ. nightmares. No use of sedatives.

Mobility: SOB ē angina p̄ walking 1 level block. NG gr 1/200 + rest → relief. Spaces activities around house. Wife manages household/ shopping tasks. Have car. Both drive.

This system also permitted us to flow along with the client rather than forcing his report to fit the tool. It was not too difficult to locate specific material in reviewing the data later.

Where the flow of the interview is impeded by writing complete findings, it may be easier to put down cue words that will serve as reminders and then fill in the remainder of the material later. This tends, however, to reduce one of the advantages of writing while interviewing and that is, saving time. The most frequent complaint we hear about making Nursing Assessments is that there isn't enough time to do them. Recording after one leaves the client would seem to reduce the accuracy of recall and increase the amount of time involved in the process.

We believe that recording data as one is collecting them is a nursing skill to be learned like any other. It can be used to enhance the client's sense of participation and to produce a climate of trust, and it can make the recording most accurate as well as economical in terms of time.

QUESTIONING AND NONQUESTIONING: DATA GATHERING APPROACHES

In a short, intense, focused data gathering interaction such as the Nursing Assessment we've found a natural and persistent tendency to use a direct questioning approach. Following role playing experiences in which participants are limited to 10 to 12 minutes for a Nursing Assessment, one hears comments such as, "I felt like it was a third degree!" or "All those questions came battering at me." "Too many questions: too invasive!" Now there is nothing wrong with asking questions. However, there are some alternatives that can be used to make the data gathering a more comfortable interchange for both parties. At first nurses report that they feel a loss of control of the flow of data, that the assessment takes too long, that it feels artificial, that it's difficult. Yet, as they have continued to work with it, role play it, and experience it as clients and practitioners they become quite positive about the value.

Let's look at some alternative forms of behavior on the part of the interviewer that will encourage the sharing of data without use of a questioning technique.

Reflection:

A technique that became so overused that it was caricatured. It is a response in which one picks up a central or terminal word or phrase and repeats it in a rather tentative tone of voice. The client says, "I've been having so much trouble sleeping at night." And the interviewer continues, "trouble sleeping. . . ." It shows that the interviewer has tuned in to the message and is interested in hearing more.

Clarification:

Restating the client's ideas in different words to allow him to hear your version and validate, modify, or expand on the ideas. The client says, "I just don't know how I can manage to rest in the afternoon." The interviewer may say, "You have too many things to do to be able to lie down for an hour after lunch. . . ." Again, the tone of voice is tentative rather than declarative.

Giving an opinion:

At times offering an opinion yields data. A lady who was inquiring about a low calorie diet in the course of discussing her nutrition patterns said she drank orange juice for vitamin C. The nurse gave the opinion that tomato juice would yield vitamin C with a lower number of calories. To which the lady responded, "But I'm on a low salt diet and tomato juice has salt in it." A whole new line of data opened up.

Sharing of yourself:

While this technique carries some risk of personal exposure for the interviewer, it can be very useful where the client is uncomfortable or the area under discussion is sensitive. Comments such as, "Being treated that way would make me angry," or "I'd be uncomfortable with such a situation . . ." "I didn't find it easy to . . ."

Describing what you see:

Putting into words your impressions permits the client to validate or modify your observations. "It seems to me you hear better on your left side." "You're rubbing your breast bone again, the pain must be returning." "It appears to me from what you've said that you're a pretty independent person who would rather not ask for things." "That joint feels stiffer than the other one."

Requesting information:

Someone once said that a question is only a disguised demand for information. A logical variation, then, would be to request information. This technique is useful in starting an interview or in shifting from one area to another. "I'd be interested in knowing about . . ." "It would help in planning for your care if you would tell me about . . ." "Please tell me how . . ." "I'd like to know more about . . ."

Rewarding responses:

Any interviewer response that shows approval will tend to encourage continuation of the behavior, for instance, such remarks as: "That's interesting," "Good," "Uhm," and "I see." Nonverbal behavior such as nodding, leaning forward, and looking interested also indicate that one is listening.

Silence:

It has been said that human beings want closure. For this reason, perhaps, people often feel impelled to fill silences with words. In an Assessment interview, pauses can encourage a respondent to continue to share information unless he is quite withdrawn, or has become aware of the technique and is playing competitive games with you.

Unfinished sentences:

The human need for closure can be used to draw the client out in another way. The nurse responds to his initial statement with an unfinished sentence and allows him to fill in the missing information. This technique takes practice, but here is an example. The client says, "I've been working the evening shift for years. I get home around midnight and unwind with the paper and a bite to eat, so I get to bed about 1 or 1:30 in the morning." The nurse then responds, "Well in the morning then you . . ." again trailing off on the last word.

It has been interesting to compare the sights and sounds as well as the reactions of group members between a first role playing of the Nursing Assessment, in which no interviewing constraints are placed on the subjective data gathering techniques, and the second version, in which any technique *except* questioning is permitted; group members look, sound, and react differently. At a glance, during the second "interview," the group looks more animated (once the initial moments are over and the participants gain momentum in their interactions). The decibel level is noticeably higher—there is more talking, more laughing. Both participants in each dyad are more likely to be leaning forward, whereas in the original interview, only the interviewer tended to do so. Nurses in the client role reported the experience as more comfortable, giving them a sense of mutual sharing: they did not feel that they were undergoing a controlled grilling. However, those in the nurse roles found the techniques difficult to initiate. They often asked questions without realizing it, and produced an unintended silence while they tried to plan a way of approaching a subject without asking a question. Yet, even those in the role of nurse found it easier once the interview gained momentum.

Obviously, these nonquestioning data collection techniques are not learned in one role-playing session or even in several client encounters. What is more, they can be just as monotonous and artificial and just as badly done as a one-track questioning approach. On the other hand, they can be practiced a little each day in *any* data-gathering situation—nursing or nonnursing, until comfort, skill, and naturalness are achieved. With these added interview skills the nurse has a choice of approaches in collecting subjective data.

SETTING THE PHYSICAL ARRANGEMENTS

Another factor that influences the general climate of the Nursing Assessment is the physical setup. The nurse has responsibility for arranging the seating and deciding on the distance between participants, controlling interruptions, and screening or managing privacy.

In some situations, such as emergency rooms and intensive care settings, or at times when the client's status requires that data be collected as care is given, the nurse will not be sitting down to talk with the client. However, as a rule, this act of sitting down is important. This allows equality of eyeline rather than putting the nurse in a position of power over the client. In fact, in one children's hospital in Canada, the nurses told us they have small chairs to sit on, so their little clients won't have to look up to them while they are talking together. This procedure of sitting down together also suggests to the client that even for a short while, the nurse is there to stay and listen, and is not preoccupied with other activities. One nurse, coming back from an interview, reported that her client said, "You're the first nurse who's sat down and really talked with me in the whole three weeks I've been here." (And, incidentally, this nurse learned some important information that helped her to deal with problems that had affected the client for at least two of those three weeks.)

Beyond the mere act of sitting, the positioning of client and nurse also has significance—whether they should sit face to face for eye contact, or both facing the same direction so that the client can see what is being written. Also, there may be some variations between.

Privacy is important, but it could be a matter of degree. In clinics or wards it may be necessary to use a curtain or screen as a shield in order to offer some form of privacy. We have known of ambulatory care settings where initially nurses were forced to do assessments in the corridors of the outpatient department or clinic, or in clinic rooms when doctors were not using them. These nurses eventually negotiated for space to be allocated for nursing contacts that offered better interview-examination quarters. And they have been able to get them. The merits of nursing management have become obvious to medical and hospital administration colleagues as has the necessity and quality of their Nursing Assessments.

Privacy also means a minimum of interruptions for the client or the nurse. It means the absence of visitors and relatives as well. Arrangements can be made with other staff to minimize interruptions during a specified period of time. Similarly it is wise to have visitors, including relatives, wait elsewhere. If it is important to talk with them, do so separately. Give the client, old, middle-aged, or young, the chance to speak for himself.

THE SECTIONS OF THE NURSING ASSESSMENT

The Nursing Assessment, whether long or short, is made up of four sections. These are:

1. the introduction
2. the body
3. the recapitulation
4. the plans for continuity in client/nurse planning

The duration of each segment may vary as a proportion of the total. Normally, 1, 3, and 4 are quite brief, while the body takes the major portion of the allotted time. Short or long, however, each segment serves a particular function which is essential to the total Nursing Assessment.

The Introduction

The introduction to the Nursing Assessment sets the stage, the expectations, the time limits, and the climate. It should answer several questions for the client. In it you should tell him:

What your name is
Who you are in this health care system
What kinds of information and data you need
What use you propose to make of the data he shares
Where it will be recorded, and who will have access to it
How long it will take
His right to consent or refuse to participate
His right to privileged communication with the nurse.

Beyond giving this information, the introduction seeks to offer a climate that enlists the client's interested participation in the activity.

As an activity, try taking an excerpt from each of the following sections to compile an introduction.

1. Hello   Miss

   Good morning   Ms.

   Good afternoon   Mrs.   } Last name

   Good evening   Mr.

   Hi   First name

                   Nickname

2. I'm   Miss

                   Mrs.

                   Ms.   } Last name

                   Mr.

                   First name

                   Nickname

3. I will be   your nurse

   the nurse responsible for planning your care while you're here

   one of the nurses who will be caring for you

   the nurse/nurse practitioner who will see you each time you come to the clinic/doctor's office

   the head nurse/clinical coordinator on the unit

   the public health nurse who will visit you each————

   the nurse who will be caring for you in the operating room/recovery room/during labor

4. I'd like to talk with you for: a few minutes

   about ———— minutes

   a while

5. About   what your usual daily routines are like

   how your life has been changed since your illness, the ways in which you've managed well and areas where it doesn't go so well

   how you see me being helpful to you while you're in labor

   how you've been managing since your last visit

   how your child was burned and his daily routines, his vocabulary, his likes and dislikes, how much you want to participate in his care . . .

111

6. In order to ... plan your nursing care

plan for your child/parent's nursing care in ways that will be comfortable and normal for him

learn how your normal routine might be disrupted by schedules here and how best to make adjustments

understand the patterns of your day to day living as a basis for seeing how illness/treatment may require adjustments and then to help you find ways to deal with these changes in the most satisfying and effective way

give you the kind of support you'll need and want while you're in the labor room/the CCU/ the recovery room/... when you're going home ...

7. I'd like to make notes ... to help me remember the important points when I make up your plan of care

to have a permanent record of information that should influence your nursing care so you won't have to tell the same information to every person who comes in

so that all the staff will have the information when they plan for your care

8. If ... you don't wish to talk with me, please feel free to say so, it won't interfere with the quality of care you receive

there is anything you'd rather I didn't write down/share with the staff, just say so and I'll keep it in confidence. . . .

9. Could we talk together now?

This type of an introduction will touch all the bases for the client in an institutional setting. In some walk-in clinics, free clinics, and the long-term clinics in which the clients come to the nurse, the introduction was much more casual: "Hello Mrs. Lynch. How are things going?" or perhaps "What can I do for you today?"

A nurse (not a nurse practitioner or midwife) at a prenatal clinic or obstetrician's office might round off her introduction something like this:

I'll be seeing you each time you come to the (clinic/office) before you have your baby as well as afterwards. Dr. Felton will be concerned with seeing to some of your health needs and those of the baby. I will be concerned with how you're managing day to day living and planning for the arrival of the baby. I'd like to talk with you for a few minutes about the ways you see this pregnancy affecting your day to day living. Then as your pregnancy progresses, I may be of help in dealing with some of the questions that arise.

The hospital nurse might finish off the introduction to the short-term client:

I realize you're going to be with us for (a very short time/ a day/ a few hours.) Still, I'd like to plan your care while you're here so that it will be helpful. Is there anything you feel *should* affect any nursing care you may receive from us . . . anything you particularly wish or do not wish?

The introduction then briefly identifies the nurse and sets the client's expectations for participating in a focused data sharing experience. It should convey the mutuality of both the process and the goals. And it should evoke an interest in the client to engage in this exchange with the nurse.

Plans for accommodating to client refusal.   The introduction gives the client the opportunity to participate in the plan of nursing care. By the same token it gives him the chance to reject this opportunity. This doesn't happen often, but it does occur often enough to warrant some advance thought and planning.

The nurse, and in fact the nursing staff as a group, need to consider how this decision of the client not to participate will be handled. Nurses have been known to say, "It's his right to say no." But we've witnessed enough subsequent subtle and not so subtle retaliation that we suggest another question, "May the client refuse to participate in the Nursing Assessment without expecting or experiencing negative feedback?" Some nurses take another tack in considering client refusal to participate. They say, "We've always gotten the information without asking them for it, just collect it as we go along. They don't notice it. So it really doesn't make much difference whether they agree to it or not." This, of course, doesn't say much for informed consent or a client's right to privacy. Our right to know is a privilege we've taken for granted for a long time. Informed consent, by contrast, is a very recent concept.

Nurses can feel rejected when they've taken precious time to talk with a client only to have him say, "If you want to know anything, just ask my doctor. He's the one who's taking care of me." Or a flat rejection, "No, I don't want to talk to you." Some role playing to get the feel of both sides of this interaction (the person who doesn't want to talk to the nurse but who may be afraid of what will happen if he doesn't, and the busy nurse whose interested offer is refused). This should facilitate development of mutually effective ways of handling such a potentially touchy situation. In addition, ward conferences or inservice among RNs and, eventually, among all nursing personnel to explore and discuss the group's values and attitudes toward the client who refuses to participate may bring to light the real working values and kinds of responses that are creeping into subsequent encounters.

The refusal of a client to knowingly share data with the nurse in a Nursing

Assessment can be a problem to the nursing staff. So it is wise to plan for dealing with it productively and objectively *before* it occurs. And, of course, the decision not to participate, or a referral to the doctor is in itself data on how this individual sees himself interacting with the nursing staff and can become a point of departure for developing the plan of care and the "relationship wagon."

The Body of the Nursing Assessment

The major segment of the Nursing Assessment is the second portion. Here the client is the expert. He can tell us what he is experiencing, what there is in his background and environment that has implications, what his expectations and desires are. His body can give us cues about how it is functioning under the circumstances. His environment can yield information about factors that influence his health. It has been suggested that if we listen to the client, he will tell us what the diagnosis is. The subjective data give his intellectual and affective impressions, then objective data can be used to validate, modify and refine these areas of diagnosis. The skill from the nurse's point of view is to pick up the cues offered, but also to direct the client's attention and recall so that he is able to share with the nurse data in areas relevant to his current care, and, if appropriate, to the long-term nursing management. Skill is also involved in the branching logic of searching for objective data to validate the subjective data, and the reverse.

The self-starters. Some clients are just bursting with information that has immediate and high priority to them. The nursing strategy here may well be to listen and make notes on these areas, noting and exploring the nursing implications and avenues for further exploration in subsequent branching logic examination. Then when the pressure of these stressful areas has been at least momentarily relieved through the initial verbalization, the nurse can direct the dialogue to assessment areas not yet covered. It shows active listening if the nurse is able not only to move on to the remaining areas of coverage but, at the same time, to tie these data areas into the ones given initial priority by the client. For example:

> An elderly man was admitted to a hospital with poorly controlled diabetes and a chronic ulcer on his lower left leg. His major concern and the focus of his conversation was that "sore on my leg." It didn't take much skill to lead his thoughts to recall the way in which the sore on his leg influenced mobility, sleep, personal hygiene practices, and management of ADL. Then, by prefacing the assessment area of nutrition with the comment, "We know that what people eat has an influence on how these sores heal. I'd be interested in what and when you eat, so we can plan together for a diet that will be best for your leg," she was able to engage his interest in talking about his eating patterns. (And, incidentally to lay the groundwork for later nursing interventions dealing with nutrition.) By the same technique, a comment that his pattern of taking insulin and related drugs and his checking of his urine was also related to healing his leg, gave him reason to talk about this area of diabetic management as well.

His desire to learn how to care for himself (by that he meant his leg) emerged clearly and became a focal point for the plan of nursing care, even though the nurse's goal was better management of the hyperglycemia and was secondarily concerned with his goal of taking care of the sore on his leg.

Had this nurse focused purely on her areas of interest and need for data, rather than couching it within his area of concern, the flow of data could have been greatly inhibited. (In fact, when a student on the unit one evening ignored the prescribed plan of care and took it upon herself to teach this man diabetes, she was turned off quite efficiently by him. "He just wouldn't listen," was her comment.)

Use what the clients give you as you move ahead in the assessment. Use their words, their focus. It lets them know you have heard them and are incorporating their interests into the plan.

The uncertain ones. Another group of clients are just the opposite of the self-starters. These people are just not certain what the nurse, "wants to hear." They are also often the ones who want to be able to give *the* right answer. Here, a more structured initial period has been found to add to their comfort and productivity.

After the introduction the nurse asks Mrs. Peterson if she would be willing to talk for a few minutes. Mrs. Peterson's timorous response is, "Well I don't know what I can tell you that you'd want to know." The nurse, not getting a definite refusal, could seat herself and say, "Well to begin with, I'm interested in a typical day for you. We could start with your telling me about your usual meals on a typical day—what and when you eat."

The nurse has started in a low risk area and has given structure even to what part of the typical day the client might focus on first.

If any comment is made by the client which shows concern about the "right" answers, the nurse should clear up this misconception. A response such as, "There aren't any right or wrong answers—what is important to me is what is right for you." Or you might say, "Just tell it like it is for you—that's what's important."

Denial. The reverse of the situation in which the client describes signs and symptoms may occur when the nurse notes objective data indicating the presence of a problem which the client does not mention. Here, the safest course is to ask general, neutral, data gathering types of questions without implying direction of response. For example: you notice that the client uses short sentences, or stops in midsentence for a breath, yet he hasn't discussed his dyspnea. You could ask, "Do you ever find yourself short of breath?" Or the individual may guard himself in a particular body area and the nurse might say, "Do you have any pain or stiffness in . . . ?" By making a neutral approach to a nonmentioned area you are freeing the client to be spontaneous in his response and to either affirm or deny his awareness to you. Remember that questions which begin with:

Don't you

Isn't it

Aren't you

or any variation of these are really saying, "This is what I think/see and I want you to agree with me." Such a slanted question format is *not* appropriate to the Nursing Assessment. Neither is the Nursing Assessment the time or place to begin to treat the denial. It is a time for neutral, objective, assiduous data gathering.

Thus when you question the client regarding an observed sign and he signals by his body English (moving away from you, dropping eye contact, restlessness, unusual stillness, or an obvious effort to disguise the identified cue), when he changes the subject at the earliest opportunity, gives a joking, superficial answer, puts down its importance, makes outright denial of any related symptoms or effects, or mentions positive body functions negating the signs or symptoms, this is noted by the nurse as data and is later integrated into the plan as client management or coping strategies. Hopefully, the nurse will also have gathered some data that will yield understanding of why this is the coping strategy of choice to the client.

Refocusing.   Many nurses have talked with us about clients who wander off on nonproductive tangents during a Nursing Assessment. With time for client assessment so limited it is hard to see it frittered away on "nonessential" discussion. Yet, in order to maintain a flow of valid data, it is important to maintain ongoing rapport with the client. Therefore it is important to know how to refocus the individual without making the transition a "put down."

When time is limited, it may be wise to make the client aware of the time limitations from the beginning. If you have 10 minutes for the Nursing Assessment, say so. If it's an hour, give the client this information. Then he can tell how much of your time he has available to him and pace himself accordingly.

However, even with this overall perspective, clients can become so engrossed in the telling of their health stories that they move into great detail or into areas that have low priority in the development of plans for immediate management of their nursing care. The nurse can make a comment such as:

> Mr. Martin, you've told me about your stomach pains, your job and your sleeping patterns. This is very helpful. We've got a few more minutes for talking together and we haven't yet talked about your eating patterns. I'm sure this is important to you too. Tell me about what you eat in a day.

Here Mr. Martin had stayed in the health/coping area and was helped to move on to an area he had not yet covered.

But suppose the client has strayed way off on a tangent that has no significance to nursing. How do you refocus this individual without seeming uninterested or making him feel foolish or guilty. Where it is possible, avoid using the word *BUT* (This word has been said to mean, "erase everything I said before the word "BUT" as in "very interesting, BUT. . . .") It is possible in many instances, if one's wits are nimble enough, to make a tie in between the tangent and another area within the assessment where you still need to go. Suppose the client shifted from talking about his dyspnea to the way it interfered with his hobby of gardening and then slipped off into a discussion of the latter topic. It would not be difficult to tie in this activity with his nutrition, mobility, or substitute diversions. An interest in animals or pets can be moved on to companionship, to support forms, to allergy, or to disruption of sleep.

In general, to refocus the client, express genuine interest or commendation for the information he has shared, and where possible, indicate some use that you will make of the data. For example, "Good, that helps me to know what kinds of activities you want to be able to get back to." Another technique is to allude to an earlier piece of information that was relevant to nursing management. Commenting first on the current subject, one might say, "That's really interesting. You know, I was also interested in something you brought up earlier. You spoke of. . . . This could be important in your care. Let's talk a bit more about . . . and the way it affects/changes. . . ." Avoid any responses, verbal or nonverbal, that could give the impression of lack of credibility. If the client feels we don't believe him or aren't interested, we are erecting effective barriers to further open sharing.

Because refocusing is not easy, and because it is a regularly recurring situation, skill in this interactive behavior is essential. An easy, available learning experience is that of role playing. Ask a partner to assume the role of a deliberately wandering client while you assume the role of a nurse who needs to accumulate a usable nursing data base in the next 10 to 15 minutes. Try different focusing techniques. After the interview has run its course for about 5 minutes, stop. Ask the "wanderer" to give feedback on which of your responses felt good and which did not. What feelings did each specific behavior engender in him? How did it do this? Reverse the roles so that you too get the experience of smooth or clumsy refocusing efforts. Try this experience with others—nurses, nonnurses, professionals, and potential consumers among your acquaintances. It shouldn't take very long to acquire a repertoire of refocusing responses and a smooth style of using them. And, to keep from stereotyping, return to the role playing to freshen your approaches and insights periodically.

Gathering objective data.   The second dimension of data gathering in the body of the Nursing Assessment is of course that of objective data. Currently, nursing practice seems to deviate from the medical protocol in the sequencing or mix of the two components. And as nurses move into nurse practitioner roles, the kind and amount of objective data collected in assessments made by nurses has begun to vary even more.

In actual practice, a physician usually takes a history (collects subjective data), and then does a systematic physical examination (collects the objective data). Currently, in nursing practice as we've experienced and observed it, the nurses' approach is a more integrated one. That is, as the client describes a condition or response, the nurse at that point begins to collect related objective data rather than to wait and do it all later. For example, when the client reports that he is short of breath the nurse begins to collect objective data on:

the rate and depth of respiration

the amount of sighing

whether sentences are shortened or interrupted to take a breath

whether chest excursion is equal

whether any accessory muscles are being used

whether any unusual sound accompanies inspiration, expiration

whether the inspiratory or expiratory phases are disproportionate in duration

whether the lips are pursed on expiration

whether the shoulders are held in an elevated position

whether the chest has increased anteroposterior dimensions

whether the nares flare on inspiration, etc.

A complaint of a stiff, painful joint may lead the nurse to inspect it for signs of inflammation, swelling, or spurs as well as range of motion and any feel of resistance to motion.

Obviously there are some risks inherent in this approach. Where nurses and physicians are both making their own type of assessments, these could be minimal. Further, in hospitals or other institutional settings, there are opportunities for subsequent observations as continued nursing care is given. In some nursing clinics, clients themselves limit the nature of physical examination. In some of the free clinics, the quickest way to drive the clientele away is to go beyond the problem they wish to have treated, the signs and symptoms they wish to share with you.

There may also be some merit, when both nurses and physicians are doing systematic assessments, for the nurses' approach to be different from that of the physician—if only to keep the patient from thinking that this is an inefficient duplication of service, second guessing among professionals, or wondering who is right when they both look for the same things in the same way. To be valid, cost effective activities, Nursing Assessments must differ from Medical Assessments in their focus. They may also vary appropriately in the technique employed.

Nurse practitioners in independent, particularly rural practice are usually involved in both nursing and medical practice. Since their medical backstop is usually some distance away and they are to all intents and purposes the lone assessors, they obviously would be safer using the medical protocol, with the Nursing Assessment as an integrated component. Whatever the sequence, or mix of the collection of each type of data, subjective and objective, the risks and advantages of each should be considered as part of making the choice.

Since whole books, both medical and nursing, have addressed the rationale and techniques of the physical examination, and since we've already devoted a chapter to the underlying skill of cue collection and inferencing, we will not presume to deal with this vast and complex subject here. Instead, we refer the reader to some texts and articles listed in the bibliography, sources which nurses have found useful in this area. This is in no way to be construed as diminishing the importance of collecting objective data in a physical nursing assessment. Quite the contrary! It is to lend to this skill the full treatment and expertise it deserves and which these expert clinician-authors have brought to it.

So do observe the cues as you interact. Use the approved techniques for obtaining covert data. Integrate or sequence the systematic physical assessment, but don't leave the client without including both the relevant objective as well as subjective information for the complete *nursing* data base whether you are using a presenting complaint or comprehensive nursing assessment approach.

Recapitulation

Once the needed information has been collected in the body of the Nursing Assessment, or the time available has been used up, the nurse moves on to the two stages of termination of the activity. The first of these, recapitulation, looks back; the second looks ahead.

Functions of recapitulation. Recapitulation serves three functions. It:

> forces the nurse to organize, prioritize and verbalize the central themes identified and supported in the interaction
>
> tells the client what the nurse heard
>
> gives the client the opportunity to validate or revise the nurse's impressions.

Recapitulation overcomes some current flaws in care planning. In the process of developing the recapitulation statements, the nurse begins the formulation of the nursing care plan. By grouping the cues and inferences into whatever combinations seem logical at that time, the central, tentative, diagnostic themes begin to emerge. Currently, the biggest breakdown in nursing care planning occurs between the data gathering and the synthesis of data into verbalized diagnoses or problem statements. A consistent behavior pattern of including a recapitulation statement in each assessment transaction will set thinking habit patterns that should eventually close this gap between collected data and its use.

A second criticism that has been levelled against nursing care plans is that they tend to be invalid and hence can't be trusted. Palison called them a ". . . Snare and a Delusion" (Palison, 1971). The immediate sharing of nursing impressions with the client should serve effectively to take care of this planning defect. If the nurse's perceptions are congruent with those of the client, then some degree of validity must exist in the care plan's foundations, at least.

Techniques of recapitulation. The process of immediately organizing and verbalizing the essence of the interaction is not a skill that many nurses today have been taught. However, it is a skill, and therefore competence in it requires practice in a safe environment. "Safe" for the reader may mean personal private practice after a Nursing Assessment, before even attempting it with a client. It may mean role playing with a safe person. Or it may mean trying to do it in the next Nursing Assessment. But critical practice is required. Eventually critiqued performance, whether by anonymous tape recordings or direct observation of performance, may be needed.

Essentially a recapitulation may sound something like this:

> "Mrs. Preston, from what you've said and what I've observed, you first had numbness on the inner leg about your ankles after your vein stripping. And now, eight months later, you're experiencing throbbing toothache-like pain, unrelieved by aspirin, but helped by Empirin Compound #2. This pain has been keeping you from sleeping for more than three hours at a stretch for over a month. It isn't aggravated by exercise or having your legs down. It's making you increasingly nervous and irritable with your husband and the children. There's no change in color in the area. It's neither warmer nor colder than the surrounding area and I can feel pulses in your ankles.
>
> Aside from this problem, you see your health as good. And from our few minutes together it sounds and looks that way to me, too. Your weight and blood pressure are in the normal range. You eat and enjoy a very balanced diet. The kids and the house and yard give you exercise and you have enough satisfying activities to keep you enthusiastic, if we can just get you comfortable and sleeping well. Have I gotten an accurate picture?"

Sometimes the recapitulation will focus on one area if the presenting complaint approach has been used. If a more comprehensive Nursing Assessment has been done, obviously it must incorporate a broader view.

Where the nurse has identified areas of concern that the client does not acknowledge, the recapitulation may also include another chance for the client to deal with these. For example:

> You've been having some episodes where your heart races for a time and occasionally you're aware that it skips a bit and is not quite regular, but you're not bothered by it and it doesn't interfere with what you want to do. Is that right?

Some areas of client deficit or concern are very obvious. If they all were, nursing and doctoring would be much easier. But life has more grey areas than black or white and so, particularly in the brief initial Nursing Assessments, hazy impressions of problem areas may occur—ones that may or may not be present. The nurse should collect more data before making any serious judgments. These are not included in the recapitulation, but are held in abeyance until they can be more definitely ruled in or ruled out.

Where the nurse has some impressions and it is obvious that the client has others, the skilled nurse may find ways to introduce to the client both perspectives.

> As you see it, then, Mr. Phillips, the major problem you're having is with your . . . .
> I can certainly see that. As a nurse I'm also concerned about another aspect, that of . . . and the way it will affect. . . .

Validating techniques. Again, as with the beginning of the Nursing Assessment, some clients will be quite comfortable in validating or modifying your summary of the data and your impressions. You will not even need to ask them. Others will be more shy, particularly about disagreeing with you. If the nurse has tuned in to the client to any degree throughout the assessment, the less aggressive, shy individuals will have been identified by this time. These persons will need the encouragement of a question, such as, "Have I got that right?" Or, "Did I hear you correctly?" Or, "I want you to tell me if my impressions are not the ones you wanted to convey."

It is important that the initial data base be an accurate one. One way to insure this is to check out our impressions with the person who gave them. This at least gives a fair start to an appropriate nursing care plan.

Setting Expectations for Future Planning Contacts

The current patterns of nursing assignments and client involvement in maintenance of care plans is so varied that there are few norms of expectations that clients can hold about any continuation of contacts with nurses. Thus, the final stage of the Nursing Assessment should give the client some realistic perspective on:

> how he will be expected to participate in nursing care planning,
> whom he should expect to see or contact if he has questions or feedback and
> whether there are any routine contacts for updating nursing care plans.

This is true whether the planning is being done in ambulatory or inpatient care settings.

In an acute care setting, then, if all nursing personnel: the head nurse, the clinical coordinator, the clinical specialist, the staff nurse, the LPN, and the aide plan care, say so. "We all plan care on this unit so you can speak to anyone who comes in and they will adjust the plan of care." Or, "We plan patient care in conference once a week when we get time." If your unit is using a primary nurse model in which one person is accountable for care planning for a particular case load, tell the client this.

> "I am going to be responsible for the management of your nursing care as long as you are with us. While I will be visiting you sometime between _____ and _____ a.m./p.m. each day I'm on duty to talk with you on how the plan is working. If you have questions or feedback at other times just tell one of the staff and ask them to let me know."

If a backup nurse takes your cases when you're off, say,

> "Miss Marvin and I work together, so when I'm not here, she'll be in and she will be kept up to date on your case just as Dr. West keeps Dr. North informed when he covers for him on some weekends."

This kind of continuity of contact expectations should be set whether the interviewer is functioning in the home, in an outpatient department, or in any setting where more than one nurse is functioning or where the person who answers the phone is not the care planner. If you want the clients to participate, let them know how best to do it in this setting.

We have done workshops with nurses from some hospitals where all nurses are expected to float and, in fact, do so regularly and unpredictably. In this case, the only constant person on a given unit is a head nurse. If this is the situation, the client ought to know that the head nurse is the only predictable constant nursing force on the unit. For maximum continuity of nursing care planning, he or she is the one the client should be told to report to—this is the only person who stands a chance of providing any meaningful continuity of care.

Successful performance of the client/patient role in relationship to the nurse role, particularly in this book's area of interest—nursing care planning—requires that the client have a realistic understanding of the role behavior expected for himself and the person in the nurse role in management of nursing care. The introduction and the finale of the Nursing Assessment serve to set these expectations for the client as they apply to his role behavior *in this specific health care setting*.

SUMMARY

The Nursing Assessment, then, is a focused, time-limited interaction between a nurse and a client with the purpose of collecting subjective and objective data needed to effectively plan nursing's participation in this client's health care management. The nurse's role in the interaction is one of directing the client's attention, facilitating recall and sharing, making observations of objective data which in turn modifies further directions of exploration. The nurse also uses it to begin the organization of the data into logical areas and to validate these impressions with the client. Finally, it is used to set expectations for further contacts and to shape the nature of mutual realistic efforts in the planning routine.

REFERENCES

Carnevali D. and D. Little. "Primary Nursing Clinic Demonstration Project," *Communicating Nursing Research*, Vol. VII, M. Batey, ed. Boulder, Col.: Western Interstate Commission for Higher Education, January 1975.

Cummings, J. "The Pressures and How Patients Respond to Them," *American Journal of Nursing* 70:70-76, January, 1970.

Enelow, Allen and S. Swisher. *Interviewing and Patient Care.* New York: Oxford University Press, 1972.

Froelich, R. and F. M. Bishop. *Medical Interviewing, A Programmed Manual.* St. Louis: Mosby Co., 1969.

Kahn, R. L. and C. F. Cannell. *The Dynamics of Interviewing.* New York: John Wiley and Sons, 1957.

Markle, G. B. "The Case for Episodic Care," *Medical Economics* 48:257-263, November 8, 1971.

Palison, H. "Nursing Care Plans Are a Snare and a Delusion," *American Journal of Nursing* 71:63-66, January, 1971.

Payne, S. L. *The Art of Asking Questions.* Princeton, N.J.: Princeton University Press, 1951.

Zola, I. K. "Problems of Communications, Diagnosis, and Patient Care: The Interplay of Patient, Physician and Clinic Organization," *Journal of Medical Education* 38:829-838, 1963.

Zola, I. K. Culture and Symptoms: "An Analysis of Patients' Presenting Complaints," *American Sociological Review* 31:615, 1966.

chapter Seven

The Content of Nursing Assessment

Assessment is the deliberate, systematic, and logical collection of data from presenting situations, together with the assignment of meaning to the input received. It is an active, not passive, process both in the search for data and in interpretation. Assessment is an initial stage and a repeated step in planning and implementation activities. It is a means to an end—diagnosis—not an end in itself (completing a form).

Within this process the nurse assesses in two areas. She has been delegated by the physician to make assessments of responses to pathology and physiologic reactions to diagnostic tests and medical therapy. Nurses have been educated and trained to varying degrees of expertise in making these kinds of assessments with or without the presence of the physician. The focus is toward assisting the physician; this, nurses have traditionally done.

However, nursing's accountability for assessment of client situations is not limited to the delegated medical observations—that represents only a portion of it. What is the focus of the nursing assessment? What are we primarily responsible for? The rest of this chapter will deal with the content that constitutes the nursing orientation to assessment.

THE COMMON CORE IN NURSING ASSESSMENTS

In the wake of the first edition of this book we saw nursing histories and assessments emerge in all variations of size, length, focus, color, and location. Each institution or agency had a different one. Sometimes each unit had a variant form. We began to wonder why it was that physicians could learn one protocol for history taking and physical examination that seemed to stand them in good stead, no matter where they practiced. This led to a search for a common core in nursing assessment. We found that this exists, regardless of the clientele, the location of their entry point or placement within the health care system. To arrive at a *nursing diagnosis* a nurse needs data in two major areas:

the health-related coping challenges to effective living in the presenting situation or foreseeable future.

and

the abilities and resources present or available to deal with the identified coping challenges.

For the youngest infant to the centenarian, for the acutely ill and those with chronic diseases, for the convalescing and the dying, for the well seeking prevention of diseases, for clients in any part of the health care system, these are the areas of data which are needed to rule out or rule in problems within nursing's primary accountability.

Data collected will be of two types. SUBJECTIVE DATA are those units of information in which the individual reports his perceptions (or what he wants the nurse to know) of what he is or what he has experienced, his responses and reactions to his status and to others around him, his expectations and desires, his perceived needs. This is the client's area of expertise. OBJECTIVE DATA are those units of data about the responses and status of the client which can be observed, described, quantitatively or qualitatively, and verified by others.

Throughout this and subsequent chapters we see the client as the *primary* source of subjective and objective data about himself. We know some clients cannot report on subjective data—they are nonverbal because of age or condition. In such situations we see others as reporting their perceptions of the client. We also see that they may serve as secondary sources about the client who can and does report about himself. In addition, they can serve as primary sources about themselves in relationship to the client.

Coping Challenges

The health-related situations and circumstances which present themselves to a client and require a modification in his use of his abilities and resources are infinite. Some will arise because a new or unusual experience is presented to the client. For example: a decision regarding surgery, sudden trauma, disability, a diagnostic test to be faced, verification of a new diagnosis, symptoms that seem significant, a change in the environment (home to hospital or hospital to home). Many others involving health *in* the normal process of birth, growth and development, maturity or aging, that present themselves to the client or to someone close to him constitute coping challenges. On the positive side, a coping challenge can occur when new insights are gained which result in a desire for a *higher* level of achievement in physical or psychosocial areas. Thus a coping challenge can occur because of a change in circumstances for one's self, someone close, or as a result of a change in one's perception.

Abilities and Resources

A second area for the data base needed to make a nursing diagnosis occurs when there has been a change in a person's *functional capacity* to engage in necessary or desired activities of daily living and/or his preferred lifestyle. In time frame, the onset may be sudden/gradual, rapid/slow. The change may be large or small. It may be predictable or unpredicted. It may involve anatomic structure and/or physiologic functioning of one small part of the body or multiple systems affecting total functioning. It may concern intellectual or emotional resources—again, with varying areas and degrees of involvement. The deficit may also occur in external support systems of any sort—personal, architectural, transportational, financial, or legal. And, of course, the deficits or changes in abilities and resources may be single, but more often than not, will be multiple. Community nurses often speak of multi-problem families. In actuality, probably most of us fall into that category; it's just that for some, the problems are more overwhelming.

Ruling out of problems will be done when the client's and nurse's assessments show that the challenges do not exceed the ability to cope with them in a satisfactory and satisfying manner. A nursing diagnosis of a need for intervention exists when the challenge exceeds or bids to exceed the identified abilities or resources in some way(s).

THE RELATIONSHIP OF THE FOCUS TO CONTENT OF NURSING ASSESSMENTS

If one accepts the belief that nursing is concerned with effective daily living as it is affected by health-related problems and issues, and if one accepts the coping equation of demand versus functional abilities plus available resources, then the focus for nursing assessment becomes quite clear. It also becomes quite distinct from the assessment of medically oriented phenomena as they deal purely with pathophysiology and pathopsychology. This distinction does not presume that each discipline will assess and diagnose only within its own primary area, nor that each discipline will use only its own data. What is expected is that the content of the *nursing* assessment, whether for infant, child, teen-ager, adult or old person, whether in home, ambulatory care setting or hospital, whether for wellness or illness, *can* and *should* accumulate a nursing data base on coping challenges and coping abilities and resources.

Coping Challenges

As nurses we need to develop an awareness of high risk situations for coping challenges. Some which we encounter regularly include: admission to the hospital with all its change in routines and the often unfamiliar "hospitalized patient" role, the decisions, the threats, the diagnostic procedures, the possibilities of new diagnoses, the wrench from supportive, familiar surroundings and personal community. And, going back home after a stay in the hospital, usually with body, and sometimes spirit, changed in some way, with one's relationships to one's family at least temporarily and tentatively modified—this too is a coping challenge.

Some coping challenges will be seen by the client and not by the nurse. These can occur because of his awareness of his own inner fears, concerns, or knowledge of his abilities, that from his perspective, may make him feel unable to meet the demands that may be made on him. For example, nurses who are routinely involved in complex diagnostic tests may not see a barium enema or sigmoidoscopy as anything to be concerned about. Nurses on a surgical unit where organ transplants and massive risky surgical procedures are done, may view a herniorraphy, appendectomy or hemorrhoidectomy as beneath concern. Where hip replacements and spinal fusions are common, removing a cartilage from a knee is an elementary problem. Nasogastric tubes are inserted every day—no big deal. But on the receiving end of these "simple" procedures the coping view can be quite different. Even lying quietly in bed with "no demands" being made may present an overwhelming challenge to some clients; we need to know that. Therefore the reality of the coping challenge needs to be documented with client data on his perceptions of what he's facing, what constitutes a coping challenge to him.

On the other side, in almost every situation we nurses, because of our knowledge, will tend to see coping challenges the client and/or his family may not perceive. We have data on the home environment, or what the proposed medical and nursing treatments will require of them. Maybe the therapy or the disease will continue longer than they expect, have a negative outcome or require abilities and resources they won't have. The nurse's perspectives are a part of the coping challenge data base too.

So, as one step of the nursing assessment, the true nature and extent of the presenting and foreseeable coping challenges need to be documented. Data should be accumulated from the perspectives of client, family, and nurse.

Abilities and Resources

The second aspect the nursing data base is concerned with is the functional assessment of the client's available abilities and resources. This may be done in a comprehensive and detailed way, if this is the philosophy of the system and the client can afford it. It may also be done in a presenting problem approach in which those abilities and resources that are involved in the presenting situation or those in the immediately foreseeable future are assessed. As with documentation of coping challenges it will contain both subjective perceptions of the client and/or his family as to functional capacity, deficits, and usable and desired resources. It will also contain objective data—cues observed that support, extend, modify, or contradict the reported client perceptions. Thus, like the medical history and physical examination, the nurse data base contains subjective and objective data in both the challenges and functional/resources assessment components.

There are standardized tools for detailed testing and assessment of certain functional abilities and developmental levels for particular age groups. On the other hand, the realities of most nursing case loads suggest that a more generalized and less detailed data base will serve their diagnostic and planning needs. This chapter will address itself to an overall assessment that would be usable with the nursing clientele under most prevalent circumstances.

CHARACTERISTICS OF A WORKABLE NURSING ASSESSMENT

There are certain criteria for developing a workable nursing assessment. It should:

1. Contain units of information that will permit the nurse *immediately* to develop a beginning, individualized, realistic plan of care.

2. Provide a baseline of information that is applicable to individualizing care of the client in *a particular setting*.

3. Be concise and permit the nurse to obtain the information in a short length of time.

4. Not duplicate information that is gathered by others on the health team unless the focus is different or the other data are collected too late to be of use in planning nursing care.

CONTENT AREAS OF NURSING ASSESSMENTS

The content of the nursing assessment will incorporate four major areas. These are: client identification, client perspective of presenting situation, functional assessment, and resources and support systems.

Identifying Information

Every health record includes client identification items. Name, age or birth date, and date on which data were gathered seem to be basic essentials. Beyond identification for recording purposes, nurses need another kind of name identification, that is, what does the person prefer to be called? Is it first name, nickname, Mr. or Mrs. _____, occupation-related titles (Dr., Sister, Father, Professor)? Modes of address can set the tone of the interaction in either a positive or negative way. They make for formality or informality, closeness or distance. Take the case of the older individual who is made angry when some young thing comes in and calls him "Gramps." Or the youngster who has been saddled with a family name of Horatio, but who is much happier being called Buz. The assessment form is the place for this kind of identifying information too.

Additional categories of information will depend on whether the nurse is working at some distance from other members of the health care system or in the midst of it, with easy access to records that contain other needed aspects of identification such as address, phone, person to contact, other parts of the health care system currently involved in care (physician, social worker, nutritionist, pharmacist, dentist) and their names and phone numbers. An essential caution is that the nursing assessment record should not duplicate information readily available elsewhere.

Client Perception of Coping Challenges

In this section of the assessment the nurse would be interested in collecting data on the client's perception of:

> his current health status and presenting situation.
>
> his goals related to his health and its relationship to his way of life.
>
> the services he needs or desires from nurses, physicians, and other health care workers to supplement and complement his own coping efforts.

Current health status. In this section the nurse's focus is on the client's health status as he sees it, and its effect on his way of life and daily living patterns. This distinguishes the nursing approach from the medical approach where perceptions of current health status are used primarily to ascertain nature and degree of organ/system dysfunction. For example, the chronically ill child or adult is reportedly wakeful at night. This presenting situation has been continuing over time. The nurse will be concerned, of course, about the sleep pattern of the sick person and how it detracts from his effective daily living. *But* she will also be concerned about what sleep deprivation is doing to the family members who constitute the client's personal support system. Or, the client may report a lack of interest in cooking and eating, with subsequent weight loss. A doctor might well branch off to dentition, stomach pains, and other factors which affect appetite and nutritional status. If the doctor is checking on potential pathology, the nurse will inquire into social antecedent events as well as previous shopping and cooking patterns, social aspects of mealtime, change of locale and marketing or cooking facilities, loss of a family member, change in prescribed diet, change in economic status, and listen for any reason why the individual might wish to shorten his life by an insidious means such as slow starvation.

Often nurses are finding that, even when a doctor is actively involved in a client's ongoing care, the data given to the nurse by the client about coping problems are different from that which he gives the doctors. A colleague told us of a 92-year-old man who was coming in for a routine follow-up on his pacemaker. The doctor had prescribed walking a certain distance each day. What was his version of his current health status? As he reported it to the nurse, "Well, my ticker's going along like a well-oiled clock, but my arches are killing me and I can't walk the way doc told me to." Asked if he'd told the cardiologist about this he said, "He's interested in my heart, not my feet. You don't tell a big specialist like him that your feet hurt." The nurse in her assessment, particularly where it complements a physician's care, is quite likely to deal more with those health problems that indeed do affect daily living profoundly, but are not seen by the clients as being what physicians are interested in. Big or little, they constitute reality to the client, and are worth reporting to the nurse. Frequently it is the management of these "unworthy" problems that enables clients to participate in long term maintenance care or to use the prescribed medical therapy more effectively. It may not be dramatic, but it can be vital.

Goals of health and lifestyle. Here the nurse is dealing with what the client really wants from his therapy and life, and if the nurse is a good interviewer, perhaps data on a fall-back position of what he expects as reasonable if his goals should prove unattainable. Data in this area give the nurse insight into sources of motivation for participation in health care as well as directions the client will tend to go, or want to go, on his own. It can also give evidence of how close the individual's desires and expectations are to the reality of the situation as the nurse sees it.

How does the nurse get at these health and lifestyle goals? Certainly a query such as, "What are your goals in seeking health care?" or "What are your goals in life?" is likely to fall flat. A more conversational gambit may open more thoughts to the client, such as, "If you could have this experience of being sick turn out the way you wanted, what would that be?" To get at the fall-back position the nurse might say, "If things were not to go exactly that way, what would you settle for?" Often data collection regarding lifestyle is not undertaken early in the interaction, but later, after the nurse has had time to get a feel for it indirectly. Then she might say, "It sounds as if you prefer. . . . How do you see your health affecting the way you would really like to live?"

A word of caution. The data gathering at this point must be limited to just that! It is a good idea to express your appreciation for sharing, but make no judgments or you'll close off subsequent disclosures. Therapy does not begin until all the initial data are in and careful nursing diagnosis has been made.

Expected health care. Every person who enters the health care system has expectations of services to be rendered. Most often these are medical services. In order to nurse these people effectively and enable them to cope with the reality of events they face, the nurse needs to know how realistic their perceptions and expectations are. Do they know what their diagnosis is? Do they know what the physician intends to do? Do they know how long the treatment will go on? How long it will take to recover? Do they know the prognosis?

Mr. Paris, for example, who has been scheduled for an amputation of his right leg in two days, states that he came to the hospital to clear up the infection in his foot. The nurse, wondering if he has been told of the surgery, phones the physician to share her information with him and to determine what the client has been told. She learns that the client was indeed told of the amputation, that it was discussed fully with him, and that he had agreed to the procedure. She does not know whether he did not understand what was said, yet agreed in overcompliance, whether he is denying the reality of this traumatic experience, or whether he is testing the nurse to see what she knows. In any instance, the nurse is alerted to a nursing care problem.

Another client may respond with goals that are unrealistic in the light of his condition or prognosis. Jerry Phillips severed his spinal cord at the level of the fourth cervical vertebra in an automobile accident, yet he states that he plans to return to water skiing when he recovers. Because the nursing history is taken early in the patient's hospitalization, this type of denying response may be quite appropriate in terms of the stages of adjustment that clients pass through in this kind of injury. However, should the denial phase continue well beyond the average duration of this stage, the unrealistic goal would represent a nursing care problem for the client. At the time of the original assessment, it may be considered a potential problem to be watched for or ruled out at a later date.

Sometimes the units of information that are elicited in response to this question indicate a lack of understanding of the treatment or diagnostic workup to be undertaken. Mrs. Worth tells you, "The doctor told me to come to the hospital to see what is causing that spot on my lung. He said I needed a good rest and it would probably clear up." At this point the nurse does not know whether the "see what is causing that spot on my lung," means to the client that the doctor plans chest x-rays, bronchoscopy, skin and blood tests, or merely further auscultation and listening with a stethoscope. Again, a possible nursing problem has emerged to which the nurse may need to attend.

It is true that many clients are not told much about their potential diagnosis or prognosis by the physician and other members of the paramedical team. Yet the nurse, who is more available, is placed in the precarious position of helping the client to accept and understand his planned therapy, diagnostic regimen or prognosis, even in cases in which at times only shadows of things to come are known. Hence the importance of the nurse's sharing with the physician the client's responses as they relate to goal expectations, and her close collaboration with the doctor in the total care plan for this person.

Two questions usually yield data on the client's feelings regarding his previous experience with nursing care. First, the nurse may ask what activities and behavior of nurses he found to be particularly helpful in previous health care contacts; second, what activities or behavior were not helpful, or were actually bothersome to him? The client's answers should provide clues to the development of a specific plan of care based on his desires as well as his impressions of non-effective nursing behavior. They also may offer some ideas as to his perception of the nurse's role, so that the nurse may foresee potential conflicts that could arise.

Histories taken using these two questions have brought forth most commonly the opinion that nurses were very busy, were wonderful, and never did anything that bothered the client. It is understandable why many patients tend to respond in this way. A hospital may be perceived as a threatening place, and the client may not wish to be labelled as a complainer who might subsequently be ignored in retaliation. Even in ambulatory care settings, care may be contingent on meeting staff expectations.

When the nurse asks these questions, she should observe how the patient responds. She may notice that he seems hesitant to express an opinion at this time, and so may not find it easy to make desires known to the nursing staff.

It has also been noted that even though the usual answers to the above questions reveal little specific information, more may subsequently be revealed by questions related to customary habits of daily living. For example, when asked about his usual habits of bathing, a patient said, "I usually take my bath every other evening, but when I was in the hospital before they made me take my bath every morning."

Needed and usable services.   In this area the nurse is seeking data on the kind of help from health care members/systems that the individual feels are *necessary* and *usable* to him. Both aspects are important. Some services may be seen as needed, but the individual or his circumstances may not permit him to accept or use them.

We experienced a recent situation in which an 80-year-old, very arthritic lady with severely compromised cardiac function wanted to visit an ailing relative in the hospital. The walk from the entrance of the hospital to the room was a long one. A wheelchair was available in the lobby. However, the lady saw some stigma associated with this. The alternative of a nitroglycerine tablet, a rest in the lobby for several minutes and a long, slow and tiring walk to the ward was chosen instead. This same lady would also dearly love to go shopping. A one-story shopping mall was close. She had transportation and access to a wheelchair that would give her the ability to shop. But again, the stigma of being seen in a wheelchair made this diversion one she could not accept.

Having nursing data on the usability of services and some data on the style of interaction that is most helpful to the client can enable nurses to be realistic in their expectations and their actions. The philosophy that the client must take what he can get from the health care system and feel fortunate to get it has not been found particularly effective in enabling clients to manage their health, particularly in long-term care situations. So much depends on their ability and willingness to participate. To say, "I've given the service," is one thing, to say, "I've given service that was used to achieve health goals," is something else.

Another example from a walk-in clinic: Mrs. Handel had come in to participate in a comprehensive nursing assessment (it was an option offered to any who were interested, whether they had a current problem or not). At the end of the interaction she was asked how the nurses could be most helpful to her in her health care. That approach drew a blank. The nurse tried a different approach. "You come across as being a very independent person who prides herself on her self-sufficiency. I wonder if you would rather that we make observations and offer a service rather than wait, expecting you to ask for it. . . ." There was a rather startled reply of, "How did you know that?" The nurse shared her observations. When she was questioned as to whether she would be able to initiate a request if we failed to perceive a need for our services, her response was affirmative, but the tone was much more tentative. Both of these verbal and nonverbal units of data would be useful in nursing Mrs. Handel in any setting.

Sometimes the nurse gleans data on a client's attitude toward medical care as well as nursing care. A strong belief in the efficacy of medications—any medications—or a strong aversion to medications—any medications—seems to predict responses to therapy. Trust or mistrust in physicians and their motives in prescribing therapy often is also shared. Data on use or valuing of nontraditional health care systems also are important.

In addition to attitudes, or religious or cultural beliefs, sometimes circumstances affect the usability of services. These may include architecture of the residence, roads, transportation, time, or money. The individual may see the need and the usability of the services but not perceive a way of making them feasible. Data on these areas can also be cost effective in making subsequent planning realistic.

Summary. The initial portion of the assessment starts where the client is. What does he see the current situation to be? What antecedent events are perceived as significant? How does he hope to deal with this situation in relationship to his daily living, his goals, and his desired or usual lifestyle? What services does he expect in terms of medical care? What does he see as needed and usable in terms of nursing care? What influences usability of available services? From these data the shape of the coping challenges begins to emerge.

Functional Assessment

To gather data on the other side of the coping equation, the nurse needs to address the abilities and resources of the client. Some of these abilities involve physiologic systems. Some involve psychosocial elements. In each area the data will be concerned not only with functional adequacy or deficit, but with its impact on daily living and lifestyle. A category system, as we have developed it, will be presented here in an alphabetical sequence. This has been done deliberately in hopes that the reader will, in practice, permit the status of the client to shape the sequence of assessment rather than some static listing.

Breathing and Circulation. Within the category of breathing the nurse would obtain any history and objective data associated with respiratory functioning. Branching logic takes the nurse's assessment to the impact of respiratory deficit on daily living. Areas of interest could and should include:

How much work is the individual able to perform?

What kind of respiratory interference does he experience?

How much must be left undone each day?

What activities would he like to do that he can no longer do?

What helps his breathing? What hinders it?

How does he accommodate to his breathing deficit?

How satisfied or dissatisfied is he with the compromises he is making?

If there are acute episodes (asthmatic attacks or paroxysmal nocturnal dyspnea) how is he managing them? What does he understand about the mechanisms of the phenomenon being experienced?

What drugs or treatments are being used? What is their effect?

The subjective data will include the perceived nature of breathing ability and its impact on activities, understanding of the phenomena, accommodations made, treatments being used and satisfaction with the present situation. Objective data on respiration will be obtained either with trained eyes and ears or by adding the use of stethescope, auscultation, and lab data to complete the data base.

Subjective data related to circulatory function could be related to any areas of ischemia/hypoxia and their relationship to activities of daily living and lifestyle. Many of the question areas related to breathing are appropriate to circulatory phenomena where these are the basis for change. In addition, one might seek data on:

What symptoms are being experienced?

Are the symptoms associated with any related events?

What technics are used to cope with such symptoms as tachycardia, bradycardia, skipped beats, angina, intermittent claudication, stasis ulcers, hypertensive symptoms?

Are relationships with others affected negatively by the invisible nature of the disability? (angina, fear of another M.I., side effects of drugs) e.g., Are inappropriate expectations being made in terms of work, attitude, sexual activity, etc.?

Because cardiovascular diseases have such a high mortality rate it is an important area to obtain data on family history (either from the doctor's history or from the client). It will be a predictor of risk, but also will be useful as a frame of reference for fears, expectations, motivation and goals.

Objective data may include: inspection of color of critical or affected body parts, taking the pulse (at rest or in activity), taking the blood pressure in different positions, observing the filling of neck veins, observing varicosities. Nurses also are using instrumentation such as the stethoscope, auscultation of heart borders, electrocardiograms, laboratory data, and other means to round out the circulatory assessment.

Elimination. Elimination of body waste products is seen by many clients as a sensitive indicator of health status, so they often monitor it closely and with concern. One of the assessment tasks here, then, is to gather data on what constitutes a "normal" response for this client, for urinary and fecal elimination. Both constipation and diarrhea have a wide range of definition among nursing's clientele, so it is wise not only to gather data on what is *usual* in their elimination patterns but also what *they* consider to be *normal*. Furthermore, both urinary and fecal elimination are treated with a vast array of dietary, folk, home, proprietary, and prescribed remedies. Again, knowing what is usual treatment or prevention is important to the nurse as well as to the medical regimen.

Also important may be deficits in control—incontinence, stress incontinence, nocturia, and enuresis. These have a high risk of interfering with an individual's lifestyle. It is a high risk in the otherwise healthy, very young and old. However, adults with spinal cord injuries and long-standing use of catheters or other urine catchment systems also have coping challenges affecting their daily living. As in previous sections, data on impact on daily living, techniques of management and satisfaction levels will be significant.

Objective data will be concerned with timing and frequency of elimination, with appearance of urine or feces, laboratory data, and equipment or architectural support systems.

Emotional and cognitive factors. Just as most nurses don't presume to be internists and surgeons, neither do they presume to be psychiatrists or psychologists, although there is no question that many with advanced education and training have competency in testing, diagnosis and therapy. For most nurses not so prepared, any assessment of emotional status and cognitive ability will be related to emotional patterns of coping that appear to be adaptive or maladaptive. In areas of cognitive ability we will seek data on education, vocabulary, and learning styles as they influence the management of health problems.

Subjective data in emotional areas might relate to:

perceived strengths and areas of needed strength
moods
needs for personal support systems
preferences for independence or comfort with interdependence or dependence
situations or times that place them at high risk emotionally
key people who are helpful or necessary to them
circumstances under which they want them excluded from knowledge or presence
areas of high need for privacy and those that offer comfort in disclosure.

Any or all of these are areas for potential nursing assessment, depending on the presenting situation.

In the learning-thinking area, the client can tell the nurse his previous experiences with health learning, his perceived need or desire for knowledge in his present situation, learning that "comes easily" or is "hard." Again, the focus will be determined by the presenting situation.

Objectively, the nurse may observe cues as to mood, body language, approach or withdrawal behavior to areas of the assessment, and responses to others. In learning, the nurse may listen to vocabulary, evidence of comprehension, ease of expression, desire to verbalize, and use of nonverbal expressions or gestures to replace words in description. The strength of cross-cultural ties or ethnicity may also become apparent in this section. These of course are crucial, even where ethnic ties at first glance appear to be tenuous.

Hygiene and grooming. In this category the nurse will be gathering data on usual practices and preferences in the daily care of one's body, such as bathing, oral hygiene, hair care, make-up, dress, or nails, particularly where these influence or are influenced by the individual's health problems and treatment. Body image and self concepts as they concern appearance, dress, and the equipment and means of maintaining appearance are involved.

Mobility and safety. Mobility and safety incorporate areas involving any form of movement and constraint on it. Physically this area may involve joint range of motion, bone integrity or trauma, pain, musculature, innervation, and any other factors that foster or limit mobility. Sense organs such as kinesthetic sense and vision may be involved. In the environment, lighting, stairs, transportation, clothing/shoes, prosthesis, equipment and money may also be of concern. The presenting situation and the skill in branching logic of the nurse will be determining features in this area. Here are two situations that we encountered which unexpectedly fell into the mobility category:

> Two single sisters were sharing an apartment in a retirement complex. One was convalescing *slowly* from a stroke; the other was a loving, devoted helper. The stroke victim, weeks after the stroke, rarely left the apartment and did not help with maintaining the apartment. There was no need. The helping sister seemed to enjoy the role of the strong one. The nurse who made an assessment saw the helper as being an immobilizing feature to the convalescing sister. A prescription was made that the client was to begin dressing, to set and clear the table, to dust, increasingly to assume responsibility for herself and do whatever she could in the apartment. The first nursing visit occurred in the apartment. The second was scheduled downstairs in the clinic located in the hobby room. Within a week of the nursing visit the client was dressing, setting and clearing the table, dusting, and, in general, doing a great deal more. At the time of her scheduled visit to the clinic, the nurse was out in the hall. She saw the client walking rapidly

down the hall, fully dressed with the sister ten paces behind. The immobilizing force in the situation had been neutralized for the moment. We then had to deal with some role realignment problems for the helper in order for it to be emotionally safe for the "victim" to continue her progress—but that is another story.

The second situation also involved an older person thought of by neighbors as an antisocial recluse because she so rarely ventured outside of her apartment. A nurse, at the request of concerned neighbors, visited to offer any services she might need. She discovered in short order that the immobilizing forces for this lady were (1) corns and calluses that made walking so painful she could not leave her apartment, and (2) insufficient funds for a podiatrist's services. Once her feet were treated and she was taught how to maintain them safely, she was neither immobilized nor antisocial.

Another dimension related to mobility and safety concerns prediction of periods of decreased mobility and safety. Here too, a nurse can be of tremendous assistance in managing challenges to the client's coping abilities. See the example in Chapter Three, p. 29. Given advanced planning the period of immobility often can be minimized and clients can safely maneuver through the demands and hazards of living with peak periods of disability.

Obviously, a variety of factors in one's life can be immobilizing and hazardous beyond those body systems we might immediately associate with movement. Some that have been identified include: decreased vision, loss of a driver's license or car (or a mate's loss of ability to drive), inadequate finances to use public transportation or to dress for "going out," or a neighborhood with a high crime rate. Mobility and immobility can take many forms. Certainly it is an area where nurses need well-developed concepts and adequate assessment techniques.

Nutrition.   Nutrition, like each of the other areas, cuts across many functions and aspects of life—cultural, geographic and religious, food and fluid likes and dislikes, patterns of eating, dentition, allergies, digestion, money, market facilities, cooking appliances and skills, shopping skills, pleasure in preparing and eating food, the meanings of food and feeding, knowledge of nutrients, social patterns at mealtime, climate, and so forth. Any assessment of a deficit in nutrition and related aspects of lifestyle and daily living, or the impact of a therapeutic diet, must take into consideration these aspects if there is any expectation that an individual will actually modify current eating patterns in terms of normal or therapeutic diets; or, if the nurse is going to discover why current nutrition is a problem.

Sensory input.   Sensory input, both that available to the client in his environment and that which is perceived and used by the client (noticed) are rarely assessed unless there are changes in the sense organs or symptoms of extreme deprivation or overload (see Chapter Eleven for symptoms). Certainly some individuals are at higher risk of either underload or overload—older people whose sense organs are less efficient and who have less stimuli in the environment can be deprived or, having been deprived, can be overloaded with normal stimuli in a new environment such as a hospital ward. The client who cannot understand the language risks sensory underload. The person whose hearing or sight is restored risks overload. These tend to be visible changes.

More subtly, each individual has a range of sensory input that is comfortable to him, each has senses that are more precise than others, each enjoys certain kinds of stimuli more than others and each can experience depatterning and distortion if prescription lenses or hearing aids are removed. Some can hear or see only on one side. Some can see only in bright light. All these units of information can and do influence coping with daily living, whether one enters a strange health care environment, becomes increasingly deprived by a style of living or is suddenly overwhelmed by a change in environment.

The nurse will be concerned with data on: the usual and preferred environmental stimuli, known deficits in sense organs, appliances used, and drugs or conditions that decrease or increase central nervous system awareness of stimuli.

Sexuality. There are times when sexuality has high priority for the client, or is at high risk in terms of the disease or treatment. If sexuality is a coping problem, all these will be areas for data gathering:

> usual patterns of sexual activity
> desire for it
> opportunities
> partner's desires and pattern of coping with deprivation
> deterrents
> knowledge of normal needs and patterns
> adjustments that can be made to accommodate to presenting situations
> resources for gaining knowledge
> a group with which to share concerns.

Sleep and rest. Patterns of usual sleep, desired sleep patterns, rituals or equipment used to enhance sleeping, usual positions, deterrents to sleep and treatments used for insomnia are all areas for data gathering where sleep is a current or potential problem. Daytime rest patterns are also needed data as a basis for predicting problems coping with changes to either more or fewer rest periods. Changes of time zones or requirements for changes of expected sleep periods from what has been the usual pattern should be assessed, e.g., the person who has worked evenings or nights for a long time and who is hospitalized and expected to sleep nights and waken early. As we mentioned earlier the nurse needs to be concerned not only with the sleep pattern of the client but, where this is disturbed, with the sleep patterns of persons who share responsibility for the care of the individual.

Summary. We have suggested some areas for functional assessment that seem to us to incorporate major areas for a data base that would permit nurses to diagnose or rule out functional capacity as a factor or deterrent to coping effectiveness in any presenting situation. Sequence and extensiveness will no doubt be determined by the client's presenting situation as will the amount of data a nurse and client can effectively use. Any assessment of a client is an invasion of his privacy; thus, only that which is essential and usable in helping him with his health care management should be collected.

Resources and Support Systems

Beyond functional capacities most individuals have external resources and support systems of varying kinds. Some are environmental, some economic, some are sociocultural, some diversional. Because these vary so widely we will speak of them more generally. We strongly suggest the use of branching logic to investigate and follow up on the relationship of specific resources and support systems (their presence or absence) to coping ability of the individual.

Environmental. Within this broad category one might consider: housing, architecture, furnishings, light, noise, transportation, working conditions, recreational facilities, distance from health care systems and facilities actually available, equipment, supplies, the nature of the neighborhood and community, emergency services, types of schools, and communication facilities such as intercoms and phones. All of these may be a part of the nursing data base, again depending on the presenting situation.

Socio-cultural. Health problems present opportunities when the dedication and steadfastness of one's personal community can be tested. Its importance cannot be overestimated. Whether the personal community consists of family, extended family and kinship networks, ethnic groups, a club or church members, friends, a pet, or whatever—these tend to form a bulwark of both moral and physical help when stresses and deficits occur. (They can also be a responsibility and, therefore, part of the coping challenge.) The nurse needs to know who these persons and nonpersons are seen to be. How extensive and what kind of a resource will they be? For how long? Do they depend on the client, or he on them? What do they *want* to be to him? What do they *not want* to be? Realistic data here, particularly in chronic, maintenance, or terminal situations is critical. The nurse needs data, primary data, both from the client as he sees the relationship and, in a separate data collecting encounter, from the other member(s) of his personal community.

Nonhuman members of the client's personal community should not be overlooked. For example, the maintenance of the skills and relationship of the seeing eye dog to his master is crucial, if the separation is to be at all extended. Acknowledgment of the role that pets play in the lives of clients is often a significant part in the therapeutic plan of coping with daily living—one we as nurses have often overlooked.

Summary. A nursing data base that has included either comprehensive or selected relevant assessment of:

> client perceptions of health-related coping challenges, goals, and needed, usuable services
>
> areas of functional abilities and deficits
>
> areas of external resources and support systems or deficits in them,

should enable the nurse and the client to arrive at a point of diagnosis leading to mutual decisions that the individual is managing quite effectively without nursing participation or that effective living and health status wll be enhanced and facilitated by nursing's participation in specified ways.

STUDENT LEARNING ASSESSMENTS VERSUS CLINICIAN'S WORKING ASSESSMENTS

Nursing students' assessments are a learning situation in which they are expected to give instructors some evidence of how they are thinking, what their store of knowledge is, and how they are using these to make decisions regarding data collection. Student assessments also serve to develop habit patterns of systematic data collection in the assessment process. Therefore, the guidelines for a comprehensive student assessment are detailed. Mitchell, in making an adaptation from several previous authors, offers a six-page outline of headings (Mitchell, 1973, 77-82). A student demonstrating her ability to complete this protocol utilized nine single-spaced, typewritten pages to submit the data she collected in these categories and sub-categories.

Each cue noticed, each inference, the rationale for combining cues into diagnostic combinations, and the tentative diagnoses that were used to set the direction for branching logic—all these indicate levels of skill which the instructor will use to further evaluate and teach a student. It is a good way to learn sound, systematic, logical assessment.

But it is not a very good way to carry out assessments in the clinical situation. This is not to say that the assessment is not systematically carried out, nor that priorities are not set, branching logic used, or tentative diagnoses tested. What it does say is that these things, if well-learned in the student experiences will be carried out *in the head* of the skilled nurse rather than being written in their entirety on the record. The skilled clinician will scan the presenting situation for cues, will set priorities of observation and recording, and will group observations in her recording in terms of categories where they will fit, rather than in the sequence they were noticed. This is true whether the assessments are comprehensive or made in terms of a portion of the presenting situation (Chapter Six, pp. 102-104). In the end, the skilled clinician will produce a concise written record of observations that include the data seen as usable, described accurately and with appropriate precision. In most instances it must be a very telescoped version of the extensive written assessment the thorough, ambitious student submits to the instructor. In the working situation few nurses would have time to write that much and few nurses would take the time to read it.

Where staff on a unit are novices at making nursing assessments, the initial learning experiences may well include more detailed guides, and systematic checklists, until these habit patterns are built into the nurse's thinking and observation. But, hopefully, as skill grows, these crutches can be discarded; the knowledge, the skills, and the systematic pattern of observation predictably will be found inside the nurse's head, rather than on the paper.

Certainly, as a profession we are wise to continue to critique the assessments we make in our ongoing efforts to grow more skillful. Let us look to the knowledge base we use, the decisions of priorities in our sequencing or observation, and the data we choose to record and choose not to record, *but* as we grow, let us also leave our crutches behind.

FORMAT OF THE NURSING ASSESSMENT FORM

As a result of having used a variety of forms and witnessing the use made of them as both interview guide and recording place, we would like to propose a fairly radical departure, an almost clean piece of paper. We have heard workshop participants leave saying, "I came thinking the forms were the important thing, now I know it's the thinking and observation skill. I can go home and do assessments and care plans on a blank piece of paper." With this experience in mind, we would like to recommend a format that specifies the identifying information and lists potential areas of assessment in a narrow column on the left side. No crutches of preformulated questions to be read off, no sequence of topics, no check lists—just a bare minimum of headings to choose from.

You might ask, "Given so much room for variation, how will one ever find any information on it?" Good question. We've tried some techniques and believe that the answer lies not in presetting the spaces by inserting headings; this gives too much for one and not enough for another. But, by having the nurse set out and underline the headings as she records. The information, while not always in the same sequence, is not at all difficult to find. And on the other hand, the nurse during the assessment interaction doesn't have to spend time looking for the right space to write the cues and data she's getting. There's always enough room and never any waste space.

We hope we have also removed the temptation to start at the top of the form and go to the bottom, regardless of where the client feels he needs to start or wants to go. We have heard the headings or questions reeled off in almost automaton fashion. Perhaps with a format that, beyond the identification stage, is alphabetical, a nurse will not feel constrained to fill in all the blanks. She will be free to look for the high priority presenting cues, she will be able to listen to what the client wants to tell her about. The focus will be on the client, not on filling out the form. She will systematically assess the person and the presenting situation and record data that she sees as being usable and needed in planning for nursing care—not merely fill out the form.

Recommended Sample Assessment Forms

On the following page you will find a blank form showing the format we have just discussed and utilizing headings we have found helpful in doing nursing assessments. Following that are completed forms in which two nurses have recorded the data which they saw as being useful in planning the nursing care of a woman and of a man who were admitted to a hospital. These will illustrate the use of the underlined headings, the identification of subjective and objective data, the variation in sequence of data categories from the alphabetical version, and the omission of certain categories where, for the present, either no data were collected or they were not seen to be needed for planning.

This assessment guide and format recommendation is a far cry from the one offered in the first edition of *Nursing Care Planning*. The former was oriented only to hospitalized clients dealing with the transition from home and the usual patterns of daily living to the challenge of changes related to hospitalization. With nursing giving growing attention to ambulatory individuals in the community as well as to institutionalized persons, and with increasing emphasis on maintenance and rehabilitation and on the care of the dying at home as well as in institutions, it was obvious that the focus was too narrow. Today a nurse's assessment guide must look to the challenges and resources for maintaining health and effective living in any locale.

Another change is obvious. The first "Nursing History Tool" offered the nurse much more structure. In the ensuing years the level of expectation for professional competence in nursing assessment has risen. Nursing assessment is being taught to the nursing students of today and continuing education is increasingly available to earlier graduates who may have missed it, so that we can expect a professional level of autonomy and creativity in nursing assessments rather than the technical skill involved in completing check lists. Granted, this approach places much more responsibility on the professional. Many will prefer the structure of the former method. We believe that a profession grows by ever higher expectations of itself.

SAMPLE NURSING ASSESSMENT FORM

Name _____ Age _____ Date _____

Prefers to be called _____ Assessment made by _____ RN

Areas	Subjective/Objective Data
Client perceptions of:	
Current health status	
Goals	
Needed/usable services	
Functional Abilities:	
Breathing/Circulation	
Elimination	
Emotional/cognitive	
Mobility/safety	
Nutrition	
Hygiene/grooming	
Sensory input	
Sexuality	
Sleep/rest	
Resources & Support Systems:	
Environmental	
Personal/social	
Other	

The Content of Nursing Assessment

SAMPLE NURSING ASSESSMENT FORM

Name _Miss Rose Stevens_ Age _48_ Date _7/7_

Prefers to be called _Miss Stevens_ Assessment made by _Mary White_ RN

Areas	Subjective/Objective Data
<u>Client perceptions of:</u> Current health status Goals Needed/usable services <u>Functional Abilities:</u> Breathing/Circulation Elimination Emotional/cognitive Mobility/safety Nutrition Hygiene/grooming Sensory input Sexuality Sleep/rest <u>Resources & Support Systems:</u> Environmental Personal/social Other	<u>Current Health Status</u>: Having severe back pain that respond to moist heat, pain ℞ and muscle relaxants @ home. A diabetic since 1957 — tends to run trace or neg on urinalyses On lente insulin. Has schedule of rotating sites — some atrophy of upper arm sites. <u>Goals</u>: Get pain under control so she can go on planned vacation trip 8/1 to France. <u>Needed Services</u>: Prefers to continue to give own insulin <u>Breathing/Circulation</u>: R-20 (uncomfortable ℞ wearing off) P. 88 reg. Color of feet and legs good / warm pedal pulses + Knows importance of foot care to a diabetic. <u>Mobility/Safety</u>: Does not want to move because of spasms. Wants help turning. No pain in using arms — hands. <u>Nutrition</u>: Diabetic Exchange Diet. Eats 7³⁰/12/ 5³⁰ Snack (Protein) @ bedtime. Knows food composition. Wt seems normal for Ht. No food dislikes or allergies. <u>Sensory</u>: Wears contacts. Sl. hearing loss — rt side. Lives alone in rural area. Teaches French in High School. Sept — June. <u>Sleep/rest</u>: Prior to back pain Slept 8 hrs. uninterrupted. For past week has slept no longer than 1-2 hrs at a time and only 4h/24 hour period. Most comf. on back uses no pillow. <u>Hygiene/grooming</u>: Grooming seems important — Hair coiffed nails manicured. Extensive toiletries. Gowns and robe well cared for — neatly packed. Showers daily @ hs. <u>Emotional/Cognitive</u>: Despite reportedly severe pain speaks quietly c̄ restraint. Describes diabetic management & experiences of back-pain with precise terminology. <u>Personal/Social</u>: Sister and her family live 20 min from hospital are available to help. Ph: 273-6410 prn. Prefers visitor restriction if in pain (except for sister) <u>Diversion</u>: Has FM radio c̄ her & some nonfiction books.

SAMPLE NURSING ASSESSMENT FORM

Name *Arthur Longbranch*   Age *47*   Date *6/22/75*

Prefers to be called *"Art"*   Assessment made by *Jill Sutter* RN

Areas	Subjective/Objective Data
Client perceptions of: Current health status Goals Needed/usable services **Functional Abilities:** Breathing/Circulation Elimination Emotional/cognitive Mobility/safety Nutrition Hygiene/grooming Sensory input Sexuality Sleep/rest **Resources & Support Systems:** Environmental Personal/social Other	*Perceived health status*: Rt inguinal hernia repair in A.M. Hosp (subj) stay expected: 3-4 days. Older brother had same surg. 6 mo. ago – no prblms. no prev. hosp admissions. Expects spinal anesthesia – some concern re aftereffects. MD told him he was in good cond. No other med. prblms. Objective: uses medical terminology *Goals*: To be out of hosp in 3-5 days, up day of surgery, To (subj) ret to job as accountant in 2 wks & to his golf game in 6 wks. *Expected care*: Dr will order R to control pain & sleep prn. (subj) Brother said backrubs @ HS → relaxation. ō limitations on visitors *Hygiene/grooming* (subj) Usually showers ā bkfst/q̄ d. shaves 2x daily ā bkfst & p̄ supper. (objective:) Trimmed moustache – long side burns Toupee *Sensory Input*: (subj) glasses for close work – none for distance, checked 6 mo ago. No difficulty hearing. *Sleep/Rest*: Usual sleep pattern 10³⁰p to 6³⁰a s̄ waking. (subj) Usual R for Sleeplessness: reading & hot cocoa sleep not often a problem unless worrying. *Nutrition*: 3 meals 7³⁰a, 12 noon 6p no snacks except (subj) coffee. Drinks 10-12 cups/day Dislikes: strong vegetables, mayonnaise, casserole dishes. No food allergies. (objective:) Ht 6' Wt 180# Looks well nourished *Elimination*: BM p̄ bkfst. q̄ d. R for constipation: 1c prune (subj) juice in a.m. No nocturia, frequency or burning. *Social/Rec*: (subj) Plays bridge 1x wk c̄ fellows in office. Plays golf 2x wk. Enjoys lake fishing, boating, reading (mysteries) Gardening – roses, orchids (objective:) Has Sports Illustrated, US News and World report, Newsweek at bedside

Nursing Assessment cont. page 2

Arthur Longbranch

Support Systems: Wife, employed school teacher. Married
(subj)   20 years 2 daughters 16 y.o. @ home 18 y.o.
away @ Univ.
Family will visit evenings.
Hospital Ins. & Sick leave.
(_Objective_) Picture of wife & daughters outside
their home on bedside stand.

Breathing: (Subj) Does not smoke. No hist. of chronic
resp. disease.
(_Objective_) R 14   No Sx of resp. infection.

REFERENCE

Mitchell, Pamela. *Concepts Basic to Nursing.* New York: McGraw-Hill Co., 1973.

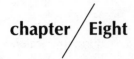

chapter / Eight

The Ruling Out Process

Human minds, like computers, have a ceiling on the informational load they can process and use. Because of this one of the first uses made of data collected in the Nursing Assessment is to rule out problems that don't exist or those the client is managing without nursing intervention.

How many of us have lightheartedly left a physician's office after being given a clean bill of health, despite the findings that doctors, when in doubt, rule in favor of diagnosing an illness rather than ruling it out, just to be on the safe side (Scheff, 1963). Yet, as nurses, we have been made to feel that every client must surely have nursing problems, or we are not good care planners. Not true. Many clients manage their health needs and associated problems of daily living very well with no help from the health care system at all. And who are we to create problems where none exist? Furthermore, with the case loads most nurses carry there is no need to manufacture client problems in order to look like good diagnosticians. There are plenty of legitimate problems.

Still, just as a physician cannot give assurance that an illness does not exist without supporting data, so the nurse must definitively rule out problems as well. This ruling out process is not a passive one of merely being unaware of situations or data—far from it. It is as active and aggressive in terms of data gathering and as disciplined in terms of critical thinking and prediction as the process of defining problems that are ruled in. When a nurse writes, "Coping well at this time," it is based on observed data indicating that one or more of three situations are present:

1. There are no unusual stressors present, therefore no coping problem exists.
2. There are unusual stressors present, but the individual has the skills and resources to cope with them and is discernably doing so, or can indicate the ways in which he will do so.
3. The stressors do not seem to be of such magnitude or of such long duration as to drain the client's resources and thus leave him vulnerable in the future.

Let us examine each of these more specifically.

No Unusual Stressors

Obviously, all of us experience stress daily. It is the mechanism by which we grow, learn and maintain our development. Each of us will have learned to cope with our own normal load of stresses by the time we encounter the health care system, except for the very young and, sometimes, the very old. Some of our clients have the capacity, skill and desire to deal with both a great variety and a fairly high amplitude of stressors. They may have done so for prolonged periods of time. It may even be their desired lifestyle. Others will not have done so. One aspect of the ruling out process, therefore, involves determining *what constitutes unusual stress for this person*. If he does not see a situation as stressful or beyond his coping ability and resources, it will not be a problem for him.

Some women, for example, do not find labor and delivery particularly stressful. We know of a woman who said she had a very satisfying experience in the delivery of her first child and a planned and uneventful second pregnancy. She also described the first stage of labor as surprisingly comfortable and felt there was adequate nursing support and medical management of the second and third stages. She said the experience was more exciting than stressful. This same individual says she experiences much more anxiety at the prospect of dental work, particularly extractions.

On the other hand, much of what become everyday mundane events to a nurse in a health care system may be highly stressful to a client. Suppose a nurse in an immunization clinic sees a group of strapping young athletes enter for some preoverseas immunizations. She has been giving injections by the dozens for years in this clinic. She is good at it and knows it. She has also experienced immunization injections herself; to her they are relatively painless. Yet three of these husky healthy young males pass out amidst the nervous laughter of the rest. A nurse must be aware of her own norms and be careful not to expect clients to share them. Objectivity and a client-oriented focus on stresses are key attributes in ruling out the absence of unusual stressors.

Another situation for consideration within this criterion is one in which the nurses' knowledge enables them to perceive problem areas that the client does not recognize. These will become client problms if or when it becomes necessary for him to recognize and deal with them. For example, it has been found that preoperative patients who coped with preoperative stress by denying the reality of the surgical procedure and the postoperative experience, had a less smooth convalescence than those who acknowledged it (Janis, 1958; Titchener and Levine, 1960). Here, then, is a situation in which the nurses' vision should be used to create a stressor for the patient so that he can mobilize his hormonal and psychological defenses for the upcoming stress peak.

But in other instances where the resources to deal with a problem do not seem to exist, either within the client or in the environment around him, it may be wiser to leave well enough alone.

> Pete Perkins is a 60-year-old transient who comes into the local Skid Row Clinic. The nurse practitioner regularly finds him to be anemic and underweight. She knows his usual housing is doorways, patches of ground under bridge abutments, or an occasional bed in a nearby flophouse when he can afford it and when there are any vacancies. (Urban renewal is fast reducing cheap beds in this locale.) The nurse knows she can't arrange for foodstamps for him—he doesn't meet current criteria of having cooking facilities in his room—he doesn't even have a room. Further, he isn't a county or state resident so he's not eligible for welfare. This time Pete has come in with a sore throat. And this time, as on previous contacts, the nurse is aware of his continuing inadequate nutrition. It is a deficit that neither he nor she have the resources to cope with, given his current desired lifestyle.

Nurses are usually intermittent figures in most clients' lives. Unless they can, within the constraints of available contacts, enable a client to deal with the problems they will bring to his attention, it may be wise to leave these problems only in the nurse's awareness, and not share them with the client.

To summarize, in ruling out the presence of an unusual stressor, nurses need data that indicate a stressor is unusual to this client, that he perceives it this way (whether or not nurses do), and that it is to the client's current and/or ultimate advantage that he be made aware of it and attempt to deal with it.

Stressors Are Within Client's Coping Resources

Another situation which calls for ruling out problems exists when data indicate that unusual stressors are present, but the client has the resources and skills to deal with them without help from nurses. Again, this is not as simple as it might seem at first glance—particularly when the client's mechanisms for coping are not those the nurse would use, understand or be comfortable with.

> A queen of a local gypsy tribe had been hospitalized for severe chest pain. She was placed in the coronary care unit and diagnosed as having had a myocardial infarction. Now the usual care in this unit involves minimizing the amount of interaction patients have with visitors. The policies permit one member of the immediate family to visit for 5 minutes in any hour. In this way, the unit hopes to help persons with decreased cardiac function to cope with the demands of daily living.
>
> This queen's fellow gypsies, on the other hand, had a different way of coping with heart trouble. They believed that her heart trouble stemmed from some wrong that had been committed against her by a member of the tribe. The diagnosis and therapy consisted of having her surrounded by members of the tribe while together they decide whether any of them had wronged her so as to remove the evil forces that were making her ill.

149

They were not to be denied. She seemed not only to survive but to thrive on their therapy.

In this criterion area the nursing skill comes in collecting data as to what the individual's physiologic and psychosocial coping resources are and their effectiveness in managing the defined demands being placed on them. The athlete with a fractured ankle and no other injuries should have little trouble with crutch walking, while an 80-year-old lady may have real problems in terms of deficits of strength, endurance and balance. The person in his middle forties or fifties who does not smoke, is normal in weight, has no respiratory disease and who is not having chest or upper abdominal surgery can be expected to cope with the effects of general anesthesia. Those older, more obese, smokers with respiratory symptoms having upper abdominal or thoracic surgery may not have the physiologic resources to prevent or even cope with postoperative atelectasis (Alexander, 1969).

In the realm of psychosocial stresses, the situation is the same. Some individuals, some relationships can tolerate the stresses of the illness experience; others cannot.

To rule out problems in this realm, the nurse collects data on both the stressors and the client coping mechanisms/resources. Where the match is adequate, even though the mechanisms or resources might not be those which the nurse would use, a problem can be ruled out for the present.

Duration and Amplitude of Stressors Do Not Exceed Resources

Many of us have the physiologic, psychosocial, and economic resources to cope with a health problem for a short period of time. However, most of us could encounter health problems that would eventually deplete our coping resources in one or more areas. Therefore a problem that may be ruled out for a period of time in terms of nursing involvement, may need to be noted for nursing intervention should it outlast the individual's resources.

> Brenda Carson was riding a bicycle down the country road when she was struck by a car. She suffered a severe head injury resulting in deep coma. Her relatives, neighbors, friends, the newspapers and the community mobilize to pitch in and help the Carson family. Mother and father take turns in a vigil at Brenda's bedside in the children's hospital 30 miles from their home. Neighbors and relatives take charge of the other children. They bring food for meals and offer to sit with Brenda so that Mr. and Mrs. Carson can get some rest. There are newspaper publicity and fund raising efforts.
>
> But the weeks roll on. Brenda remains comatose—some improvement, no longer critical, but still nonverbal, still not recognizing anyone. Costs mount. Money runs out, the volunteer child care runs out, the siblings' patience with lack of normal parental attention and fun runs out, hope runs out, and Brenda continues.

150

What holds true for duration also applies to the amplitude of the stressor. Again, many of us can cope with minor health problems that are acute, but most of us could become victims of short duration health problems of sufficient intensity in their stress to us that we would find it difficult to manage. The nurses' task is to gather data on whether *this* stressor constitutes an above-and-beyond coping situation for this person.

As an example, on a busy surgical unit in a teaching and research hospital a man in his thirties is admitted for elective knee surgery. The nurse learns from him that he has accepted both the inconvenience and pain of his "trick knee" for five years before finally deciding to have surgery, that if he hadn't been so heavily sedated he would have changed his mind at the last minute, and that the postoperative immobilization was beyond even what he had expected, driving him close to panic. Here is a very intelligent man having what is, in the era of open-heart surgery and transplants, minor surgery. Certainly, this is stress of short, predictable duration. Yet it was almost beyond this man's coping resources.

Again, as it does in terms of what constitutes a stressor, the nurses' attitude toward the magnitude of stress generated needs to be open. Familiarity may breed contempt for experiences of high stress potential. The net result may be that nurses could so minimize the experience as to fail to collect data on its meaning to the client. Or, they could by their attitude make it impossible for him to reveal his true perceptions of the anticipated experience and his inadequate coping resources. Maintaining this openness and neutrality to clients' versions of stress is not easy—not for physicians, or social workers, or nurses. It is, however, essential if clients are to be enabled to give valid data on coping abilities and deficits.

TESTING YOUR RULING OUT SKILL

To test your ruling out skill, do a Nursing Assessment on a client in your work setting. If you're not working, try the activity with someone who could be a client—someone with potential or actual health problems. Then, away from the client or whomever you have assessed, and away from the work setting too (for who has time for contemplation at work?), quietly think through the data you have received. Identify client- and nurse-perceived stressors and client and nurse versions of coping skills and resources. Then write down the areas/problems you would rule out from nursing management because the client seems to have the ability and resources to cope with them. Under each area, jot down the data that support your judgment. Then put this piece of paper away in a safe place and ignore it. Later, when time has translated predictions into fact or fiction, take your paper out and see whether your predictions were accurate.

This is an effective first time activity to practice the new skill. Obviously, you cannot do the ruling out for each client you assess in this way—at home, on paper. Much of the ruling out must be done in your head both while and after you are doing the Nursing Assessment. But it is also true that ruling out does take time and concentration in the beginning. You may need to supplement your on-the-job thinking with some at-home contemplation as well until experience and skill grow.

In addition to being an effective introductory activity, this technique is also a good way to check up on increasing skill as well as a means of keeping yourself from going stale. Efforts at maintaining freshness too are a part of the nurse's continuing self-development.

RECORDING PROBLEMS RULED OUT

Nurses have asked us at many workshops, "Must you have a problem on every patient?" Obviously no nurse should create problems to make the care plans look good, nor to meet audit requirements. If the nurse has assessed the stressors from the point of view of both client and nurse, if the nurse has assessed the coping skills and resources also from both points of view, and if there is a good match, the Kardex should show something to the effect, "Coping adequately/effectively at this time." If there is some concern for the future, another clause might be added, "but watch for . . ." Here any area of possible future concern could be noted.

The legal record might receive a fuller treatment, particularly if the Nursing Assessment forms are not a part of the clients' permanent records. Here the nurse might record:

"An experienced diabetic, manages diabetic regimen, diet, exercise, surveillance, and accommodation to life changes well. Spouse also well-prepared to deal with any diabetic emergencies if client incapacitated."

or

"Has realistic expectations regarding the downward course of the disease and is working through the grieving process with the family. Both client and family are open in their relationships. They care and are hurting, but they are managing and prefer no outside intervention."

or

"Has mastered crutch walking around the home. No small rugs or slippery floors. No stairs to climb. Has transportation to store and help for emergencies from neighbor in apartment next door. Has portable intercom unit."

These notations tend to focus on particular areas where stressors currently exist for these clients. Realistically, it does not seem reasonable to expect recording of all areas where problems may be ruled out. It does seem reasonable to expect that nurses will have taken most areas of consequence into account in their thinking and be able to make a summary statement that takes data and priorities into account. In addition, Nursing Assessments should include notations of strengths and resources where they exist, as surely as notations of deficits.

SUMMARY

The first step in using data being collected in the Nursing Assessment is to rule out problems. This calls for nurses to focus on ability and resources and to match them with demands being made. Ruling out is an active, not a passive, process. It is not to be equated with failure to collect data or failure to recognize problems. It requires a balance of viewing the situations—both stressors and coping skills/resources—from the client's point of view as well as the nurse's. It is no crime for a client not to need a nurse, and not to have a nursing problem. It is professional negligence to impose the nurse's coping style on the client, and thus create a problem, or to minimize a stressor because the nurse constantly encounters greater, more exotic health problems, or more dramatic diagnostic-treatment modalities. Maintaining sensitivity to cues and open neutrality of manner that permits the client to share his honest perceptions and, having a broad enough vista to understand and incorporate the many styles of coping—these are the integral skills of the ruling out process in the field of nursing.

REFERENCES

Alexander, Ardyth. "A Study of Nursing Measures for Improved Ventilation Following Surgery." Unpublished masters thesis, University of Washington, 1969, 67 pp.

Cummings, Jonathan. "The Pressures and How Patients Respond to Them," from Hemodyalisis—Feelings, Facts, Fantasies. *American Journal of Nursing* 70:70-76, January, 1970.

Janis, Irving. *Psychological Stress.* New York: John Wiley and Sons, 1958.

Scheff, Thomas. "Decision Rules, Types of Errors and Their Consequences in Medical Diagnosis," *Behavioral Science* 8:97-107, April, 1963.

Titchener, James and Maurice Levine. *Surgery as a Human Experience.* New York: Oxford University Press, 1960.

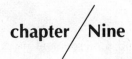

chapter / Nine

The Nurse and the Diagnostic Statement

Once the ruling out process has taken place, often the nurse is still faced with data indicating that all is not well in health-related areas and that assistance is needed. This may be the case where the client is not managing effectively, is not happy with what is happening to his lifestyle, or is likely to be unable to manage effectively in the foreseeable future.

Nursing problems must be diagnosed and ruled in when the client's daily living is made ineffective or unsatisfying as the result of at least three major factors:

> coping ability is reduced due to health-related stressors,
>
> new coping demands outside of present coping skills or resources are emerging from changed health status or situation, or
>
> the nature and direction of health-related stressors and potential resources lead the nurse to predict that there is risk of ineffective coping in the future.

In order to get more of a working understanding of what these factors mean in everyday nursing experiences, let's look at some common examples in each of these areas.

Examples of reduced coping ability or resources might include:

> diminished strength and endurance after a bout of pneumonia, anemia, or sleep deprivation
>
> inability to ambulate due to pain from a severely sprained ankle
>
> lack of desire to live because of grief over loss of a child
>
> reduced participation in social life due to hearing loss
>
> stretching a marginal, fixed income during a period of inflation

Examples of new demands for coping skills in health areas might include:

> carrying out routine demands of daily living as a new hemiplegic
>
> being a new parent

moving away from home and being on your own for the first time

learning that your illness is terminal

being hospitalized for the first time

becoming a resident of a nursing home or a state institution for the mentally ill or the retarded

being a new widow/widower/single parent

retiring or aging

being a new diabetic

enduring ongoing hunger while on a long-term low calorie diet for obesity.

Examples of high risk of future coping deficits:

persons who experience malnutrition over prolonged periods of time leading to predictable risk of premature babies, higher infant mortality, and subsequent learning problems

parents who have been abused as children with their high risk of coping with child rearing frustrations by abusing their children in turn

workers in high noise environments who face future hearing loss

persons growing old who face the risk of loss in a variety of areas—functional capacity, peers and family members, status, money, control

drug addicts who face high risk of returning to addictive patterns once they return to their former environment

persons with chronic respiratory disease or cardiovascular disease who face predictably increasing losses in strength and endurance.

These data on resources, on deficits, on stressors, on daily demands, and on the directions of change in any dimensions need to be organized into explicit working diagnostic statements. This step is as crucial to the practice of nursing as it is to medical practice, so that a predictably therapeutic plan of management can be achieved.

WHAT'S IN A NAME?

To date, these statements of client nursing situations have been given a variety of titles: concerns, needs, problems, nursing impressions, and nursing diagnoses—to name those most frequently used. Some authorities recommend differentiating them, others are tending to use them interchangeably.

In this chapter we propose to concern outselves not so much with the name applied to the statement as with the expertise needed to communicate clearly to the diagnostician/planner and others exactly what the focus of the client's nursing management is to be. We look for a statement, by whatever title, that will call to mind the associated diagnostic concepts and relevant knowledge base, which in turn suggests the logical scientific rationale involved. Therefore we will be content for readers to call this statement what they will as long as, in the end, they create an accurate, precise, neutral view of the client's presenting situation as it relates to *nursing* management.

For consistency within this chapter, we have decided to label this statement a "nursing diagnosis." We do this with the understanding that when the exact nomenclature for nursing diagnosis is standardized and accepted by the profession it may emerge in a somewhat different format and taxonomy from that described here.

THE COMPONENTS OF THE NURSING DIAGNOSIS

The definition of nursing which involves health-related situations and their influence on effective daily living by the client must in turn determine the nature of the components of the nursing diagnosis. It suggests that at least two areas, and often a third, must be covered in the diagnostic statement. These components are:

> the area(s) and nature of the coping deficit(s)
>
> the area of impact on day to day living and/or desired lifestyle
>
> the stressor that is the major contributor to the deficit (this may be a more optional component at times).

The nursing diagnosis, then, is *a concise, precise, neutral statement of client response to a stressor or potential stressor in the health area and an identification of the area(s) of impact on his lifestyle.* An example of a diagnostic statement for an outpatient who has a cardiac problem might be:

> Depression secondary to loss of independence in cooking, shopping, and care of apartment due to Grade III cardiac disability.

The stressor is the Grade III cardiac disability that is reducing the client's strength and endurance. The specific pathology is not spelled out, but the Heart Association's taxonomy of levels of activity and disability gives a relatively precise idea of the degree of disability. The area of impact on daily living is the loss of independence in activities of daily living, specifically—cooking, shopping, and caring for the apartment. A further coping deficit is indicated in the affective response to the loss of independence in ADL and that is the response of depression. Stated in this way, the nursing diagnosis suggests the dynamics of the disability, the areas of concern to the client as well as the outcome, namely depression. From this it would be possible to develop plans for nursing management that deal with the precise factors involved in the situation, much as the physician is enabled to deal with precise pathophysiological phenomena as a result of an accurate medical diagnosis.

WHAT THE NURSING DIAGNOSIS IS NOT

Having taken a short initial look at what we see as the nursing diagnosis, it may be helpful to look also at the surrounding territory that we believe falls *outside* the area of nursing diagnosis. We do this because over the years we have seen these areas used as nursing diagnosis with some resultant inadequacies in nursing management. Each of these areas obviously has a direct relationship to the nursing diagnosis. However, since we are suggesting that they are not synonymous, let us examine what the relationship really is.

Nursing Diagnosis Is Not the Medical Diagnosis

The nursing diagnosis is not a reiteration of the *medical diagnosis*. The primary focus of nursing management is not treatment of the cirrhosis of the liver, the pneumonia, the schizophrenia, the Down's Syndrome, or the pregnancy, even though nurses will carry out delegated medical treatment functions. The nursing diagnosis and subsequent management will emerge from the change in style of living demanded for each day, whether temporary or permanent, that results from these conditions. Later in this chapter we will explore in more depth the relationships of the medical diagnosis and management plan to nursing management.

Nursing Diagnosis Is Not the Diagnostic Test

The nursing diagnosis is not the *medical diagnostic regimen*. It is not the cardiac catheterization, the psychological or developmental testing, the laparoscopy, the pelvic examination, the barium enema. A nursing diagnosis can, however, arise from the client's response to the anticipation and/or actuality of these tests should they be stressors in the psychological, physiological, financial, or sociocultural areas of the individual's life.

Nursing Diagnosis Is Not the Medical Treatment

The nursing diagnosis is not the *medical treatment regimen:* the restriction to protective isolation, the group therapy, the colostomy, the salt-free diet, the daily insulin injections, or the periodic dialysis. But, again, the nursing diagnosis may develop from the adjustments in daily living and lifestyle for the individual and those close to him as they try to live with these treatments and the dislocations that sometimes come with them.

Nursing Diagnosis Is Not the Equipment

Just as the nursing diagnosis is not the treatment regimen, so also it is not the equipment. It is true that an indwelling catheter may cause problems in daily living, so may the cast, the dentures, the hearing aid. It is the physiologic, the psychological, sociocultural, and economic problems generated by the presence, use of, or need for the equipment that are the focus of the nursing diagnosis. It is the crystal formation on the tube, the infection, the discomfort, the immobilization, the embarrassment of the indwelling catheter. It is the cost, the discomfort, the change in body image, the dissatisfaction with chewing ability or distortion of speech related to wearing dentures. It is the immobilization, the itching, the embarrassment to circulation from tightness or lack of support from looseness, of the cast. It is the static, the discomfort from inability to tune out sounds, the cost of batteries, the danger and isolation when the hearing aid is not in use, the dissatisfaction with observably changed body image. The nursing diagnosis is concerned with the specific effects on daily living generated by the equipment or the lack of it, but not the equipment itself.

Nursing Diagnosis Is Not a Concept Label

Closer to the nursing diagnosis, but still not synonymous with it, are the concepts that are used to explain the presenting situation. One often sees these broad general concept labels used as a nursing diagnosis: anxiety, grieving, constipation, hypoxia, malnutrition, pain, immobilization or frustration-aggression. Concepts are, by their very definition abstractions, not specific presenting situations. Unquestionably, these concepts are essential as an aid in deciding what to observe and in organizing data received into meaningful, identifiable clusters. Furthermore, once a situation has been identified and labeled, the concepts involved will be most useful in arriving at an understanding of the dynamics of the situation. Nevertheless, a concept label alone is not sufficiently specific to give either the diagnostician or the implementer the knowledge of relationships and precision in describing the presenting situation needed to plan nursing care or to understand the reasons for the specific orders written for this person.

Here is an example. If one were to say that the nursing diagnosis was "Immobilization," this label could apply to any number of clients in one's case load in some form or other. No one who read this diagnosis would know

the area of immobility (physical, social, emotional, intellectual)
the degree of immobility
the cause
the direction
the risk of sequelae needing preventive management, or
the area of impact on daily living.

Many of these elements would need to be stated either explicitly or implicitly in the working nursing diagnosis in order for a therapeutic individualized plan of nursing management to be developed and understood. Each of the following statements concerns some form of immobility, yet they are so different that the plan of management for one would be entirely inappropriate for another:

Frustration over inadequate grooming and diff with other ADL 2° 45° contracture of rt. elbow.

Immobility in all ADL 2°. inability to choose between radical surgery for Ca of jaw and certain death from failure to have Rx.

Loneliness 2°. Sm. pension + ↘ eyesight → immobility & ↘ social life.

Beyond these examples, just think of persons whom you have nursed who legitimately could have been labeled as immobilized in some way. Think of the questions you would have had to ask if "Immobilization" were the only diagnostic statement made. This, then, is our rationale for suggesting that the use of a concept label alone is an inadequate working statement of the nursing diagnosis. It would be the same as if a physician were to say, "Neoplasm" without indicating the type, location, and the rate and amount of growth. A working diagnosis in either field must be sufficiently specific to permit a rationale for appropriate therapy.

It may be that for later classification and recording purposes, working diagnoses will be categorized in summary problem lists that will use concept labels for coding and computerizing records. Concept labels for problems have also been used in problem-oriented charting to highlight the nursing management and client responses in various problems being recorded on nurses' notes. For example:

Pain—requesting MS q̄ 3 h. Comf for 2 h p̄ Rx. Immobile when in pain.
Sleep—sleeping restlessly 2 h period. Cx nightmares. Afraid to go to sleep again.

Neither of these problems would have been verbalized in a nursing diagnosis as just pain or sleep, but the label is quite useful in discussing ongoing recording, where the total diagnostic statement is unneeded. In the statement of the nursing diagnosis as in every other aspect of the nursing care plan, **the format should serve the need to which it is being put.**

Nursing Diagnosis Is Not the Nurses' Problem with the Client

Despite years of so-called "patient-centered nursing care," many diagnostic statements still project nurses' problems in coping with clients and turn them into clients' problems. True, if the nurse has a problem with the client, the client may soon have a new problem in coping with daily living that was not there before. However, that is hardly the purpose of nursing care—creating new problems for the clientele.

Areas of high risk. There are some areas of high risk where nurses as human beings with human frailties may safely predict that they will have problems with clients as a result of their own coping difficulties. For example:

the client takes more time than the nurses feel they have available

the client's way of communicating with the nursing staff is not acceptable;

his speech is "foreign;" he is unable to communicate verbally; alternative means are time-consuming or inadequate; he speaks too slowly; he gives double messages

he does not wish to participate in the health care workers' goals for him or the treatment regimen; he is passively or actively uncooperative

he does not respond to the medical or nursing treatment plan; he continues to have pain; or he has the side effects without the desired effects; he makes us unsuccessful and usually continues to be around so that health care workers have ongoing reminders of their inadequacy, lack of success, and of the client's disappointment or lack of satisfaction

his ways of coping with problems of daily living are not the ones we would use or choose for him; the more deviant they are from those of the nursing staff, the greater the risk that the nurses will have problems with him

he is in an emotional state that is communicable and causes discomfort/uneasiness or outright hostility in others; he is hostile, anxious, unpredictable, sexually aroused, denying, depressed, projecting

his knowledge or skill in the health care area are potentially or actually greater than that of the persons caring for him, e.g., the coronary care specialist who becomes a patient in the CCU; in some way, because of knowledge, skill, or position there is threat related to continued contact and exposure of the health care workers to the scrutiny of the patient

he is dull and uninteresting, but is due to stay around for a long time

his family wish to participate actively and regularly in his care (particularly if they do so in ways disapproved of by the staff).

These are but a few examples of clients who are labeled "difficult." No doubt, if pressed, each of us could think of other areas where clients are difficult for us to enjoy or even with whom it is difficult to maintain a neutral type of caring. These clients actually engender negative feelings which in turn can be translated into a projective type of nursing diagnosis.

Diagnosing nurses' problems with clients. In order for nursing diagnoses to be effective they must deal with the *client's* situation and coping deficits. There is need therefore to *separate and legitimize* the staff's problems in coping with clients. There is the same need to assess, to diagnose and to treat the staff's problems. The same skill and finesse should be addressed to the problems of the staff as to those of the clientele. The data should be as well-collected, and the diagnosis should be based on these data and precisely, neutrally, and accurately stated. Then a plan of management can be developed. In several settings we know of, clinical nurse specialists, and occasionally psychiatrists, are being used to deal with the staff's problems with clientele. This area of difficulty is expected, it is viewed as normal and it is dealt with as a legitimate *staff-oriented* diagnosis—not a client diagnosis.

Summary

It may seem that we have belabored the topic of what the nursing diagnosis is not, rather than what it is. However, there is a reason for this seemingly negative, round-about approach. Over the years, each of the areas discussed here has been substituted for the nursing diagnosis. They have been areas of confusion. We hope that by specifically citing the nonnursing diagnostic areas and showing how they explicitly relate to the actual nursing diagnosis, we can decrease future confusion.

From our own experiences in transition from a medically oriented model to a nursing model, and in teaching nursing diagnosis to other practicing nurses and students, we have become aware that the movement in thinking away from the medical/task/equipment orientation is neither easy nor rapid. It takes day-in, day-out thoughtful comparisons and critiquing. This is true especially for nurses whose education has been based on the medical approach to both medicine *and* nursing.

If we as nurses are going to project a clear image of the area of nursing expertise, the focus of the nursing diagnosis becomes extremely important. How else will our clients and our colleagues in other disciplines know when it would be productive to consult us? When we are functioning in the nursing area, let us make nursing diagnoses. If we as nurses are needed to make medical diagnoses let us do that too, but let us be very clear on which is which. And let us remember —time it finite; thus, time spent doing the doctor's work of medical diagnosing is not available to spend in nursing diagnosis.

THE RELATIONSHIP OF MEDICAL DIAGNOSIS AND TREATMENT TO NURSING DIAGNOSIS

While there are situations in which nursing's clientele may have no medical problems, for the most part, both medical and nursing diagnoses will exist concurrently. So, although we believe that they are not synonymous, we do believe that they are closely interwoven. Ways of integrating medical diagnostic labels and concepts into nursing diagnosis and plan of management must be made *explicit*. We also believe that the reverse should be true and that **nursing diagnoses and plans of management need to be explicitly incorporated into medical plans of management.** It's a two-way street. First let us examine the explicit and major ways in which the medical diagnosis and treatment plan articulate with and influence the nursing diagnosis.

The Medical Diagnosis as a Stressor

The medical diagnosis, in and of itself, can be identified as a stressor and therefore can generate the need for coping responses. Let us look at an example where this may be the case.

Suppose that the medical diagnosis is that of a metastasized malignant neoplasm.

The client is given this finding. A stressor has been added or confirmed in terms of a major threat to his existence. This stressor of knowledge exists quite apart from the need to cope with the symptoms and pathophysiology, and the financial and emotional strains which the treatment and progression of the disease will produce.

The nursing diagnosis will be concerned then initially with coping with deficits that may fall within the categories of:

courage
desire
knowledge
support systems.

These are all areas of coping skills and resources that must be present in order to cope with the new awareness of the verified presence of a metastatic neoplasm in one's body.

In a somewhat similar vein, diagnoses of diabetes, moderate hypertension, as well as initially relatively asymptomatic diseases that will alter the person's self-concept and/or desired lifestyle require new coping efforts to assimilate this idea into one's identity. This assimilation and modification of self-concept will be an early goal in *living* effectively with the disease or with dying. In any of these situations and many others the medical diagnoses are themselves stressors with which the client may need assistance in mobilizing or developing the necessary coping skills and resources.

Medical Diagnoses as Explanations of Coping Deterrents

The medical diagnosis enters into the nursing diagnosis in another way. It offers the explanatory pathophysiology or psychopathology that leads to understanding of:

1. the mechanisms of changed coping resources
2. the constraints on coping resources
3. the prognosis or direction and duration of these changes

For example, knowledge of the pathophysiology of diabetic retinopathy can enable the nurse to predict continuing vision loss and hence the need for compensatory coping skills and support systems. Because it is progressive with poor prognosis for sight, it also suggests the need to seek out and adjust to a changing lifestyle, preparing gradually for the changes that are occurring.

Understanding the mechanisms of presbycusis—the deafness of aging—would lead the nurse to recall that: (1) the loss of hairs in the lower end of the cochlea and the decrease in adequacy of neural transmission of impulses lead to loss of clarity, not improved by mere increase in volume; and (2) background noise and the use of higher pitched sounds only contribute to decreased usable auditory input. This knowledge suggests some decreased and changed coping behaviors, the need for some new ones, and some environmental modification. On the other hand, the *onset* of any kind of deafness has been found to result in changes in socialization patterns. Participation in groups larger than dyads is particularly difficult. In addition, there is high risk of development of psychological coping deficits with any deafness in which paranoid tendencies are characteristic.

The respiratory system is afflicted by conditions both acute and chronic among young and old which affect body oxygenation and, therefore, physical strength and endurance. Knowledge of the physical and chemical mechanisms interfering with the oxygenation process can enable the nurse to determine whether the experience will be mildly or severely discomforting and anxiety producing, whether the changes involved will be severe or slight, of short or long duration, what actions will help and what actions or conditions in the environment will aggravate it. How much is being lost in usual coping resources? How much will demands have to be reduced, delayed, or spaced out? How much assistance will need to be provided within the support systems?

Looking at a less physiologic problem area, any medical diagnosis that threatens loss of life, loss of function, or loss of a cherished body image should lead the nurse to examination of the dynamics of grieving—the stages, the normality of vacillating from one stage to another, the variations in duration of stages, the signs and symptoms associated with each stage, the possibility of arresting at one stage rather than moving through to acceptance and restitution. All this understanding of the mechanisms of grieving is essential to diagnosing the coping behavior of persons experiencing losses of any significant nature. The medical diagnosis or therapy identifies an actual or potential loss of some significance. The coping response to that loss situation is the area of nursing diagnosis.

Thus, the medically diagnosed phenomena relate very intimately to the nursing diagnoses and management. It would be fair to say that where medical problems are present, nursing diagnoses related to coping cannot be made effectively without understanding the dynamics of the pathology with which the individual must live. Therefore one explicit way in which medical diagnoses articulate with nursing diagnoses is in the area of associated pathophysiology and psychopathology and their impact on coping resources and ability.

Medical Treatment as a Genesis of Nursing Diagnosis

Not only does the awareness of a diagnosis as a stressor and knowledge of the pathophysiology involved become a part of the nursing diagnosis, but so, at times, does the medical treatment. Iatrogenic diseases (treatment-related health problems), are becoming increasingly prevalent as more potent medical treatments upset the normal balance within the individual. Drugs reduce sodium and fluid retention and reduce blood pressure, but they also produce potassium losses

163

which cause ongoing coping problems—dietary difficulties as well as deficits in strength, endurance, and the feeling of well-being. Other regularly used anti-hypertensive drugs that produce impotence are generating major marital problems. The commonly prescribed salt-free, fat-free, low calorie, low cholesterol, and bland diets create dissatisfaction in the daily enjoyment of food. Regularly prescribed, seemingly innocuous medical treatments (like exercise for those who abhor it, or emotional calm for those addicted to excitement) upset the *status quo* of living for the client and those close to him. High risk areas of disruption of daily living from pharmaceutical or other treatment regimens and their side effects and also the more subtle influences on daily living, are areas of vital concern in nursing diagnosis.

In fact, one physician interviewed regarding the role of the nurse practitioner in an outpatient department, said he referred many "difficult" cases to her. When asked what a "difficult" case was, he described them in general as medically diagnosed, currently stable clients on long-term management who were unsuccessful in remaining on the prescribed medical treatment and thus were being admitted intermittently for exacerbations resulting from falling off the treatment wagon. The nurse practitioner's success, he noted, was in diagnosing the ways in which the client could successfully incorporate the medical regimen into his patterns of daily living. This, he suggested, was quite a different art from diagnosing the pathology and prescribing the treatment of the disease. The nurse's management plan in turn shaped aspects of the medical treatment plan.

The articulation between medical treatment and nursing diagnosis may be most prominent in maintenance care of clients with chronic illness or conditions. But it is also crucial in acute short-term medical treatment.

Summary

Medical diagnosis and treatment, while not synonymous with nursing diagnosis and treatment, are integral forces in shaping nursing diagnosis and management. It is important for the nurse planner to know how each segment of medical diagnosis, pathology, and treatment patterns articulates with the development of the nursing plan. The medical and nursing management are symbiotic in their relationship—neither one works as well without the other.

To test this for yourself, try to recall any clients for whom the medical plan could stand alone with no nursing diagnosing or intervention of any form. Try also to think of clients for whom nursing diagnosis and management could proceed unimpeded without medical diagnosis and management. There undoubtedly will be some cases that fall into both categories, but the bulk of them will tend to fall in the middle where both medicine and nursing are involved to some degree. We have addressed the way in which the medical diagnosis and treatment become a part of the nursing plan—now try to reverse the pattern and consider just how the nursing diagnosis and management should relate to and influence the medical diagnosis and management.

Having examined the definition of a nursing diagnosis and some of the related areas, let us move into a fuller exploration of the focus of the nursing diagnostic system and the techniques of developing the *working* diagnostic statement.

AREAS OF FUNCTIONAL COPING DEFICITS, A POINT OF DEPARTURE

Medical diagnoses designate particular kinds of pathology/dysfunction applicable to any body system. Nursing's taxonomy may well be built in a similar pattern. Our foundation will rest, not on pathology, but on key functional coping deficits that, like pathologic processes, could be applied to any area of living or coping. In the medical models, the phenomenon of inflammation communicated by the suffix of "itis" can be applied to any anatomical area. In the nursing model, coping deficits also can be applied to any area of life where they deter effective living.

Sometimes these coping deficits will be the result of medically labeled phenomena, sometimes not. And, obviously, as we have just noted, any underlying pathology which contributes to a coping deficit will have to be taken into account in both the nursing diagnosis and in planning for the management of these functional deficits. But, the pathology constitutes only a component of the coping deficits and is not the focus of the diagnosis.

As a point of departure for building an overall category system of coping deficits that could be widely applied to any health problem or area of living, let's examine some rather common areas to which nurses address themselves. Our clients can experience difficulty in attaining or maintaining effective living—on their terms or ours—if they lack one or more of the following resources.

Strength Strength is the ability to engage in physical, mental, or emotional work at a given point. It may be sufficient neuromuscular ability to breathe, to move, to chew, to cough, to walk . . . the emotional reserves to face a necessary encounter . . . the mental ability to engage in a presenting task requiring thought.

Endurance Endurance is staying power—in terms of physical and emotional stamina. A person may have the energy to do only a limited amount of work, to walk only a certain distance, to lift a fork only twice without rest, to chew only soft foods. Frequent fatigue or exhaustion interferes in varying degrees with daily living and desired lifestyle on his own terms and/or that of society. He may have the emotional reserves to tolerate demands for an hour, a day, a week, or a month but no more.

Sensory Input Marked underload or overload of available and/or usable sensory input resulting from changes in sense organs, the central nervous system, or the internal or external environment can modify the individual's ability to live effectively. The deviation is from the individual's normal input in the components of kind, variability, amplitude, and quantity, not from any standard. It may be acute/sudden or slow/chronic. Each will result in both physiologic and psychological responses that deter effective coping/living.

There is high risk of his coping deficit being present when

- there is sudden change in the status of one or more sense organs making them either *more* or *less* functional
  - trauma or pathology that leads to deafness or vision loss
  - cataract surgery
  - surgery to restore hearing
  - hearing aids
  - paresthesias
  - large casts
- central nervous system changes occur
  - LSD ingestion
  - organic brain syndrome
  - sleep deprivation
  - encephalitis
- the internal environment changes
  - anxiety states
  - depression
  - pain
  - aging
- changes in the external environment in terms of kind, amount, or amplitude of stimuli
  - the teen-ager with hi-fi addiction being placed in an isolation unit
  - the retiree who has lived alone being placed in a busy 4-bed ward
  - the widow who clings to her home while her children move away, while finances or disability prevent her getting out, her peers die off, neighbors are busy, and TV and radio break down
  - the loss of taste and texture in food when a diet restricts salt, sugar, spices, or certain food textures

Knowledge It is difficult to live effectively with phenomena, with diseases, with health maintenance, or with new roles when the dynamics and responses that are occurring or likely to occur are not recognized or understood. The day to day management of diabetes, paroxysmal nocturnal dyspnea, angina, ulcers, depression, arthritis . . . require knowledge of the pathophysiology and the rationale of the knacks of management. The new roles of—sick person, hospitalized patient, postoperative patient, disabled person . . . all require knowledge and often experiential knowledge as a basis of participation quite aside from any associated skills.

Desire A deficit we as nurses have often dealt with ineffectively is desire: the deficit in the wish or wanting: to know—to participate—to manage—to change—to live. We have tended to misdiagnose this as lack of knowledge despite the fact that the number of addicts to nicotine, food, and drugs among the knowledgeable of the medical and nursing professions should have disabused us of this idea long ago. They have the knowledge, but not desire. Perhaps we cling to it because it is easier for busy nurses to teach than to deal with clients' lack of desire to participate in health workers' versions of health care. These are the clients we diagnose as the "won'ts," the "difficult patient," the "uncooperative person," the "turkeys." These people keep abandoning the treatment regimen—not because they don't understand, but because they don't want to participate for any number of reasons. (Our therapy or at least our response has frequently been punitive, shaming, or attempting to product guilt.)

It is time we as nurses face this difficult nursing diagnosis and label it neutrally. Where desire is the deficit, let us so diagnose. Then let us try to understand the

166

dynamics of this concept as openly and as sensitively as we do others and build appropriate treatment options.

Courage   Another area of deficit, often misdiagnosed, is the lack of courage. Here, the individual may have no deficit in knowledge, or even desire, but lacks the bravery to participate in effective daily living. There is high risk of this deficit where there has been a change in body image that is visible and disfiguring or which is seen by the individual himself as being disfiguring to his self-image. A second high risk situation occurs when an individual is required to accept predictable pain or inflict pain on himself. A third would be the situation where there is some risk to self-concept or body integrity related to the decision or the response.

Again, we do not have very effective therapeutic interventions to help our clientele deal with this deficit. It is another area of nursing knowledge and skill that requires more research and effort. But this should not deter us from making an accurate differential diagnosis in this area and continuing to seek effective specific therapy.

Skill,   All of us have experienced times when we had plenty of head knowledge but when
Dexterity   it came to translating it into skills, we were clumsy dolts. We have seen awkward nurses, doctors, clients, whose heads were better than their hands, feet, or interpersonal skills. Deficits in skill and dexterity need to be differentially diagnosed and treated differently from deficits in knowledge. In the end, skill deficits must be treated with opportunities to safety, repeatedly and critically practice the behavior. It may mean practicing giving an injection, crutch walking, using a prosthesis, or an IPPB machine, log rolling. Or it may mean practicing giving vent to internalized anger, assertive behavior, observing, playing a new role with a safe reciprocal role partner. Skill and dexterity require assessment of different variables and different treatment regimens than do other deficit areas and therefore must be differentially diagnosed.

Support   Persons experiencing health problems may cope effectively if they have external
Systems   support systems in the forms of helpers (professionals, family, friends) insurance, transportation, equipment, supplies, architecture, positive caring attitudes from important others, etc. Where these are missing, though the individual may have no other deficit, he still may not be able to live effectively.

Let us take an example of a post-myocardial infarction client who understands his pathology and the treatment regimen, accommodates to the angina, has increasing endurance for the exercise and work, has adequate finances and is willing to modify his diet in terms of cholesterol and sodium. But if his wife continues to cook a high cholesterol, high sodium diet, is disparaging of his changed physical status and highly anxious that each episode of chest pain means a fatal attack, denies him sexual intercourse for fear of precipitating another attack, this man is lacking in important external support systems. The nursing diagnosis of this deficit must be made and therapy directed toward the wife as well as the husband if effective living is to take place.

Summary

Undoubtedly there are other major areas of deficits in coping that fall within the nursing field. Those we have suggested can be a point of departure. They have been deliberately divorced from body systems and the medical model of diagnosis of pathology in order to focus nurses' thinking on the nursing model—coping with daily living. In each instance, any underlying pathophysiology or psychopathology that contributes to the deficit or prevents personal management must be taken into account. For example in the area of knowledge, the dynamics of the knowledge deficit and its treatment must take into account impediments to acquiring needed knowledge (learning). Such impediments might be: IQ, toxicity, level of consciousness, available language, previous conflicting knowledge, cultural mores, belief systems, age, and intactness of sight and hearing. Each category of deficit will have associated factors which determine the nature of the person's ability, his resources, and the constraints which in turn must modify the nurses' intervention. These factors may be related to pathology or treatment as well as to a variety of other factors.

Right now we do not have prefixes and suffixes which designate the categories of functional/coping deficits and which could in turn be affixed to words or stems indicating the area of impact. However, eventually nursing may seek to develop a taxonomy and a vocabulary to communicate these ideas in a shorthand manner. Or, it may be that we as a profession will choose not to develop a separate jargon. We may continue to use words that everyone understands; and that would be a new twist for a scientific discipline, wouldn't it?

CATEGORIES OF COPING DEFICITS

Strength   Ability and resources to handle physical, mental, emotional work at a given point in time

Endurance   Stamina, staying power with a work load (physical, intellectual, or emotional)

Sensory Input   Abilities and resources to maintain an adequate, satisfying sensory environment

Knowledge   Status of acquired content in the relevant area to be coped with and level of ability to use that content (e.g., recall, comprehension, application, etc.)

Desire   Will or motivation to participate

Courage   Risk-taking capacity

Skills   Psychomotor, dexterity, communication, interpersonal

Support Systems   Ability to recognize, obtain, use, maintain and (enjoy?) support systems such as equipment, people, systems, etc.

THE IMPORTANCE OF VERBALIZING THE DIAGNOSIS

Over the years since the inception of nursing care plans, competent clinicians have said to us, "I know what the problem is; I just can't put it into words." This is a bit like a physician saying, "I know there is something wrong here; I just can't tell you what it is." This formative stage of diagnosing is just that—a beginning.

Plato wrote that thinking was the mind talking to itself. So, thinking, like talking and writing, does require words. Therefore, nurses may no longer rationalize their inability to put the diagnosis into words. There is no alternative to words, either in private thought or in communication to others. Without words there can be no nursing diagnosis.

It is true that not all nursing diagnoses are written. At this time many of them remain in more or less nebulous form in the minds of nurses who, together with the client, function to deal with living on the basis of these personally held impressions. For us to progress to increased skill and professionalization as a discipline and to function more precisely on the client's behalf, it is essential that in our thinking, as well as in speech and writing, we verbalize our diagnosis, neutrally, accurately, and precisely.

GUIDELINES TO EFFECTIVE DIAGNOSTIC STATEMENTS

The nursing diagnosis is the crux of the whole plan of nursing management and often the arbiter of the style of nursing care given. It focuses the attention of the diagnostician as well as others on certain areas while relegating other areas or problems to the background. The attitudinal tone of the diagnostic statement can shape both expectations of client response and the behavior of health workers toward the client. It can be so vague as to give only a fuzzy image of the presenting situation. It can be so narrow as to foster tunnel vision of the problem. On the other hand, it can be accurate and sharp, offering sound priorities of attention and a neutral or positive tone.

The Difference Between the Data and the Diagnosis

The verbalizing of effective diagnostic statements (in thinking, speaking, or writing) is a critical thinking skill of a high order. In a way, making a diagnosis is like baking a cake. The cake is made up of raw ingredients, but is quite different from them because of the mixing and exposure to heat. Just so, the nursing diagnosis is made up of the ingredients of cues from the assessment which are thoroughly mixed with relevant explanatory concepts. From this thoughtful mixing, emerges a concise statement that incorporates all of these components, yet is different in appearance from any of them.

In cooking, there are beginning cooks, there are Cordon Bleu graduates—and there are many levels of skill and creativity in between. Some can only follow recipes, some can branch out to combine ingredients creatively. And so it is with nursing diagnoses. There will be varying levels of expertise from the most simple skills in putting small amounts of data together to arrive at a problem statement for each area all the way to higher levels of thought synthesis. Here, the diagnostician is skilled enough to look at the commonalities represented in all of the presenting data and to combine them into more encompassing diagnoses that will offer a sound basis for management of the sub-problems. Such a plan of diagnosis and management will still deal with the multiple problems cited by the less skilled diagnostician, but will do so in terms of nursing orders that are tied to the main diagnosis.

> For example: A person may have a pervasive problem of need for independence and activity in a situation where dependency and inactivity are prescribed. This person may also have: pain, need for fluids, skin care, dietary management, and so forth. Yet each of these areas of needs can be dealt with in nursing orders which incorporate the desire for maximum independence and activity permissible in any given area.
>
> In another situation, a client's culture and language are different from those of the physicians and nurses. Here, an overall problem is not desire for independence and activity, but understanding and being understood across cultural differences. The nurse again might deal with pain, fluids, skin care, and diet, but the style of nursing prescribed in managing these demands of daily living would be related to the cultural and language orientation rather than the independence/activity frame of reference.
>
> Both, of course, would incorporate knowledge of the specific pathology and medical therapy involved into the plan of nursing management.

This is not to say that either the multiple problem approach or the central problem approach are the only "right" way. Some nurses will be able to handle diagnosis in one way, some in another. Where there are commonalities among the problem areas, or central diagnostic themes, it is the more skilled diagnostician, the more experienced one, who will recognize them and incorporate them into an identified style of nursing management for the sub-problems.

There will also be honest differences among nursing diagnosticians wherein the same information is combined in differing ways to arrive at different diagnostic statements. Such differences must be seen as "normal" and ways to accommodate to these differences must be found. A recent cartoon showed a patient in bed looking somewhat disconcerted as four physicians stood, heads together, and looked at the record. One turned back to the patient and said, "That's democracy, Mr. Jones. Four doctors, four diagnoses." Obviously, another of the health disciplines has not quite solved the problem of diagnostic differences either, so we'll be in good company as we try to deal with it.

However, while acknowledging that there will be differing levels of competence, different approaches to diagnosis, and a high probability of variations in diagnostic perspectives, there are still some basic characteristics of diagnostic statements in nursing. And there are some technical aspects that will facilitate the writing of diagnoses at our present stage of development in making nursing diagnoses.

Effective Diagnoses Are as Precise as Data Allow

An area where we have noted that current nursing diagnosing tends to break down is in precision. Any diagnostic statement should be as precise as the data allow. Of course one may not go beyond the data, but on the other hand one must seek, incorporate, and synthesize all of the pertinent information available.

Anxiety or pain or weakness may be a problem to many clients in a nurse's case load. It's nice for the next nurse to know that six persons on a unit are experiencing pain, but if that is the only degree of precision in the nursing diagnosis offered, the focus is too ambiguous and consequently less useful. For a physician, the diagnosis of "Infection" is less useful than one of "Viral Pneumonitis," or "Far Advanced Tuberculosis" or "Pneumococcal Pneumonia." Each suggests an area, the nature of the organism and the disease process and the appropriate direction of treatment. Similarly, nursing diagnoses must offer sufficient precision to suggest avenues of productive, specific nursing management.

In the same way, a nurse might offer a diagnosis of "Constipation" but more precision, and hence more understanding of the actual situation, would result if the basis of the term were indicated. Is it constipation related to

desire to have a bowel movement daily regardless of intake?
long standing laxative or enema pattern?
loss of rectal sensation?
loss of abdominal strength?
fear of precipitating an M.I.?
hemorrhoidal pain?
inadequate bulk?
inadequate fluids?

Each more precise diagnosis of constipation suggests differing patterns of nursing management. In turn, the need for precision in diagnosis suggests the obligation to collect enough relevant data *to permit* an effective working diagnosis related to constipation.

Let's take another area common among clients facing surgery, that is, preoperative anxiety or fear. It is a recognized necessary force in readying the body's physiologic and psychological defense mechanisms to cope with the stress, so the absence of working anxiety is not desirable. However, some clients' fears are unfounded and they worry needlessly. Effective coping requires minimizing the nonworking, needless worrying.

171

Example

An older man facing a transurethral prostatectomy is highly worried about dying postoperatively. Data: his father died within 24 hours of the same surgery twenty years before. There were multiple postoperative clients on the same unit for him to visit. There were survival rates from TUR's that were very promising. There is information on new techniques used to control bleeding, etc., that have markedly reduced risks. There were data on his own physical condition, quite different from that of his father, making him a good surgical risk where his father was not.

Dx: Fear of death p̄ TUR 2° to lack of knowledge re ↓ risks.

Example

A 45-year-old man is facing his third spinal surgery for intervertebral disc disease. On both previous surgeries he recalls experiencing postoperative choking. Once he was alone and almost died, according to his memory of it. In this institution there is a recovery room, with the clients under constant surveillance. A nurse in this unit who will be on that date is available for a visit to discuss his previous experiences and assure him that she and others will be alert for any signs of respiratory distress and they have skill and equipment to manage.

Dx: Fear of recurrence of p̄ op choking & inadequate nsg. surveillance 2° to prev. choking experiences.

Example

A 50-year-old woman with a vascular frontal lobe brain tumor will surely die without surgery and may well die during surgery. She knows this and is responding with gallows-type humor and behaving oppositely of requests made to her.

Dx: Realistic fear of dying → 3+ anxiety & ↓ ability to cope c̄ preop role DDL*.

The nursing diagnosis, in order to be most productive of effective nursing management, must be as precise in the nature of the coping deficit and the area of life involved as the data permit. It should communicate *this* client's situation at *this* time. It should differentiate for you and for anyone sharing the information just how this person's situation is unique. This needn't take more time either. It is a lifestyle in thinking, not time, that is involved (although it takes some extra mulling and verbal practicing to get the knack in the beginning). Nurses can train themselves to diagnose precisely (or generally). Precision is not easy but it is essential. Appropriate precision is more productive!

Effective Diagnoses Locate the Common Denominator

With the case loads that most nurses carry these days, regardless of setting, there is little merit in stating ten discrete problem areas for a client *if* a common denominator can be found that will offer perspective and a unifying theme. Such

*Demands of daily living.

an approach can help in recall of the overall situation while not diminishing the implementation of nursing orders which deal with the specifics. For example:

> An elderly lady had suffered a fractured hip. It had been pinned two days previously. She reports having always been fiercely independent. At 81 she still lived in her own home and maintained herself with little help from her family or neighbors in the small town. She wants very much to return to her former living arrangements and is worrying that she will not be able to do so. She is vehemently angry when the words "nursing home" are mentioned. She has told the nurse she would like to be able to brush her own teeth today.

Now, the diagnosis could be stated in terms of her desire to brush her own teeth (and actually was so stated initially). It could also be stated in terms of her loss of strength, her discomfort, and a variety of other aspects of her situation. However, her history of independence, the desire for continued independence, combined with the knowledge that her strength and endurance are predictably diminished by the trauma, the surgery, and the bed rest at her advanced age—all these could be combined in a diagnostic statement that focuses on the common denominator that threads throughout the presenting situation. For example:

> Usual independence $\downarrow 2°$ fx, pinned hip, $\bar{p}$ op. pain $+$ wkness $+$ old age $\rightarrow$ anger $+$ fear re future lifestyle.

This type of diagnostic statement will in turn act as a force that can shape *every* nursing transaction of the day whether it be:

> basis of motivation for her to participate in range of motion, deep breathing, or muscle setting to diminish further losses
>
> making it possible for her to do a little more for herself in a variety of activities each day rather than doing for her
>
> emphasizing the normality of the current deficits that frighten and threaten her in terms of her goal of independence, or
>
> giving encouragement by calling attention to gains she is making by identifying specific achievements from day to day.

The skilled nursing diagnostician will locate the essence, the central core, of the presenting situation in the diagnosis. And this will in turn shape the management of specifics in the goals and nursing orders. In looking for directions of professional growth, one might expect the novice diagnostician to deal with a variety of smaller problem areas while growing skill should be evidenced by greater synthesis of data into diagnostic statements within the applicable concepts. While this characteristic may seem paradoxical to the previously mentioned one of precision, it is possible to achieve both the essence and the precision. That should be the nurse diagnostician's goal.

Diagnoses Are Concise

Another area where we as nurses have not been particularly sharp is in the skill of conciseness. We seem to omit communications, write ritualistic banalities that are so general as to communicate nothing or write long entries on supposedly compact records.

Most work loads of nurses and most client record forms do not permit a nurse to take many lines to write a nursing diagnosis, nor do most nurses' memories enable them to recall paragraphs on each client. So, while we still have not come to the point where we can encapsulate our diagnostic statements within a word or two as the physicians currently can, or in a number, as the computer scientists would have us do, still, we can teach ourselves to be concise as well as precise. With a vivid, adequate, descriptive vocabulary and the use of meaningful symbols and abbreviations, nurses can teach themselves to think and communicate concisely without loss of precision.

Symbols save space. Nursing diagnoses are concerned with stressors and responses, with direction of responses and demands of living, with timing. There are symbols that quickly communicate some of this in minimal space.

leads to	⟶	before	$\bar{a}$
resulting from or secondary to	⟵ or 2°	after	$\bar{p}$
		with	$\bar{c}$
increased	↑	without	$\bar{s}$
increasing	↗	equal	=
decreased	↓	unequal	≠
decreasing	↘	degree of	o
greater than	⟩	complains of	c/o
less than	⟨		

Abbreviations. There are also commonly used abbreviations that can communicate quickly. It is important, of course, with both symbols and abbreviations to be sure that they do communicate. If there is any doubt, a glossary of commonly used abbreviations and symbols should be available in an easily located spot in the area where nursing records will be read.

Some of our abbreviations will come from the medical field. SOB meaning (usually) short of breath, is a common basis for coping deficits among persons with cardiac and respiratory problems. CHF, congestive heart failure, may be used to explain underlying phenomena of a variety of coping deficits and indicate both prognosis and duration of coping problems. Cx, complaints (subjective data), diagnosis (dx), prescription (℞) all may be useful. Nursing, too, has its established set of abbreviations. One that is frequently used in the coping orientation to nursing is that of ADL, activities of daily living or DDL, demands of daily living. No doubt others will be forthcoming as we focus on our own bailiwick. It would be wise for nursing to approach these as systematically as we seem to be approaching the development of a taxonomy for nursing diagnoses. Hopefully the professional organization will assume some responsibility for coordination of standardized abbreviations as well as nursing diagnoses.

Let us look at how some diagnostic statements can be concise, yet retain their precision by use of symbols and abbreviations.

> Suppose Mrs. Frandsen, aged 70, living in her own residence, has shortness of breath with even short periods of activity demanding minimal physical effort. It has been increasing noticeably. Previously an energetic person who moved through her daily activities quickly, she is bothered by what she sees needing to be done and is discouraged by her obvious decline. How could we communicate the essence of her coping deficit and her dissatisfaction with the resultant lifestyle in minimal space? Try it, then see how it compares with our diagnostic statement.

> ↘ endurance for min. ADL 2° to SOB → ↗ frustration & despair

This diagnosis completely spelled out should read, "declining endurance for even minimal activities of daily living secondary to increasing shortness of breath is in turn leading to growing frustration and despair."

Or, take a different situation, also involving strength and endurance as well as an affective state.

> Mr. Johnson, married, 48 years old, lives in a condominium with his wife. He has a job that is within his recent post-myocardial infarction capabilities. He still cannot undertake strenuous activities without experiencing some chest pain or shortness of breath, but he senses improvement. What he really misses is being able to return to his weekly golf games.

His diagnostic statement might read:

> p̄ M.I. ↘ angina & SOB + ↗ endurance for routine ADL → encouragement but frustrated re golf restrictions.

This should communicate:

> Post-myocardial infarction healing with decreasing angina and shortness of breath, together with growing endurance for routine activities of daily living, is leading to encouragement but still some frustration at not being able to resume his golf games.

In each diagnostic statement, the use of symbols and abbreviations saved about two to three lines of writing without loss of essential meaning. You may see a different way of stating the diagnosis, given the data that have been presented. Try your hand at it.

Conciseness means that unnecessary words are omitted. For instance there is never a need to write the words "client" or "patient" in the diagnosis; that is implicit. On the other hand, words that increase the precision of the diagnosis should not be omitted for the sake of brevity. An example here would be including the words "usual" or "unusual" to signal a baseline. Learning to think and write concise but sharp nursing diagnoses is not easy. The development of a taxonomy would help. In the meantime we are faced with the task of learning to walk a narrow line between really sharing an accurate diagnosis and not taking too many words to do it.

Neutrality in the Diagnostic Statement

The statement of the diagnosis initiates a point of view for seeing the client. Therefore, its degree of neutrality is important. Emotionally colored words such as: won't, uncooperative, overbearing, demanding, time-consuming, enjoying illness, denying, or labels such as "difficult patient," "turkey," "crock," "hypochondriac," and "gomers" (grand old men of the emergency room), will all make planning care and responding therapeutically more difficult for the diagnostician and those who read the diagnosis. Negatively value laden diagnoses also tend to generate punitive or distancing nursing orders.

The importance of the nature of the diagnosis as a well-spring for the plan of care cannot be overemphasized. (See forces influencing data collection, Chapter Four, pp. 63-64.) Let us take a situation that has the potential for several options of diagnostic statements and look to see how different versions could result in differing approaches, despite the fact that the data which generated the diagnoses were identical.

Mrs. Dawson is a 45-year-old diabetic single parent of 2 teen-age sons and a married daughter who lives in another state. She is currently hospitalized for an above the knee amputation for gangrene of the left foot following an accident in an institutional diet kitchen. Cards from the children, pictures, flowers, and gifts crowd her bedside stand. She speaks frequenty of her "kids" and talks with them on the phone daily. Her daughter has just traveled back home to help manage the situation till her mother has convalesced. Mrs. Dawson is very worried about one son who is out riding in the family car instead of attending school.

Physically, Mrs. Dawson has been found to be rapidly losing her sight. She weighs 180 pounds and is 5 feet tall. She received an immediate prosthesis following the amputation and is regularly attending PT and making excellent progress. She is expected to go home in another week.

The nurses on the unit are quite concerned that Mrs. Dawson seems to know very little about her diabetes and to care less. A registered nurse student developed a clear and interesting scheme for teaching some of the important aspects of management of her disease. Mrs. Dawson was polite, lay quietly in bed as the nurse tried to engage her in conversation about the ideas, avoided eye contact and changed the subject whenever possible. She asked no questions and repeated that the amputation was the end result of poor medical care after she cut her foot on "that glass." She expressed interest in keeping her kids well-fed but turned off any other discussion of her own nutrition or diabetic control.

Now, Mrs. Dawson's diagnosis could have read

"Uncooperative in learning diabetic management."

There were also some cues tending to indicate that she was coping with diabetes by rejecting or ignoring its impact on her lifestyle. So, one might also diagnose the situation as

"Denial of diabetes → lack of control."

Given this diagnosis the nursing care plan would deal with the denial, since the focus of the diagnostic statement in turn sets the focus of the plan and the management.

The nurse in this case, instead, decided to focus on Mrs. Dawson's priorities in her diagnosis and to use the closeness of the family and the availability of the daughter as resources to deal with the management of this chronic illness—perhaps the affection bonds of the family could be harnessed to help Mrs. Dawson manage her diabetes more effectively. Her diagnostic statement read:

Concern for family well-being > priority than self-care → ↓ attention to modified ADL & management of ↗ diabetic pathology.

Mrs. Dawson's concern for her family was much more acceptable to the nursing staff than were lack of cooperation or denial. As a result, more positive plans of care and attitudes toward the client could be generated.

Where there is the possibility of stating the diagnosis in such a way as to cause the diagnostician or others to view the client from a negative point of view, examine some different options or versions of wording. Try to state the diagnosis from the client's perspective and see what emerges. It is not likely to come out negatively if one uses the client's point of view as a point of departure.

Focus in the Diagnostic Statement

Another factor to consider in the diagnostic statement is the placement of ideas within the diagnosis. Placing the prime target for nursing attention first highlights it. If sleep deprivation is leading to irritability and fatigue, it would be important for "sleep deprivation" to appear first in the diagnosis. On the other hand, if worry about family or health is a deterrent to sleep, "worry" should appear first. Or, should sleep deprivation in family members erode the support system to the client, this should receive the prime position in the diagnostic

177

statement. Look at the elements and decide which is to be the focus of nursing management.

SUMMARY

At this point, we could present a group of cases and some model diagnostic statements. In fact, we considered it. However the reader's world is full of real live case material just waiting to be diagnosed. It will not matter whether the diagnostic practicing focuses on one's own situation, a clinical situation, or those around us—the process, the vocabulary, the synthesis will be the same—so, practice diagnosing and developing diagnostic statements regularly on anything and everything around you. Share them. Then get others to tell you what you really communicated. When you have communicated what you intended, congratulate yourself. When you have not—it's back to the drawing board. In clinical units, set up inservice to try to improve diagnostic statements. Critique colleagues' statements. Try as many variations on a diagnostic statement as you can—just to keep yourself from grinding out narrow stereotypes like so much sausage meat.

> Be accurate
> Be precise
> Be objective
> Be concise

And remember, the situation out there is always changing, so don't fall in love with your current diagnosis. Nursing diagnoses are like doing dishes—there are always more to be done.

chapter Ten

Client–Nurse Goals

Whenever a nursing diagnosis is made there is an implication that the current situation and its outcomes are not satisfactory either to the client or the nurse. If a different outcome were not desired by at least one of the parties there would be no reason for the client to accept help, or for the nurse to offer it. The different outcome that is desired is the goal. Thus, goals are present for the client and the nurse in every encounter, whether they are recognized or not.

Given such a commonplace situation, then, one might wonder why this task of stating goals should be so difficult. One experience that has cooled many practicing nurses on the idea of making goals explicit in client care has been a sudden mandate from on high in the establishment (usually immediately prior to an accreditation visit) that, "There must be a goal for every patient on the Kardex." Sure enough, within 24 hours, each Kardex card has been adorned with an appropriate gold-plated platitude in the space marked "Goal," or "Objective." The tried and true classics that can be produced almost without effort are:

"To return to health."
"To die with dignity."

and occasionally, when nothing can be done, but the client is not going to die either,

"To accept his disability."

They sound good; they meet the letter of the law; they serve the establishment's needs. And they don't interfere with what we were doing in the first place. No wonder nurses become cynical about the hypocrisy of the care planning process.

The trouble with the platitudes we have just cited is that they are too general. They could be used for almost every client. True, they do give a sense of general direction, such as, we are going north, or south. But, on the other hand, there is a lot of territory in any of these directions and no sense of what the precise destination is, how long we can take to get there, by what style, and by which particular route. A useful goal statement needs to:

be realistic (no pie in the sky)

take client wishes and circumstances into consideration

set a direction

specify an outcome

possibly indicate some dimension of time for accomplishment.

Put together then, a client–nurse goal would be: *a statement of a desired, achievable outcome to be attained within a predicted period of time, given the presenting situation and resources.*

Throughout this chapter, these characteristics of care plan goals will be incorporated. Look for them in your goals too.

AGAIN, WHAT'S IN A NAME?

In a previous chapter we discussed the fact that the term "nursing diagnosis" has been given many labels. In the concept of goals, too, there are a host of synonyms. In education-ese, goals are called objectives, and there are some who separate goals from objectives and use both terms. In clinical practice we are usually lucky to have either one. Our clients, on the other hand, might use any of the following words when they are communicating their goals to us:

hopes

aims

desired outcomes

aspirations

needs

targets

desires

ambitions

purposes

wants

wishes

desired end results

By whatever name, the goal is a desired outcome, one hoped for by the client and/or the nurse.

THE NATURE OF NURSING GOALS

Goals in the plan for nursing management of client's health problems emerge from the *nursing* diagnosis just as medical goals derive from the medical diagnosis (e.g., in the diagnosis of pneumonia the goal is resolution of the inflammatory process and maintenance of adequate oxygenation until normal functioning is restored). In nursing, *the goals in most instances will be closely related to the specific coping deficits and the impact on the person's lifestyle.*

The Fundamental Directions of Nursing Goals

NURSING DIAGNOSTIC AREA		GENERAL NATURE OF THE GOALS
Client Resources	*Lifestyle/Demands of Living*	
Identified coping ability and resources.	= Optimum lifestyle and/or essential demands of daily living.	No Nursing Goals—the person is coping without assistance or intervention.
Coping resources and ability are identified as being available or potentially available but not fully used.	≠ *NEW* OR *INCREASING* Health-related demands in daily living.	Help the individual to develop or more effectively use the potential resources and ability identified as being available.
DECREASED OR *DECREASING* Coping ability or resources in identified areas.	≠ Unchanging demands of daily living or possibly new/increasing health-related demands in daily living.	Reduce the demands in daily living. and/or a) substitute for the lack of ability and resources b) supplement the client's current inadequate ability or resources with other source (nurse, another person, equipment, etc.).

As shown in the chart above, nursing goals can focus on two major areas. They may focus on helping clients to more effectively use their own potential or to obtain more resources so that they can function at a higher level or cope in new areas. On the other hand, where resources are diminished or inadequate, they may concentrate on modifying the demands of daily living and usual lifestyle to bring these into line with changed coping ability and resources or supplementing them with outside assistance.

It's a bit like a seesaw. The game is to keep the weights and forces at either end in sufficient balance so that the client may move up and down within a desired and possible range and is not stuck either up in the air or on the ground in a fixed position. Often it is the nurse who can assess the situation, help the client to creatively reorganize the resources and demands, and restore balance and mobility.

The nurse and the client, as they consider the desired outcome options, may look to either end of the seesaw, the client's coping ability and resources at one end, demands of daily living and desired lifestyle at the other. When they go out of balance, one or the other, or perhaps both, will need to be adjusted in a satisfying way. In addition, if it can be predicted that they will go out of balance immediately (as in elective surgery) or gradually (as in increasing disability), preparation for future goals is obviously essential.

To illustrate these two ends of the equation a bit further let's examine some situations nurses encounter frequently in which clients either have new or increased demands made upon them, or have diminished resources for living their lives. New demands come so often in our lives that we tend to take them for granted, but some do require new skills, more energy, or new knowledge—many of these in health-related areas.

Often we find our clients:

> becoming a parent for the first time
>
> going to school, or to a new school
>
> leaving home
>
> having a sick or dying member of the household or family
>
> perceiving threatening signs and symptoms in themselves or someone they care about
>
> undergoing diagnostic tests
>
> being labeled with a diagnosis
>
> undergoing major medical treatment (or even minor treatment, for that matter)
>
> getting married, separated, divorced, becoming a widow/widower
>
> becoming old

You can undoubtedly think of many more circumstances your clientele experience where new, or increasing, demands of some sort become a part of their lives by choice or circumstances.

On the other end of the balance, what are some examples of decreasing or decreased ability or resources? Again, we encounter regularly:

> decreased decision-making ability among the unconscious, the confused, those on sedatives or mind-altering drugs
>
> decreased potential for action and participation related to hypoxia among persons with respiratory and circulatory pathology
>
> decreased ability to respond to reality among the mentally disturbed
>
> decreased mobility among the aged, those with fractures or paralysis, those with sight inadequacies
>
> decreased ability to communicate among the aphasic, the retarded, the confused, the laryngectomized, the cross-cultural groups, the unconscious, the very young, the very old, the very hostile
>
> decreased ability to maintain a viable personal community when one ages, lost financial resources, residence in a high risk neighborhood

The list could go on and on, but you get the idea.

When the nurse or the nurse and the client determine that the individual has the coping resources and ability available, obviously the goal will be to make effective use of both resources and abilities to creatively meet any new or increasing demands in living and, hopefully, to maintain the client's desired lifestyle in the process. This would be true for both long- and short-term goals.

On the other hand, when the nurse or the nurse and client determine that the individual will not or does not have the abilities and resources to accommodate to the demands, present or foreseen, then obviously the direction in goal setting will be a different one. One may deal with the demand side of the seesaw in one way by setting goals of reducing these demands appropriately (and, hopefully, in a way acceptable or desirable to the client). The nurse also has a goal option of contributing to the coping abilities, that is, adding to what the client brings, or where the client can bring nothing to bear, substituting for him. For example, if the client can feed himself only half the meal, someone else will be needed to provide the power to feed the remaining portion. If the client can make only little decisions, then bigger decisions will need to be broken down to little ones that he can deal with, or someone else will have to deal with the larger ones. If the client cannot void, a catheter can be inserted, if he cannot breathe, a respirator can be used. If he cannot shop for food or clothing, these must be provided in some way.

Thus, the major directions in goals will deal with management of demands or lifestyle, the enhancement or substitution/supplementation of coping abilities, or both.

COMPONENTS AND TECHNIQUES FOR GOAL STATEMENTS

Having examined areas within which goal statements can be organized, the next logical step would seem to be that of noting any particular styles for stating goals. Since most nurses have more than enough to do, with goals as with any other communication, it becomes important to communicate quickly and with appropriate precision. Get the specific message across in the fewest number of well-chosen words, whether those words are in your head for you or on paper for others.

Goals Are Stated in Terms of Client Outcome

Goal statements are made in terms of the client's behavior and outcome, not the nurse's. We have noticed in our own activities with goal setting that when goals were stated in terms of the client, it caused us to pause and reflect on whether what we have considered is really what the client wants. When we recognized that it has not been, we noticed that our next thought was how to make a goal we saw as valuable to the client compatible with those goals we have found the client wanted. This is quite different in both valuing and process from having purely nurse-centered goals.

183

Any goal statement that starts out with: *enable, facilitate, allow, let, permit* or similar verbs followed by the words "client" or "patient" is a nurse-centered goal. It cites what the nurse hopes to accomplish. Such a statement may have a place in the nurse's head, but not on the client's plan. The nurse is functioning in lieu of the client.

You might ask, "Well, what if the client's goals are inappropriate, meaning that they are wrong for him?" In the long run, a goal the client can't or won't buy won't work anyhow, so it is false economy to waste time writing goals the client will not agree to live with unless he is going to be institutionalized and, therefore, under the power of those who are setting goals for him indefinitely. How much better to try to set congruent goals.

Goals Are Stated Concisely

Getting rid of unnecessary or redundant words is obviously a good place to start in making goals concise. We still often see goals stated as, "The patient will. . . ." If the goal is for the client, this should be obvious without having to make an explicit statement. So, perhaps one guide should be that, unless otherwise stated, the goal refers to the client. Then we would need to include an indication of the clientele in the goal *only* when it involved family, friends, employer, school teacher, or someone other than a focal individual. This omission has an additional bonus in that it confronts the reader (or thinker) with an action verb as the initial attention-capturing force in the statement.

This is not the only way to reduce words. The trick comes in striving for economy of words without loss of precision or impact—at all times. Never use two words where one will do.

Use Specific Action Verbs

Start your goals with a specific action verb. The placement of an action verb at the beginning of the goal statement gives it immediate impact, by focusing the attention of the reader on the behavior that will announce that the client has achieved the goal. It tells what to look for, what the nursing orders are going to enable the person to achieve.

When the client is observed to:

Plan	Sleep	Turn	Speak
Identify	Drink	Cough	Sing
Walk	Report	Help	Read
Run	Laugh	Initiate	Share
Eat	Confront		

anyone who is aware of the goal will be able to realize that the goal has been achieved. This behavioral approach to goal statement with an action verb may have some limitations, particularly in long-term goals when one may not wish to be as behaviorally precise; but for many goals involving short or intermediate time spans, this format is the best.

Modifiers Add to Specificity

In addition to the action associated with the goal, there is, more often than not, a style with which that action is carried out. One walks slowly, steadily, quickly, or without limping. One eats with satisfaction, or with someone, or slowly or steadily or within a time span. In each instance, there is greater precision in the expectation that is related to effective coping and satisfaction with the outcome.

Content Area Is Essential

The content area adds the finishing component to the goal as we noted in discussing goal areas. It indicates what the person is to identify or what he is to plan, the area of subjective experience he is to report, the persons he is able to confront, the risks to be taken, the projects to be worked upon, the food or fluid to be consumed or avoided, the activity or knowledge to be learned. Just as with the action verb, the content area should be defined with *appropriate* precision.

Time Elements Are Identified

Time for achievement of the goal may be stated explicitly or implied. Often in long-term goals the time is not specifically identified.

Suppose a client who is dying has indicated that he wishes to be able to talk over what is happening to him and his reactions with someone who won't withdraw or make judgments about his way of dying. He indicates that having this type of dependable, nonjudgmental, and caring listener will provide support to him in this stressful experience. The goal then might state, "Shares the experience of dying in a way that is consistently satisfying to him." No time has been indicated, yet any reader knows that death will terminate the goal. On the other hand, the preoperative person who must learn the log-rolling turn effectively before surgery would need an identified time element to suggest the pace of learning activities. So this goal might read: "Performs log-rolling turn correctly and easily by Tuesday A.M." The diabetic or the one in the household who will be responsible for cooking and dietary management as soon as the client goes home needs a certain competence in the rudiments of preparing a diabetic diet in x number of days. The goal should identify that time explicitly where this is important.

Summary

Goal statements describe the observed response the client will make when the desired outcome is achieved. Such a statement specifies: the action, the style with which the action occurs, the content involved or context within which the action will take place, and the time within which the outcome is expected to occur. It is always stated in terms of the client's behavior, not the nurse's. Technical skill is directed toward communicating to any reader (or oneself) as quickly, forcefully, and precisely as possible what the desired outcome is to be.

GOALS AND COPING DEFICITS

Whatever diagnostic taxonomy nursing eventually develops and accepts, goal systems will obviously be closely related to it. As an example, let us use the categories of functional coping deficits to illustrate how goals can coordinate with a diagnostic classification system.

Strength and Endurance

Despite the fact that strength refers to the capacity to engage in a particular activity while endurance is concerned with staying power (stamina), many potential components of the goal statements will be similar. Goals for **both types of coping deficits** will deal with:

> kinds of activities
> the amount of work involved
> its frequency
> the duration of an activity
> rest periods—frequency, duration
> consistency of participation in activities
> pleasure in participation
> ease, style, and vigor displayed in activities
> the pace
> comfort with constraints or capacity
> inventiveness with resources that supplement
> limited personal abilities.

Some clients will have potential for *gaining additional strength and/or endurance.*

Examples: Obese clients engaging in exercise program gain both strength and endurance as they work on physical fitness. Their eventual coping resources in these areas may well exceed those they began with. Sedentary persons who suffer coronaries and subsequently join jogging or physical fitness groups may also achieve a degree of vigor they did not have prior to their heart attacks.

Some clients will be concerned with *restoration of losses that have occurred.*

Examples: One of our local basketball pros experienced a bout of viral pneumonia during the season and was assiduously (albeit gradually) pursuing the goal of regaining his midseason strength and endurance. Elderly persons who experience transient illness are often very concerned about the slow pace of regaining their pre-illness strength for single tasks and endurance for the ongoing demands of daily living.

Many clients have goals of *maintenance of present levels of strength and endurance* even as disease or age bid to reduce them.

Examples: Normal aging takes its toll in loss of thickness of bone cortices, less flexibility of connective tissue, loss of muscle mass, decrease in cardiac output and in the ceiling of heart rate the person can achieve during the stress of work. All of these tend to reduce the capacity for work on a single task and endurance for work over time, particularly in taking on peak loads of work. Thus, even without disease, maintenance becomes a goal. Given chronic illnesses such as joint disease, and cardio-pulmonary diseases, and so many others, the goal of maintenance can be very challenging.

At times the goal of maintenance is not feasible and must be changed to that of *slowing losses*. Where losses must or do occur, the goals may well relate to *adjusting to the body image and self-concept of being less strong, having less stamina*. With that comes a concommitant goal of *adjusting both demands of daily living and lifestyle* to the reduced resources and *finding satisfactions in the new way of living*.

Where the strength or endurance involve emotional fortitude and persistence, the areas of goals will be similar but of course will be concerned with those activities which primarily tax the spirit of the individual more than they make physical demands upon him. The components listed in the first paragraph of this section lend themselves to these goals as well.

SAMPLES OF GOALS RELATED TO STRENGTH AND ENDURANCE

Strength   Grasps utensils without dropping them
Lifts arm till elbow even with shoulder within 2 weeks
Accepts (or seeks) help in moving heavy objects
Initiates full program of isometrics AM & PM with growing enthusiasm

Endurance   Walks _____ level blocks this week without discomfort, to _____ next week.
Plans personally acceptable schedule of ADL to include rest periods $\bar{p}$ meals.
Enlists help of relatives to care for child 2 afternoons/wk.

Management of Sensory Input

Goals in the management of sensory input will concern themselves with both *available* and *usable* stimuli. *Available* stimuli would refer to those stimuli in the internal and external environment that are accessible to or impinge upon the receptors of the individual. *Usable* stimuli are those which are actually perceived by the individual, the ones which get through the central nervous system threshold to affect the individual. Goals in this category must also concern themselves with the comfort range and the usual norm of the client (*not* the health care worker), in any sensory dimension. The dimensions or components of goals in the area of sensory input will be concerned with:

> Awareness of areas of deprivation, risks of deprivation at various periods in life and in differing life situations
>
> Ability to obtain/maintain devices (glasses, hearing aids, etc.) to minimize sensory distortion or diminution of available stimuli
>
> Control of overload or resources to enrich an impoverished sensory environment in meaningful/acceptable ways
>
> Management of stimuli in the environment to prevent sensory deprivation despite loss of sense receptors or their efficiency
>
> Prevention of overload despite hyperaresthesia or sudden correction of sensory defect (e.g., stapedectomy for otosclerosis)
>
> Self-sufficiency in providing for own sensory environment
>
> Successful management of pharmacologically based sensory deprivation (sedatives, narcotics) or overloading (mind-expanding drugs)
>
> Development of acceptable techniques for accommodating to or overcoming reduced effectiveness of sense receptors while maintaining a desired lifestyle.

SAMPLES OF GOALS RELATED TO SENSORY INPUT

Arranges with other residents to share supper meal to avoid loneliness this week.

Using ear plugs/cotton to screen out noise/music/ . . . from adjoining apartment/room at night.

Increases size of light bulbs in reading lamps.

Purchases (accepts gift of) pet/fish/bird for diversion.

Knowledge

Goals concerned with knowledge will have two dimensions. One aspect will be the content to be acquired. The second will be the level of cognitive skill to be attained in organizing and using that content.

Content might be concerned with symptoms, techniques of prevention, resources for assistance, the nature and action of drugs being ingested, the ways of working with or around a system, developmental tasks, indicators of normal growth and development, role expectations, the normality of what is being experienced, and so on. The list is endless. It can include anything and everything an individual needs to recognize and understand to cope more adequately with life in terms of his health status.

The skills needed to use the content in living will be addressed more fully in criteria for evaluation. However, in brief, three major levels of skill in use of knowledge will probably be most frequently employed with three other levels to be attained in some instances. These levels include:

Recall
being able to remember specifics, processes, methods, or patterns when the situation calls for it.

Comprehension
being able to give the ideas and facts in one's own words, give life illustrations, explain these ideas/facts, compare them and predict possible relationships or outcomes.

Application
applying the content to concrete situations as a basis for understanding them and making decisions or taking action.

The possibly less frequent areas of achievement would be:

Analysis
breaking down situations or communications into component parts and reorganizing them for greater understanding.

Synthesis
putting ideas together in such a way as to come out with something new or different—using the content creatively.

Evaluation
using the content to set standards or criteria and collecting data related to these standards, then applying the standards to measure and make judgments about findings.

Goals of knowledge, then, will have to incorporate both the area of content to be acquired and the skill in using that content at the level needed.

SAMPLES OF GOALS RELATED TO KNOWLEDGE

Identifies agencies available to Senior citizens and their services.

Relates sx of hypoglycemia to experiences of ↓ food intake, emotional stress ↑ physical activity, illness.

Explains how central pooling of blood can lead to shortness of breath at noc; & how extra pillows or putting legs in dependent position prevents/relieves sx.

Speaks at ostomy club meeting to share knowledge of ostomy management with others.

Desire

Goals related to a diagnosed deficit in desire will be in an affective area. Nurses who have diagnosed a lack of desire will undoubtedly be seeking to generate a spark of interest, initiative, eagerness and enthusiasm; or at the very least, a neutral toleration of a treatment regimen, a state of affairs, or a way of life.

SAMPLE GOALS RELATED TO DESIRE

Says he wants to lose weight.

Creates a system for losing weight while eating from family/dorm menu.

Jogs 1 mile $\bar{q}$ a.m. regardless of weather.

Discusses enthusiastically the achievements in returning to normal schedule $\bar{p}$ M.I.

These goals will be concerned not only with the level of will and interest but must also identify what the person is to be interested or involved in. Some examples might be

Wants to learn/participate/live/help others/relate to others/or whatever the activity may be

Actually participates with/without encouragement in . . . with reported/observed tolerance/pleasure

Takes initiative to find opportunities to participate in . . . .
Engages others or enables others to participate in . . . .

More specific observable manifestations of interest or desire to participate will be covered in criteria for evaluation. At times these could be incorporated into goal statements if the goal is to be quite specific or limited.

Courage

Goals related to courage may take several forms. They may be related to the recognition of risks involved in a situation. They may also be concerned with assessing the actual nature of the risks. In activity-oriented goals, the focus may be on testing the risky behavior in safe situations or experiencing the sense of vulnerability associated with the threatening situation—again, in a mock or role-playing setting. Eventually, however, goals for courage must involve decisions or performance in the real life situation requiring genuine risks. If it is an ongoing encounter with a continuing threat, then some degree of comfort would also be a necessary goal for effective living.

SAMPLE GOALS RELATED TO COURAGE

Admits he's afraid to inject himself.
Submits to injection by nurse.
Injects insulin with minimal delay or overt nervousness.
Reports fear of injection no longer a problem.

Skills

Goals related to skills may be concerned with psychomotor skills and dexterity. They may also relate to interpersonal skills, communication, decision making, or priority setting, to mention other areas. Goals here may well need to identify the environment or situations within which the skill must be performed. If speed is a factor, then this too must be incorporated into the goal statement. At times, skills and procedures must be adhered to rigorously (not touching certain sterile surfaces, following prescribed sequence in steps of initiating dialysis, etc.) and at other times, improvisation and creativity are the desired outcome. When there are constraints or outcomes of this nature, the goal statement should call this to attention.

SAMPLE GOALS RELATED TO SKILLS

Describes techniques found effective in interacting with hostesses/hosts to avoid eating (high Na, high COH . . . foods, alcohol, or whatever substance must not be ingested) at a variety of social occasions (parties/restaurants/cookouts/picnics/pack trips. . . .

Prepares and injects correct dose of insulin quickly, smoothly, and with asepsis in any of the rotating sites.

Develops system for maintaining rotation schedule for injections.

Devises more effective tool for . . . .

Communicates with minimal discomfort his changing behavior to family as he moves from dependent/ill role to independent/healthy role.

Support Systems

The goals in the deficit area of support systems will incorporate the resources involved and the ability of the client to:

> recognize
>
> obtain
>
> use
>
> maintain
>
> enjoy them (possibly)

At times, adjustment to dependence on an external support system will be a primary goal; at other times, just locating a resource and making it financially feasible will be a focus. When the support system is another human being or group of human beings, the goal may well have a dual focus—one related to the client and his skill and comfort in using this support system and another focusing on maintaining the person or persons in their relationship to the client. Some examples of goal areas related to support systems might be:

Aware of areas of support that humans require/how these may vary with age, culture, circumstances

Knows of resources for acquiring and maintaining support systems—personal, community, mechanical, financial, etc.

Maintains and uses personal community effectively

Accepts/or has varying degrees of initiative/skill in gaining support systems

Creates/participates in support systems for others with similar circumstances or those in need of support systems

Adjusts to dependence on external support systems
Adjusts to refusal to accept dependence on support systems and the lifestyle this decision generates
Generates positive feedback from persons in the support system used.

SAMPLE GOALS RELATED TO SUPPORT SYSTEMS

Acknowledges need for resources outside self to maintain ADL.
Phones FISH (volunteer transportation resource) for transportation to doctor for next visit.
Uses walker regularly around the house.
Reports less discomfort in accepting help from . . . or using crutches/prosthesis. . . .

GOALS RELATED TO SPECIFIC SYMPTOMS

The foregoing are samples of goal areas related to a functional coping/living style category system. They are not exhaustive, nor are they offered as models, just samples of categories of goal areas that you and your clients may consider as a point of departure for your own creative thinking.

One of the gaps that may seem to be present in this particular approach to nursing diagnoses and goals is that it deals with coping phenomena and impact on daily living more than it does with the underlying conditions that have contributed to the deficit in the first place. However, just as symptoms as well as diseases can be identified and treated in medicine, so particular symptoms or conditions generating coping difficulties can be identified with separate goal statements. The appropriate coping difficulty can be used as the organizing heading. For example, loss of endurance and its impact on daily living may derive from loss of sleep over time for one or more reasons. A goal, then, may be directed toward improved sleep patterns through decreasing interruptions, modification of the environment, or controlling pain. Other examples of contributing conditions requiring specific goals might be: dyspnea, dehydration, muscle spasms, anorexia, itching, baldness—the list is endless. Obviously, there is no reason why goals should not be developed in relationship to specific phenomena as well as to the major areas of coping and the impact associated with them.

The important point is to have a logical system for organizing goals so that multiple unrelated goals are not strung out willy-nilly in our thinking or our recordings. With normal case loads, disorganized goals tend to get lost. Hence, a system is needed for organizing problems and goals into larger units for easier recall, and for ease in recognizing potential relationships among phenomena and responses.

TIMING OF GOALS

As was suggested in the previous section on the techniques of writing goals, time is a feature in every goal. Some are long term, perhaps never achievable, but always there as a source of motivation and direction. Others are of shorter duration, points of arrival along the way. A further exploration of time as a force in goals and goals as a force in management of our nursing time may be helpful in developing our skills in creating goals.

Long-Term Goals

It is with long-term goals that nurses run the greatest risk of dealing in platitudes. It need not be this way. If goals are deliberately developed from data given by the client on his hopes and wishes combined with the nurses' knowledge of the reality of the presenting situation, and the predictions of both coping demands and resources, then there is no way that clichés can result. Data on the client's health-related goals and desired lifestyle should be as much a part of any assessment for long-term care as is the heart and lung examination or the family history to the physician. Using the data base and one's knowledge, it is possible to discover and create genuine working goals that will be as variable as our clientele. These will be intriguing goals that will be a challenge to our nursing skills, interesting goals that can capture our attention, client-centered goals that will keep us focused on them rather than merely meeting establishment or accreditation requirements. We can just as easily deal with the true spirit of care planning rather than the letter of the law.

> Maintain maximum independence in face of congestive heart failure and normal limitations of age (82).

Intermediate Goals

Intermediate goals serve an important purpose, both for the nurses and the clientele. They are identifiable points of achievement or movement on the way toward the long-term goal. It is essential that both the client and the nurse be able to identify them, particularly when the long-term goal is truly distant, and slow to be achieved. Both parties need a sense of achievement and intermediate goals do make this possible.

Let's take an example. A person who has been directing anger inwardly without knowing it for all of his life, is not going to be able to move directly to the awareness, values and interpersonal skills that will enable him to harness his feelings and energy in a productive fashion. Both he and those who interact with him (family/friends) can benefit by and be assured of identifiable progress when a series of recognizable, predetermined intermediate goals are aimed for and achieved (or not achieved). The angry client may begin with the goal of:

recognizing when he is experiencing or has experienced anger.

He may progress to:

identifying the event or person that triggered the feeling of anger.

talking about the feelings and the triggers with a "safe" person (one not involved).

A more advanced intermediate goal may be achieved when he:

confronts the object of his anger not too long after the encounter and experience of anger, either partially giving vent to his feelings or exploding in such a way that large amounts of negative feedback result.

A still later intermediate goal, perhaps a final desired outcome, may be that he will:

express himself in ways that are currently congruent with his internal feeling state yet not disrupt the overall productive relationships with the person(s) involved.

All of these would be stations on the way to the long-term goal of using anger as a productive force.

In the article "Blossoming of Ruthie," the long-term goal was that Ruthie, a retarded child, would learn to communicate verbally, to undertake productive daily activities including play, and to relate to others in spite of her retardation. To do this, Ruthie had to learn verbal and task skills. She had to harness her energy and hyperactivity that was currently resulting in temper tantrums and destructive behavior. She had to learn how to relate to others in an accepted manner. Even some of these sub-goals seem pretty long term. In such a case, it may be productive to make intermediate goals even shorter term. Cullinane reported that Ruthie did learn to help with the linen and washing sinks on the unit and other activities. She did learn to play with a push-pull toy. She learned to speak, first words, then short sentences. Points of achievement to give satisfaction to all concerned, even where "normality" was never a possible long-term goal (Cullinane, 1968).

Persons who become diabetic don't learn to live successfully with diabetes in a week. There are skills to be mastered, meanings of symptoms to be learned experientially and understood, relationships of events to blood sugar levels and outcomes, techniques of managing a controlled diet—at home, in restaurants, at social gatherings. There is the assimilation of the concept of diabetes as a physical condition with predictable sequellae to be incorporated into one's self-concept. Each of these areas needs to be dealt with in terms of achievable intermediate goals in a given reasonable time limit—long enough to permit expectations of accomplishment, but short enough to maintain motivation and momentum for those involved, including the nurses.

Short-Term Goals

Short-term goals are those involved with this week, today, this encounter. The focus is the hope of immediate achievement. They serve the purpose of specifically shaping nurse (or client) behavior in a given encounter, including the observations of responses as the interaction or activity is taking place. More than any other time span, these goals are probably the most concrete and tangible, since they deal with expectations and hopes for the here and now.

> Participates in coughing-deep breathing routine effectively
>
> Shares current knowledge and feelings about illness of her child
>
> Shares his usual way of treating this illness and the ethnic beliefs and folk-ways associated with it
>
> Drinks 6 glasses of fluid/day
>
> Sleeps satisfyingly without sedation
>
> Discovers satisfying and effective ways of communicating (e.g., when speech is denied him or is different from that of the health worker)
>
> Performs a developmental test
>
> Reports gains in insight in responses to—authority figures/parents/children/spouses.

Making explicit the short-term goals is a many-times-a-day experience. As one nurse reported when she first tried it, "You've mixed up my whole nursing life-style! I used to be able to pop into a patient's room, pass the pill, turn him, chat with him—whatever, and then go on. Now I have to hesitate at the door and think about what I want from this contact, what he might want and how I can accomplish these things in the few moments we have together, to say nothing of thinking about how I will recognize whether either of us is meeting these goals. My nursing is clumsy and self-conscious all of a sudden." This is not a surprising outcome. It is for this very reason that we strongly recommend limited initial trials of this goal setting nursing behavior, building up expectations of quantity as tolerance and comfort for the behavior develop. You could, for example, set a short-term goal for yourself of being explicitly goal directed in one encounter or with one client today, or for a part of today. Then, as you become more comfortable and skilled, you will no doubt be able to increase the numbers of encounters and persons (both clients and staff, as it is appropriate) where you can be consciously, explicitly goal directed. It can become a behavior you can choose and use as long as it is desired and productive.

Summary

Goals involve differing time spans—long, intermediate, and short time periods. While each is involved with a common desired outcome, they all serve differing purposes. The long-term goal sets the final desired endpoint and the overall direction of behavior. Intermediate goals set shorter range desired achievements and so influence more specifically the tone and nature of the interaction and activities. They also serve as forces for both motivation and momentum, or pace, in the flow of the activities and interaction. In addition, they can be sources of satisfaction of achievement and points for interim evaluation. Short-term goals, dealing as they do with the immediate here and now, are specific guides to action, to climate, and to criteria for making ongoing observations.

A LOOK AT GOAL SYSTEMS

Being pragmatists, we have discussed first the "what" and the "how" of stating goals in planning for nursing management of client's health problems. However, the most effective use of goals by individual nurses and nursing care systems also involves an understanding of how goals can serve them, as well as the client. It has been said that we are all self-serving in the midst of our service to others. It stands to reason, then, that if we can see how goal setting will do something for us, we may be much more willing to learn the skill and implement it.

Beyond this is the basic consideration of the nurse's value system and its pervasive influence on goal-setting behavior. Unless the nurse understands the values held about clients' rights and responsibilities in determining outcomes in their health and lifestyles, there will be conflict and confusion in the process of developing client-nurse goals for health care. For this reason, we intend to explore the relationship of values to goal setting.

Finally, because we do not believe in rote behavior, we intend to introduce some alternatives to diagnosis-goal statements: some times and ways in which they may be productively combined rather than stated separately as we usually do. To be creative about care planning, one must be flexible and use plans in the most productive ways—even if one changes the protocol to do this. The process should serve the person, not the other way around.

With this introduction, transition, and rationale, we hope you are ready for the rest of the chapter.

WHAT ARE THE FUNCTIONS OF GOALS IN THE CARE PLANNING SYSTEM?

Goal setting serves four functions necessary to maintain the vitality, the momentum, and the professional quality of nursing care. These include giving:

> a sense of direction and perspective to nursing activities
> a sense of pace of activities with each client
> a sense of achievement
> a basis for criteria for evaluation of response.

ALL of these are essential to the well-being of the clientele *and* the nursing staff. In this section, we will discuss the first three, leaving the last for a fuller treatment in the chapter dealing specifically with evaluation.

In some instances, goals orient one to the future, in others, to the present, while in still others, to the past. In their future orientation, they serve as compass points and endpoints that offer *direction* and *perspective* to our activities, to those of the client and to his personal community, in some instances.

In their current orientation, they can set the *momentum* or *pace* of activities. For example, if an individual must learn certain skills before surgery in order to perform competently as a postoperative patient, obviously the timing and pace of the teaching-learning activities are determined in part at least by that deadline. If a person on limited hospitalization must learn how to cope with diabetes before he goes home in order to care for himself (a situation presenting itself with increasing frequency as third party payors determine what they will support as a "normal" duration of hospitalization for any given diagnosis and treatment), then high priority learning experiences must be introduced and accomplished within that time span if it is at all possible.

In a current, and perhaps a past orientation as well, goals have the function of offering a sense of accomplishment—acknowledgment that certain achievements have been made. Notice that we did not say gains, but achievements. The achievements may well be having maintained present status in the face of poor odds, having minimized expected losses, or having coped effectively with losses that occurred.

How can these functions of goals apply to situations in which clients have short- and long-term contacts with nursing care?

Functions and Nature of Goals in Short-Term Contacts

In short-term health care the goals will naturally tend to involve short time spans, perhaps single encounters. These goals will have a tendency to be quite concrete. What can the nurse and the client achieve in a one-visit encounter—with the person having a VD checkup, with the transient in the Free Clinic, with the young woman in the Abortion Clinic or Family Planning Clinic, with the school child coming in with the sudden fever from the classroom? Nurses can settle for doing the obviously necessary tasks, or they can inject another goal of trying to behave in such a way as to increase the client's valuing of the potential of nursing care to his health. They might have a goal of building trust between client and nursing staff—attitudes that could modify later practices in utilizing health care services in general and nursing services in particular. Here the nurse's skill and emphasis is concentrated on determining what is *possible* in the short duration health encounter balanced by what is desirable beyond the skill of carrying out the task. A technician in many instances can quite adequately perform the task. The professional looks to the goals of what can be done *while* the task is being performed.

Functions of Goals in Long-Term Care

In long-term care, in maintenance, and in terminal care, as well as in prevention, goal setting has very important functions related to:

1. the directions of care,
2. the motivation for care, and
3. the ongoing satisfaction of both the client and the nurse with their efforts.

How does the elderly person in the nursing home, the young retarded person in a large institution, the person at home or in an institution for long periods achieve any sense of accomplishment if goals aren't identified and achieved? Where do the nurses, other personnel under their supervision, and other caring persons involved find the zest and rewards to keep them truly nursing professionally and caring personally if they too cannot recognize when they are achieving goals with these people. Skilled, professional goal setting may mean the difference between humane professional care and routine custodial care for clients and their close personal community.

Goal setting, whether it be in the mind of the nurse or communicated in speech or writing is an important professional function of the nurse, particularly in long-term care, institutional or community based. It is safe to say that professional nursing care cannot be accomplished without the functions that goal setting serves.

WHO SETS GOALS IN THE SYSTEM?

When individuals are playing on the same team, it helps if they play in the same ball park and aim their coordinated plays in the direction of the same goal lines. Any person who seeks help from a health care system has some desired outcomes that he is unable to achieve unassisted. On the other hand, we know that health care workers have goals that may be quite different from those of the client, or even from each other. The fact is that the client, his family, the doctor and the nurse, as major parties in health care, may each be playing in different ball parks. Or they may be playing in the same park but aiming at opposite goals. For instance, the placing of persons with high risk of fatal emergencies "on code" (to be automatically subjected to cardiopulmonary resuscitation and other emergency lifesaving measures), is a recurring situation in which the goals of individuals tend to vary. The clients may wish release from suffering, may even have a "living will." The family may also wish for the individual to be permitted to die without additional suffering and physical indignities. The medical group may desire to sustain life to avoid risk of malpractice suits. The medical students may have a goal of gaining experience in the techniques of resuscitation—certainly a worthy professional learning goal. Nurses often serve both as client advocates and supporters of the goal to preserve life. We are caught in a dilemma between client goals, medical goals, and our own goals for the person and his family.

When differences in goals between clients and health care workers are ignored, one can predict that no one will be happy with the outcomes. If the client behaves (or tries to behave) in terms of his own goal, the nurses and doctors are likely to label him as the "difficult" or "uncooperative" patient. He is the one who doesn't take his pills, or takes too many, or too many kinds; fails appointments; eats the wrong foods; sees multiple doctors; gets up when he is supposed to stay in bed; or is obstinate about getting up when ambulation has been ordered. On the other hand, the client is probably no happier with us, finding us unfeeling, lacking in understanding, or just downright mean!

But suppose each party were to take the trouble to learn what the other's goals were, to share their perceptions and notice differences. We could acknowledge that these differences are real and that each of us is behaving in terms of our own goals. In the end, we still might not agree, our activities to achieve our own goals might well continue, but at least our behavior would be comprehensible in the light of acknowledged goals. It would surprise neither party that until a compromise was reached, each would march to his own drummer. And it might mean that working for an acceptable accommodation or articulation between client-nurse goals would have early priority.

THE PROBLEM OF CONFLICTING GOALS

Wherever there are people, there are bound to be differences. It is both the delight of variety and the despair of conflict. The setting of goals in health care management is no different. Clients and nurses are going to have different value systems, different backgrounds and experiences, and from this will arise desires for different goals. The resolution of these differences is one of the skills associated with goal development in the nursing plan. In the past, we have sometimes played the ostrich about client goals that differed from those of the nurse, feeling perhaps that if we ignored them long enough they would go away. Sometimes in the rush of giving all this nursing care we just said client goals were not important, not as important or as "good" as nurses' goals. We would like to have you look at some other options in dealing with differences in client-nurse goals. Of course, first one must recognize that differences are present in the situation, so let us look at how to recognize when these differences are occurring.

Recognizing When Goals Are Differing

There are cues in our behavior that can tell others when conflicting goals are operating in an encounter. Since we are concerned with nurse-client situations let us take our examples from this category. When the client is not interested in the nurse's health care goal the nurse may notice:

a lack of enthusiasm for ideas or activities

an absence of questions

nodding compliance

failure to take any initiative

failure to contribute any ideas about how to fit actions or desires into the proposed plan

expressions of guilt at failure to comply

forgetting to carry out prescribed activities

carrying out activities despite requests or "teaching" toward not engaging in them

lack of enthusiasm in encounters with the nurses

distinct coolness toward the nurse

avoidance of the nurse

hostile responses to suggestion

changing the subject

avoidance of eye contact

missed appointments.

Some of these behaviors represent withdrawal from the nurse and the nurse's goals. Others may represent attacking behavior. All suggest lack of enthusiasm, to say the least, for the goal directed behavior of the health care worker.

Nor is the nurse immune from sending out cues to the client when there is disagreement with the client's goal directed behavior. Some of these same manifestations may appear in the nurse's behavior. And there is an additional behavior seen in health workers trying to achieve their goals in the face of some type of opposition from the client. This is the response of trying to produce fear, shame, or guilt in the client in order to achieve compliance with the nurse's goal.

201

When either the client or the nurse can be observed, or observe themselves giving cues in these areas, one could predict that differences in goals interfere with their mutual achievement. There is, then, a need to try to explicitly identify the differences and to mediate them in some way before proceeding.

Differences, Not Rights or Wrongs

You may have noticed that we have not alluded to right goals or wrong goals, nor to any other value judgments. We have spoken of differences, a much more neutral concept. Naturally, each of us is going to think that our own goals are "right."

It helps in nursing, however, to keep things in perspective if data on goals and goal-related values and behavior can be viewed with the same objectivity one associates with laboratory values and other cues. This objectivity should be applied to data on nurses' goals and behaviors just as surely as it is to those of the clients.

Differences in Goals Based on Nurses' Greater Knowledge

There can be no question that at times nurses have more scientific knowledge and insight than do clients. They are able to formulate goals that clients cannot even envision until they too have the knowledge and insight. In such situations the differences in goals and the basis for these differences need to be recognized. Then, intermediate and immediate goals can be set up wherein the client can be helped to gain the knowledge and insight needed to make responsible choices in the goals he sets for himself in health care areas.

By the same token, however, there are times when it seems that clients have greater insight into the needs of their own bodies than nurses, who are not experiencing the symptoms, can have. It does not pay to let this "wisdom" of self-preservation go unheeded either. Nurses and lay persons have written in nursing journals and other magazines of situations in which they were aware of their needs and set goals for themselves as patients or clients, but were frustrated in achieving them because the nurses caring for them "knew better." Sometimes nurses do know better, sometimes clients know better. The skilled professional listens to both voices.

Goal Setting Behavior of Nurses for Clients—for Patients

It is in the area of goal setting—discrepancies of goals between nurses and consumers of nursing care, as well as in priorities of goals in nursing care—that the nurse's philosophy of nursing is a significant influence. It is here that the concept of "patient" or "client" is a real force. For example, if the nurses believe that persons with whom they are working are in a patient role ("a person who *receives* the action," "enduring . . . trouble without complaint") they may believe that the nurse knows best and is obliged to set the health care goals (Webster,

1968, 1078). In such a relationship, it is quite likely that the consumer's goals may receive rather superficial attention or be negated if there is a conflict in goals. On the other hand, if the consumer is seen as being in a client relationship to the nurse, that is, one who employs the services of a professional, then the nurses' role in goal setting would be to enable the consumer to recognize and understand his own goals and the range and options of goals available to him under the circumstances. This would be done in order to enable him to make a responsible choice, whenever his mental and physical capabilities permit it.

As we (the authors) worked with the ambulatory elderly, we chose the "client" rather than the "patient" concept since these retirement apartment residents were the ones who took the initiative in consulting and utilizing our professional services. Our nursing goals often were at variance with the operating goals of these older folks. Our interaction became one of making them aware of their current goals and the other goals they could hold, then exploring what they might choose and the implications for their health and lifestyle. It was quite different from some earlier nursing both of us had done when we cared for hospitalized persons in a patient role. Here, we had behaved primarily in terms of treatment-oriented goals with only secondary regard and priority for clients' goals when they were not congruent with those of nursing.

TECHNIQUES FOR LEARNING CLIENTS' GOALS

Since goals determine direction, there is a need early in the health care encounter to understand what the client/patient's operating goals really are (and that means deliberately collecting data on them). This is not always easy to do. If the consumers' goals are divergent from those of the health worker, a certain amount of trust must be established before they are likely to be shared. We have also found that clients do not easily verbalize their explicit goals. More often their goals are implicit in their actions rather than explicit in their thoughts and words. Sometimes these goals are nebulous and therefore hard to put into words. It may take some astute observation and listening—picking up of cues—to learn the goals of the individual. Then it is the nurse who may have to put them into words and do a perception check to see if she is correct in her conclusions. For example:

> A man was admitted for a stay of a couple of weeks in a hospital to have his abdominal pain diagnosed and treated. He had for many years held jobs in which he was in control of the situation. If one had asked his goal in seeking health care, the initial statement would have been, "To get rid of this pain." But after a few days it became very obvious that it was, "To get rid of this pain, but also to maintain maximum personal control over my daily living and environment while under treatment."
>
> Actually, the two goals were not incompatible, nor did they conflict with the specific nursing goals. However, this nonverbalized, acted-out goal had

to be defined by the nursing staff and validated with the client in order to incorporate it into the plan of nursing management. When the nurse had put the cues together she said to him, "You know, Mr. Ranger, you've held very responsible positions for so long, ones where you've made many of the day to day decisions, not only for yourself, but for a lot of other people. It must be difficult to be here where so many are being made for you." He looked rather startled and then responded, "You'll never know how hard." With some further validation, they went on to find ways in which he could maintain control, those instances where he couldn't—and why he couldn't. Then they planned for the style of nursing staff-client interaction that would be used in the delivery of both the nursing care and the delegated medical care. It took no more time. It did not much modify what was done. But it did change the style of the interaction that accompanied the activities.

SELF AWARENESS AND NURSES' WORKING GOALS

Clients are not the only persons who are not aware of their working goals. At times nurses, too, carry on activities and relationships in which they have little awareness of desired outcomes, other than those of getting the delegated medical or administrative functions accomplished. Thoughts may even be elsewhere as hands and feet carry out familiar tasks.

Since it is easier to look at others than ourselves, we might begin by looking at others' interactions with clients to try to ascertain the goal that was actually accomplished in the encounter, and perhaps speculate on what was intended. Are either of them the goals you would have set? How did they relate to what you know of the client's goals? Of course, eventually, it is wise to look at ourselves in current or past nursing activities and ask:

> What am I achieving in this activity/behavior?
> What do I really want to achieve with this person?
> What do I think he wants from this encounter?
> Could I behave in such a way as to accomplish these mini-goals?

Four questions about one encounter seem like a lot when they are read in print. Yet, like so much of nursing process, it is the thinking that accompanies one's activities that is so crucial. Thoughts flow rapidly. It is not at all impossible to consider one's explicit goals as one nurses.

Both nurses' and clients' goals are involved in the planning and giving of nursing care, to say nothing of other health care colleagues. Sometimes nurses and clients may hold very congruent goals. Sometimes we may differ, but agree to disagree. At other times, the nurses' goals are a result of greater knowledge and insight than the client has available at a given point in time. He cannot hold that goal yet. He is not ready for it. But he may be, once he understands the factors and the options.

In each instance nurses need to set themselves to determine in some way what the client's goals are, and what their own are. Acknowledgment of identified goals of both parties then becomes an integral part of subsequent planning and care.

VARIATIONS IN APPROACHES TO GOAL STATEMENTS

As in every other field of endeavor, there are a variety of approaches to stating goals and some philosophical differences. Some people prefer to specify observable behaviors, while others will identify broader outcomes, leaving the specifics of observable behavior to short-term goals, or even reserving them for the criteria for evaluation of response.

Combining Goals and Barriers in Diagnostic Statements

Another area where variation can be seen in the approach to stating goals is in the relationships between goal and diagnostic statements. We have seen forms which require the separation of the diagnosis and goals. Actually, there are times when the goal is encompassed by the statement of the diagnosis or problem. Then it seems rather ritualistic to indicate that goals must be specified twice, merely to meet the demands of the system. On the other hand, if goal setting is in a fledgling state for the staff, there may be merit in requiring separation to heighten awareness. It is helpful if the system can accommodate to both levels of sophistication.

To illustrate how long-term goals and problem statements can be meshed, here are a few examples.

A teen-age boy was abruptly and mandatorily hospitalized for tuberculosis of lungs and kidney. He found that overnight he had lost control over his lifestyle in areas both large and small: he was confined legally to a compound outside of the city limits and, in fact, limited to a small, rather barren room. His mother signed a surgical consent form while he thought he was going in for diagnostic testing under anesthesia. He was required to take multiple pills at certain hours. He was wakened to wash at an early morning hour, was offered food at set hours, was told when to rest and sleep, was restricted from seeing his girl friend, was deprived of any modicum of privacy in his room or in his bodily functions—no one knocked when they entered and he was told how his room was to be kept.

Now, the normal development task for a 17-year-old male and one which most will undertake with vigor, if not finesse, is that of moving into the independence and sexual identity of the adult male role in the society in which they live. At this crucial point, this young man was surrounded by female authority figures in the form of nurses and even the doctor, while

205

his peers were older male patients. He was deprived by the contagious nature of his disease of any contact with his former peers—male or female. And, further, a permanent nephrostomy tube was placed during the diagnostic surgery, adding to his uncertainty about his sexual abilities (justified or not).

In this instance, it would be quite possible and profitable to encompass the major nursing goal and the barriers to it into one working diagnostic statement:

> Movement into independence and adult male role frustrated 2° loss of control over daily living, loss of trust in adults, and presence of nephrostomy tube.

The "movement into adult male role" specifies a long-term goal encompassing a time span of years. Its placement into the diagnostic statement in conjunction with the barriers to achievement gives it the perspective of this client's presenting situation.

In dealing with this situation, the nurses also developed some specific intermediate goals. One was to help him find a way of coping satisfyingly with daily living, some areas of which had to be restricted; a concomitant goal for themselves was to discover areas of living where he could, without harm to himself or others, have greater control. (They were able to find quite a few.) They also set a goal of assessing and dealing with areas where they could rebuild his trust in adults. They set a goal of moving out of the mother-surrogate roles into more adult relationships that were still compatible with the nurse-client relationship in a long-term care situation. This was geared toward facilitating his skill in managing adult to adult relationships. And, of course, an attempt was made to actualize all of these intermediate goals as the medical management of his tuberculosis was being carried out.

In format, these nurses departed from a pure style of stating a diagnosis and then separately stating goals. They combined the long-term goals and the barriers in the statement of the working diagnosis. Then they created explicit intermediate goal statements and short-term goals supportive to the overall goal.

Another situation in which the goal and problem could be combined in the statement of the working diagnosis is that of the elderly Scandinavian lady we discussed earlier—the one who wanted to return to her own home and previous independent lifestyle following treatment for her fractured hip. It could be stated as:

> Desired return to usual, independent, solo lifestyle threatened by fx hip and old age.

Again, placing the client's goal in juxtaposition with the barriers to it gives perspective to all of her care, both nursing and medical. Shorter term goals can be developed within this.

Nurses in a children's hospital told us of another example in which goal and problem readily combined. Parents of a 13-year-old girl who had sustained critical brain damage in an auto accident were denied access to accurate knowledge of her poor prognosis for weeks. They were coping with her continued coma and the life-sustaining therapy by a combination of anger and denial. They were hostile toward the nursing staff, which generated negative feelings in them in return. They continued to plan for the child's future, including the purchase of a new winter coat despite their limited funds. The physician would not inform them, nor permit them to be informed, that she was being kept alive by mechanical means and that possibility of return of cerebral function was virtually nil. The nursing staff had goals for the parents as well as the child. Their combined problem-goal working diagnosis was:

> Lack of knowledge regarding negative prognosis—arrests the grieving process at denial/anger stages.

The implied long-term goal for the parents was to work through the eventual loss of their daughter as they lived daily with her dying. As these nurses worked through their problem/goal statement, they were able to set immediate goals in terms of encounters with both the physician and the family. They reported interactions became more productive and satisfying.

Thus, it is possible to combine problem/goal statements advantageously at times, at least in terms of long-term goals. Sub-goals of shorter duration undoubtedly need to be made explicit in thinking and/or writing as a basis of productive use of time and resources with clients.

SUMMARY

Goals need to be recognized in order to understand the dynamics of behavior —ours and that of others. They need to be created explicitly in order (1) to serve as guides to behavior, (2) to set the pace of the interaction and activities, (3) to offer a sense of progress and accomplishment, and (4) to serve as the foundation for criteria setting and evaluation.

Nurses' and clients' goals may be identical, they may be different but not incompatible, or they may be diametrically opposed. The nurses' data base must eventually include information on the client's goals in health and illness. Since explicit goal identification is difficult, nurses may need to infer the client's goals from presenting cues rather than direct statements and then validate them with the client. On the other hand, nurses too have unrecognized goals and it is equally important that these too be identified honestly and openly.

Goals are time-oriented; therefore, skill in goal setting must incorporate timing which offers high probability that goals are accomplishable within the time spans set or agreed upon. The achievement of goals often implies movement or change, but it can also involve lack of change, slowing of undesired change, or living in some form of acceptance of what cannot be modified.

We have considered goal setting within the context of the client-nurse relationship. In actuality, this is only a part of the larger aspect of health care management. Therefore, client-nurse developed goals must become a harmonious part of an overall health care goal. For, while each discipline involved in contributing to the well-being of a client will have goals related to its own area of expertise, none should be contradictory to the overall health goal that has been set. Of course, this demands interdependent relationships among the health care disciplines involved in helping the client. Those of us who have participated in this type of shared planning have found a bonus in the growth of insight on possible goals (even as we may have been frustrated by the differences that undoubtedly will occur). As we learn from clients and colleagues, we can also communicate nursing's vista, expertise, and contribution to health care. It is an opportunity for growth for each participant, and it certainly challenges us as nurses to create and communicate goals that will command the respect of client and colleague alike.

REFERENCE

Cullinane, M. "The Blossoming of Ruthie," *American Journal of Nursing* 68:112-124, January, 1968.

Bloom, Benjamin, et al. *Taxonomy of Educational Objectives, Handbook I: Cognitive Domain.* New York: David McKay, 1956.

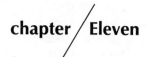

chapter / Eleven

The Nurse and the Prescriptive Process

When the problem areas have been defined and the client/nurse goals determined, the next step in care planning is to select the actions that are expected to achieve the goals. This constitutes the plan of nursing management. Its basic unit is the nursing order.

Again, an adequate knowledge base and skill in verbalization are vital. This is true regardless of whether the order is to oneself and, therefore, communicated in thought only, or whether it is communicated to others in speaking or writing. The rationale should also be as sound whether it forms the basis for personal action or for the actions of others. Beyond these basic skills, one needs to consider the practicalities of the situation. An action that is seen as unacceptable by the client will be unlikely to achieve either his or the nurse's goals. A prescription that does not take into account the feasibility of implementation in terms of staff, supplies, equipment, and money is also doomed to failure.

NURSING ORDERS, WHAT THEY ARE AND WHAT THEY ARE NOT

Nursing orders are directives for specific behavior on the part of the nurse or others, based on a known scientific rationale whenever possible. The expectation is that the prescribed behavior will benefit the client in a predicted way related to the diagnosed problem and accepted goal.

The nursing order has the intent of *individualizing* care to give maximum health benefits to a particular client at a particular time. It is this quality of individualization (based on collected data) that differentiates the nursing order from some other closely related plans for health care, plans that nurses may be expected to use.

Standard Nursing Plans Are Not Nursing Orders

Standard plans for the management of nursing tasks or observations associated with certain diagnoses or treatments have often been labeled care plans. True, they are plans. True, they involve care a nurse gives. But they deal with what is to be done or observed and with techniques that constitute COMMONAL-ITIES of care.

Nursing orders, by contrast, do not communicate what is to be done the *same;* instead, they indicate how approaches must be *DIFFERENT*—modified to suit this client's needs at this time. How would your delivery of "standard hysterectomy care" to Mrs. Brown differ from the way you deliver "standard hysterectomy care" to Ms. Rust?

Standard plans are excellent, efficient ways of communicating expected actions to a staff when staff capabilities require this kind of reminding. They can be duplicated on small cards which can be slipped into the Kardex together with the client's card—Tracheostomy Care, Radiation Implantation Care, Preoperative Care, Postoperative Care. . . . What is important is that nurses don't waste time copying standard orders, or presuming that these take the place of individualized care plans. Machines can duplicate these. Instead, nursing talents should be invested in what machines cannot do. Use the plans as a point of departure for creating individualized plans of nursing management based on the current data and nursing judgment.

Delegated Medical Functions Are Not Nursing Orders

Originally Kardexes were used as a convenient way of communicating delegated medical care. They are still effectively used to do this. In fact, Nursing Kardexes in many places are more effectively communicating medical care than nursing care (Ciuca, 1973; Pankratz, 1974). Now, there is no question that nurses legitimately implement medical plans of care. It is part of our current role.

But we do need to separate one from the other in our minds so that clients do not suffer through neglect in the nursing area as a result of our thinking that medical management and nursing management are synonymous. They are, and should be, complementary but not identical.

In many Kardex forms these days we notice that nurses are separating the space for Medical Orders from the space for Nursing Orders. In fact, some places are not even including any medical orders on their Kardex. This certainly serves to alert the staff to the absence of nursing orders since it does not permit the same space to be occupied by the medical plan of care. If there are no nursing plans, that Kardex is bare.

As with the standard plans for nursing care, the complementarity of planned nursing care to medical care becomes apparent in the *style* of carrying out the medical order or in the additional nursing actions that may accompany it. These nursing actions might deal with related teaching, discussion of dietary implications of a potassium-losing diuretic, techniques for preventing the spread of the infection for which the individual is receiving treatment, drug side effects, or contraindications of other drugs (particularly across-the-counter drugs), ways in which the individual might modify the treatment at home, and so forth. On the other hand, they might deal with quite different approaches to the client that could be carried on while the medically prescribed treatments are being implemented. Or the nursing orders may be carried on in the absence of any delegated medical functions.

In the article "The Blossoming of Ruthie," the order to sing to Ruthie and other orders that teach her to talk, to play, and to learn to deal with her hyperactivity in increasingly effective ways are examples of nonmedically oriented nursing orders that will be carried on in the presence or absence of medical care (Cullinane, 1968). Other orders complementary to medical care might deal with the provision of adequate and appropriate kinds of sensory stimulation, helping the client to find mechanisms to deal with loneliness (Hood, 1974), with loss of sleep, with transportation deficits, with activity schedules, or with other aspects of daily living in hospital, home, school, recreational and industrial settings.

Naturally, we should continue to collaborate with doctors and implement their medical plans of care, but not confuse nursing and medical prescriptions.

ACCOUNTABILITY IN NURSING ORDERS

As nurses we have been much sloppier in our expectations for accountability, for currency, and for precision of prescription of nursing care than we would ever tolerate in the parallel performance of our medical colleagues. Delegated medical care is not carried out by nurses unless it is prescribed, preferably in writing, and signed by a doctor who is then accountable for the outcomes resulting from his decisions. It is expected that medical orders will be reviewed and updated periodically. In fact, in some areas of treatment, orders must be updated every 48 to 72 hours or they will not be acted upon at all. Nor do we tolerate an order so ambiguous that we would have inadequate guides for the actions involved. For example, no nurse would accept an order of:

> "Give a broad spectrum antibiotic, a few tablets several times a day, for a while."

We require precision from the physician or no care is implemented.

Once medical orders are transmitted, we have an elaborate system to assure that they are carried out, implemented, and recorded. There are chart flagging systems and special personnel to transcribe the orders and to incorporate them into the various systems involved. We have recording systems of implementation. We spend a great proportion of the change of shift report communicating the medical plan of care in our acute care institutions (Copp, 1972). Further, when medical orders are not implemented for some reason or other, it raises a real ruckus including incident reports, and often confrontation.

In contrast, nursing apparently has considered its own contribution as unworthy of even a portion of such expenditures of energy or such an elaborate system. Maybe we do not see it as so important, or perhaps we do not have clinicians skilled enough in diagnostic and prescriptive nursing skills. On the other hand, we may not wish to give up our individual freedom to nurse in any way we as individuals see fit, leaving it to the client to make the adjustments (Palison, 1971; Trasker, 1970, 34). Prescription implies the control of one person over the responses of another. Certainly, our current system of assigning nurses to constantly shifting case loads, hours, and floors in institutions does not permit any personal sense of accountability for more than immediate shift-oriented care. Our strong belief that all individuals are created equal seems to result in a corollary that everyone, therefore, must prescribe nursing care or else an elitist system will result. As a consequence, in many settings, no one really coordinates the nursing management of the client's care and in the end no one person is accountable.

But for whatever reason: time, skill, interest, opportunity, confusion as to content area, beliefs in democracy or in the fact that clients have gotten along so far without all this folderol, the fact is that nursing orders are not effectively written, and where written are often ignored in a great many health care settings.

We believe that when nursing is seen as making a significant contribution to the well-being of clients' health, we as nurses are going to insist on nursing's accountability for coordinated, consistent, prescribed nursing management.

KNOWLEDGE AND THE NURSING ORDER

Prescribing nursing actions or behavior is not as simple as it used to be. There was a time when we just "knew" what needed to be done and we did it. With our maturation into a more truly professional approach, intuition becomes much less acceptable. More often now, nursing actions are expected to be deliberative and purposeful. They are taken because the nurse has data on what is going on and on desired changes. There is knowledge of the underlying mechanics or dynamics of the phenomenon as well as the effects certain options of intervention should predictably have. In other words, when a client is having ventilation problems you do not automatically order, "Stay with the patient while he deep breathes 10x q̄ h.," without having information in some of the following areas:

Is there any pathophysiology interfering with ventilation?
What does deep breathing accomplish in the face of this?
Why not prescribe yawning? Or sighing? (Alexander, 1969; Cahill, 1973.)

Is any position more effective during the maneuver? (Alexander, 1969.)

Why choose the number 10 x?

Why choose the interval of one hour between the activity?

What attitudinal dynamics do you expect to modify by being present during the activity? How will your presence accomplish this?

The body of scientific principles embodying the prescription of nursing care must be used as logically as that buttressing medical therapy. We would want it for ourselves. We should want it for our clientele.

NURSING ORDERS AND THEIR COMPONENTS

We have deliberately chosen the term "nursing order" in preference to such alternatives as "approaches," "suggested approaches," "activities," "actions," and "interventions." Our rationale is that the term "order" carries with it a sense of accountability for the one who gives the order in terms of its correctness and outcome. Also, it extends accountability to the reader/implementor to carry it out.

Nursing orders are made up of five components:

> Date
>
> Precise action verb and possibly a modifier
>
> Content area
>
> Time element
>
> Signature.

No nursing order is complete without the inclusion of all of these.

Date

Written nursing orders are dated. They are reviewed regularly within specified intervals in terms of client response. They are then discontinued, renewed, revised and updated.

The interval specified for review and updating will of course vary with the clientele. Certainly, any order may be revised at any time, but there should be a maximum time limit set for an order to be in effect. In a clientele which changes very slowly, perhaps a month or even longer is an acceptable interval. During the research project in which nurse specialists cared for chronically ill men, the goals, orders and client progress had to be evaluated, progress notes written, and the plan renewed or revised monthly. We found, of course, that many orders had been modified, deleted or added within that time span, but this was the overall review period for each case. Obviously, in an acute care setting, such a time span would be absolutely inappropriate. Daily or weekly reviews are needed. In intensive care units, emergency units, walk-in clinics with few repeaters, and similar situations, a review deadline may not be appropriate at all. But in most settings, it maintains the continuity and momentum of the nursing care as well as evidence of evaluation and progress of the client in the nursing dimension.

Whatever the system of renewal, each order should be dated or timed. It offers perspective to the one who reads it and to the one who carries it out.

Action Verbs and Modifiers

Each nursing order begins with an active, not passive, verb communicating the specific behavior to be engaged in by the implementor, whether that person be oneself or others. Even more precision may be achieved by adding a modifying word or phrase.

Some common examples of imprecision. Examples of imprecise verbs used in nursing orders abound. We have all used them when we were too lazy to find the right word, or did not have enough data to know what the precise action should be. Let's look at some examples:

"Have the client . . ."

Does this prescriber want you to:

> Ask the client if he will?
> Request the client to . . .?
> Demand that he . . .?
> Remind him to . . .?
> Observe to see if he carries out the activity without reminding?
> Acknowledge when he remembers to . . .?

Each of these behaviors is quite different and each could be productive or counterproductive with a given client. It is therefore the responsibility of the prescriber to decide which behavior is likely to be the one of choice for this client at this time and to make a decision by ordering the precise behavior, not using the word, "have."

Reassure

Does the prescriber wish you to:

> Pat the client on the shoulder and say soothingly, "Don't worry"?
> Give reality-oriented data on observed progress? On lack of decline?
> Listen to him?
> Stay with him?
> Touch him? Refrain from touching?
> Stay away so that he knows you trust him to take responsibility for himself?
> Inform him of your belief in his capability?
> Introduce him to others who are coping effectively, given similar stresses and deficits?

Reassurance is generated by many forms of behavior, but they are not synonymous nor interchangeably effective. Again, the prescriber must decide which behavior is appropriate for this client now and communicate this.

Teach

When this action is prescribed are you to:

Tell	Reverse role play
Explore	Interpret
Listen	Draw
Show	Require
Demonstrate	Identify
Observe	Discover
Critique	Ignore
Evaluate	Provide
Role model	Share
Role play	Reward

These behaviors and quite a few others could result in learning, or in some situations could just as well be nonproductive. Choose, be precise, and take responsibility for your choice.

These are but three of the very broad verbs we often see in nursing care orders. They are words which do not communicate expected behavior very precisely. Think of others you have seen that left you wondering what the prescriber intended.

To gain skill in achieving a broader working vocabulary of verbs that will be useful in prescribing care and in thinking in terms of specificity rather than generalities, undertake individual activities, ward conferences or inservice conferences in which you select one of the global terms currently in vogue. Then list the operational terms that would be more precise, hence, more useful. You could expand on the three cited already in the chapter, or begin with one of the following:

support

encourage

do (as in range of motion)

counsel

force (as in fluids)

provide (as in TLC)

ambulate

observe

cough and deep breathe

give

reinforce

In practice, ask a colleague who has used a general verb to tell you what she/he wants you to do, what has been done, what has been working. Then try to place the behavior into the most descriptive verb form. Be sure to compliment those who do prescribe specifically and whose orders are easy to follow. Make specificity the goal and the norm, not generality. Create both the skill and the climate for precision in prescribing actions.

Modifiers. In addition to the word prescribing the action, precision may be enhanced by adding modifiers. Words such as gently, aggressively, pleasantly, firmly, slowly, quickly, softly, loudly, neutrally, vigorously, actively, passively, and a host of others, give more of a sense of the style with which an action is to be performed. Sometimes phrases instead of words may be used such as: with humor, in accordance with her mood, with resistance, and the like.

Content Areas

The content area deals with the substance, the "what" and "where," of the order. Which joints are to be exercised? What fluids are to be offered? What subject is to be discussed? What skills are to be demonstrated or observed? Where is the person to ambulate? What activity is to be engaged in? What position is the person to be moved to? What is the location of the materials? What is the person to wear?

If an order has been written telling the person caring for a mentally retarded child to sing to him, the content would deal with what is to be sung. Now, if this week, he particularly enjoys "Old MacDonald Had a Farm" and is currently able to follow along with the sounds of the verses about the ducks, the cows, and the dog, then this content area should be indicated. Repetition may be important to his achieving progress in his verbal skills. Where continuity is desired and repetition or variety is important, the content area becomes significant.

Again the quality of specificity should prevail. For example, a prescription to, "Teach diabetes" is less than helpful. Diabetes is a vast area. As we have already shown, teaching can involve a variety of very different behaviors. Has this client worked through his feelings about a changed body image and lifestyle, so that it is content, not attitudes, that is to be the focus? Or both? Are we currently dealing with skills of insulin injection? Or urine testing? Or diet? Are we to prescribe modifications of usual/expected eating patterns that will result in variety and satisfaction? Can the client fit the diet into his budget? Prescribing content and action needs to focus the reader's attention.

Time Element

The time element indicates when, how often and how long. It may be as precise as a clock hour (9-1-6). It may be associated with certain nursing actions such as: when you enter the room, or while you are giving the injection, when you are putting him to bed. . . . It may be associated with a client response: when he has a temper tantrum, when the output is below . . . each time he mentions pain, if he begins to. . . .

Such time prescriptions as: frequently, ad lib, q̄ 2 h, and prn are less than helpful. Data need to have been collected so we know when ad lib is likely to occur, when the action tends to be needed, and which two hours.

A common nursing order is, "Turn q̄ 2 h." To demonstrate what a miserable order this could be if it were not tailored to the patterns of the individual, we have asked groups of nurses to assume that they were going to be our clients, clients who are not able to turn themselves and hence are in need of a turning schedule. Now, tailoring a turning schedule so that it is comfortable to the individual involves collecting data on a few key variables such as:

> *Are you right-handed or left-handed?* (Data needed to know which hand to keep free during mealtimes if they can't assume a supine position.)
>
> *What hours of the night do you sleep best?* (This should influence the time periods when the turning schedule might be held in abeyance in order to enhance normal sleeping patterns.)
>
> *What is your preferred sleeping position?* (A combination of the preferred sleeping position during the preferred sleeping hours is a happier grouping than a disliked position during these hours. Save the less preferred positions for hours when they don't sleep well.)
>
> *When do you expect visitors?* (Visiting hours is the wrong time for the prone position.)
>
> *Is there a time when you really want to watch TV or engage in hand work or reading?* (Again the wrong time for prone position.)

Not being able to move yourself is bad enough. Being placed by others into positions which are undesired or uncomfortable, and being moved at the inconvenient times makes the situation even worse. To prescribe, "Turn q̄ 2 h," or "Turn frequently," carries with it high risk of creating an ineffective living situation. Further, people who cannot turn themselves are often going to be institutionalized for some time, so the time spent in getting answers to these five questions could be considered cost effective to say nothing of humane. It does not take long to note the turning schedule in terms of times and positions on a card and tape it to the bed or bedside stand. This, together with a timed treatment card (indicating the hours of turning but not the position schedule), can be given to any person caring for the client on any shift and this should expeditiously and economically result in the most satisfying care for the client—in one dimension at least.

The other dimension of timing is duration—how long. One client, when asked what she wanted most in nursing care said, "If I could just be sure a nurse would be in to sit down and talk with me for five minutes on each shift, it would make me feel so much better." In another situation where a client was becoming utterly fatigued from too frequent attention, the time element concerned the duration of an interval in which he was *not* to be visited or contacted or cared for unless he signaled.

Appropriate kinds of timing are essential to an effective nursing order. Look for the time designation on the orders you think of, write, see others write or hear. Critique them. Improve your timing skill.

Signature

The final element of a nursing order is the signature of the prescriber. It is another manifestation of accountability—personal and legal, if the record becomes part of the permanent document. It permits nursing colleagues to give feedback on the effectiveness of the order, to explore the rationale of an order, to obtain clarification. And *if* the situation should persist where everyone writes orders, a signature at least enables the reader to judge the level of expertise that formed the foundation of the prescription.

RECORDING NURSING ORDERS

Nursing orders are only recently coming into their own as a legitimate part of the health care record system. Many nurses have not believed in them; and this lack of conviction did not generate much interest in them or sense of importance for them in other parts of the health care system. Even the labels—Suggested Approaches or Actions—had a slippery, elastic quality that negated accountability for either the prescriber or the implementer.

However, there is growing awareness that nursing management (even more than medical management among some clientele, in some settings, or during some stages of illness) is the key to survival, maintenance, rehabilitation and prevention. With this acknowledgment, the need for legal evidence, quality control and accountability has become increasingly urgent. A corollary of this is that plans for nursing management cannot be kept in some nebulous state within the nurse's head, but must be documented explicitly and publicly in a permanent form.

This does not mean that all nursing orders will appear on client order sheets or on a Kardex. It does mean that any significant efforts at nursing management, whether carried out by a single individual or shared with others, should appear on the client's legal, permanent record, either on an order sheet, the Patient Progress sheet or the Nurses Notes.

Regularly scheduled nursing actions may also be documented on the medicines and treatment page together with the record of implementation of regularly scheduled delegated medical functions. This not only gives documentary evidence of the nature, quantity, and perhaps quality of nursing management, but it also increases nursing's visibility in a real and pragmatic way that is essential in establishing a genuine working colleague status and relationship.

Having said that nursing orders should be recorded somewhere, we should now examine criteria for deciding where this recording should take place. The criteria we have found helpful are simple, few and pragmatic.

1. Include documentation of nursing management undertaken and client response in all relevant charting on nurses notes and/or progress sheets. This should be done regardless of whether one nurse or more are dealing with the problem or the care.
   Record, tick off, and initial regularly scheduled nursing activities on the Medicine and Treatment sheet to give efficient yet legal evidence of the quantity and nature of *regularly scheduled* nursing contacts and actions.
2. Include on the sheet devoted to orders (and this may be an integrated Patient Orders form in which medical and nursing orders are combined, a separate Nursing Orders sheet, or the Problem Oriented Progress Notes and Orders sheet using the S-O-A-P format), any prescribed nursing orders *you or your colleagues* will carry out.
3. Include on the Kardex *only* those diagnoses/problems, goals and orders that *should* involve other nursing staff in either their perspective for observation and interpretation or in carrying out the prescribed actions. For example: You would not write "Teach TCBD" (turning, coughing, and deep breathing). Imagine how the preoperative patient would feel if all nursing personnel who came in to him for 24 hours preoperatively literally acted on that order.

Nursing Orders Not Placed on the Kardex

Personal prescriptions. Nursing orders can and should be developed in one's thoughts to prescribe personal behavior when only one nurse will deal with the client in any particular diagnostic/problem area. Making explicit the kind of behavior to be personally engaged in should involve the same rigor that is expected when nursing orders are written to modify the behavior of others.

Personal orders are verbalized in thought rather than in writing. However, nurses who are in solo practice (Public Health, clinic, office, school, industry) or independent practitioners should record nursing orders as a basis for perspective in continuing contacts, legal evidence, and data for quality control.

Whether the personal prescriptions are thought or written, the individual should require the same precision of thought. The verbs should be explicit, the content area focused, the timing acknowledged. Developing thinking habits of this type sets the pattern and develops the skill that are the antecedents to committing the orders to writing. If you can't think it, you can't write it. If you can think it, the action of writing is relatively simple.

This pattern of thinking before carrying out nursing actions is a behavior associated with the professional nurse role. Just as one learns the difference between social and therapeutic communication in early nursing classes, so one must learn to differentiate between *spontaneous* and *prescribed* nursing behavior.

Each has its place, but the productive use of each must be differentiated (Rogers, 1955; Peplau, 1969).

One-time orders. One-time orders, carried out by the nurse or someone else, do not need to be recorded on the Kardex. However, if a problem-oriented form or nursing orders sheet is part of the client's legal record and nursing is functioning other than as an implementation system for delegated medical activities, then one-time orders should be recorded on these sheets for documentary evidence of nursing decisions. Some examples of one-time orders that would not appear on the Kardex would be: client referral to a dietitian or social worker, the teaching of knowledge or skill the client learns in one session, preparation for a one-time test or treatment, or discharge planning done by one nurse.

Implementation of such orders together with notable client response are of course recorded on the progress sheet or nurses notes—wherever the nurse charts nonroutine events or care.

Orders Implemented by Others

In most settings, at least institutional ones, nursing orders that are intended to influence the behavior of others are recorded on Kardexes only. However, with increasing frequency they are becoming a regular component of the client's permanent, legal record so that evidence of both medical and nursing management is preserved. Where the nurse's prescription is made initially on the client's record, some mechanism similar to that used for doctors must be developed to get the nursing orders into the system. The decision on whether expensive professional nurses spend their time copying their own orders in all the necessary places—Kardex, treatment cards, and so on, or some less expensive support person takes on this task is an administrative one that will need to be made in each system.

Certainly, most nursing orders are communicated in writing via the Kardex, but that is not the only way. In nursing homes, bedtime rituals and turning schedules are being placed on cards that are issued to the person giving the care on the appropriate shift. Placement of articles in a consistent location on bedside surfaces for the blind or prone-positioned clients is communicated via labels affixed to the surface of that piece of furniture. Placement of furniture in a room for blind persons could be marked on the floor. In other words, the nursing orders are being located in the place and in the manner which will result in the most consistent effective implementation. Both creativity and logic are being focused on doing just this, rather than accepting a single approach such as total reliance on the Kardex.

For example, where the client is assuming the major role as planner and the nurse is the supporting consultant, the plan or contract itself might well remain in the client's possession. Only those orders influencing the nurse's behavior need be noted on the nursing record or Kardex.

Nor are the nursing orders always communicated in words. While working with nurses in institutions for the mentally retarded, we learned about pictorial nursing orders. In these settings, other residents who can't read are frequent implementors of nursing orders on dressing, undressing, and hair combing. The nurses developed color-coded line drawings that indicated what a particular resident could do by himself, with some help, and those activities where the helper had to do it all. One pair of figures (dress/undress) was created for boys, another for girls. (See illustration for a facsimile.)

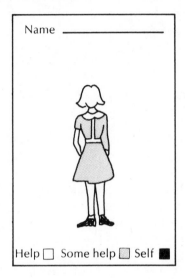

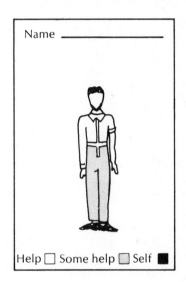

As nursing is becoming more creative, we are weaning ourselves from blind rituals. We can make nursing orders functional without constraints. At the same time, the legal record of decisions on plans for nursing management and strategies for effective communication of these decisions for implementation must be handled now and in the immediate future. Nor can we overlook the importance of the computer in nursing as well as medical records; it, too, must be creatively handled to foster individualized nursing care.

BARRIERS TO ACCOUNTABILITY IN NURSING ORDERS

There are several barriers or conflicts in the development of effective nursing prescriptions. The territory of medicine and nursing offers many grey areas in which nurses tend not to prescribe. The avoidance of these grey areas results in gaps in health care management, while active prescription within these areas can result in interprofessional conflicts. A second major deterrent to accountability in prescribing nursing care is the current institutional staffing patterns. Finally, there is the frequent practice of group planning—a very expensive approach which ends

221

up with no one person having the responsibility or accountability for the effectiveness of the plan. Let's look at these three barriers more closely.

Conflicts in Areas for Nursing Orders

When any two disciplines are closely related and serving the same clientele, there are bound to be disagreements over the boundaries of responsibilities. Such, of course, is the case with medicine and nursing. At a somewhat earlier time, nursing was even in retreat from areas where it *had* held responsibility. This occurred when staff made errors within these areas of responsibility; then, decisions would be made to place these nursing judgments within the domain of the physician.

Now, as nurses are seeking to achieve more professional approaches to the services they give in order to improve health care delivery, they are seeking to appropriately increase the territory of their accountability. They want to include judgments which their contacts with clients and their preparation place them in the best position to use in offering effective health care management. For example, in institutional settings, nurses are often the first to know that a client normally uses a bed board and therefore needs one, or that he has a fluid imbalance and, therefore, intake and output records or weighing need to be initiated. They have more data on eating patterns and can modify diet textures or substances within prescribed therapeutic diets. Nurses may be the first to note a sign or symptom that suggests the need for a lab test, wound culture, the checking of vital signs at a particular time or rating the level of consciousness. They know of the home situation and the need for home *nursing* supervision or assistance through a public health referral. Yet, policies dictate that most of these areas must be prescribed by physicians. And, further, any service that is billed, a sheepskin, a public health referral, a laboratory test, must be physician-signed if the cost is to be reimbursed. Not only in institutional settings are the nurses placed in narrow boxes; school nurses, public health nurses, industrial nurses also are in constraints that minimize areas of legal prescription.

Yet, despite the legal, bureaucratic, and financial pressures to maintain a physician-centered medical care model, many nurses are vigorously testing the borders of nursing territory. They are writing nursing orders as individuals. They are working as groups within institutions and agencies to legitimize areas of practice where nurses have the qualifications and the need to be accountable for nursing care. They are also working through their professional organizations to develop interprofessional liaison committees and to achieve legal changes through legislation on state and national levels.

Obviously, with any new territory of accountability, comes a parallel need for the knowledge base and prescriptive skills to deal with problems safely and creatively. It also means that nurses consistently must maintain quality control over the areas of their accountability in prescription of nursing care, so that once again these are not lost to other professions through incompetence. Beyond this, we need to learn how to assume responsibility for our decisions when they are questioned, or when they appear inappropriate (and some of them will be). In the areas covered by nursing orders, we need to behave like professionals.

Staffing Patterns, Assignments, and Accountability in Nursing Orders

We still have a way to go when it comes to normalizing accountability for nursing management. In most institutions currently, nurses fill slots rather than carry responsibility for case loads. These slots are best filled by maintaining maximum flexibility and "floatability" of the staff from assignment to assignment and unit to unit. No wonder the nurse feels responsible to the task and not to the client. As one nurse told us, "I never know when or if I'll have the same patients again, so what's the point in my trying to do assessments or individualize their care? What's important is that I get all the assigned care done on my shift." When this built-in pattern of transiency is the norm, an attitude of shift-limited, task orientation is a predictable result. Non-acute care institutions and solo practice nurses of course do not have the same situation. Our current staffing practices affect about 70 percent of nurses, those who work in acute care settings. Yet these same institutions' accreditation standards say that there will be planned care.

In recent years there has been a growing effort in some institutions and by some nurses to change this orientation from slots and tasks to client management case loads where staff have cases for whom they have the responsibility of planning, if not total implementation of the care. Primary nursing, as developed by Manthey in a Minnesota hospital, was "alive and well" when last heard from (Manthey, 1973). A decade earlier pairs of nurse specialists were managing the care planning for case loads in a chronic disease hospital (Little et al, 1965). Other places are currently using nursing care coordinators, clinical coordinators, patient care coordinators, and clinical specialists who have round-the-clock responsibility for planning the nursing care for clients on an ongoing basis. On some obstetric units nurses are taking responsibility for coordinating the nursing management of the mother, the infant and the family. Some HMOs and OB clinics are seeking to have nurses involved in the prenatal care, attend the mother during labor and delivery, and then supervise the post partum nursing management, not only in the hospital but also in the extended period. Similar patterns of responsibility for management of client and family needs are seen in pediatrics.

If personal accountability is to come, styles of utilizing nursing personnel and continuity of assignment of case loads must be reexamined. Flexibility/floatability are incompatible with accountability for client-oriented management and continuity.

Group Planning and Accountability in Nursing Orders

Now, what of the practice of planning for the care of clients by committee? In many places nurses tell us that care plans are developed in nursing care conferences. Here decisions are arrived at by consensus after all the data collected and the inferences drawn have been reviewed.

This would seem to be a pretty expensive way of planning care. If one multiplies the minutes consumed in developing each plan of care by the hourly rates of the persons involved, it mounts up. Try it and see. Furthermore, there is often real difficulty in gathering the group together regularly enough to maintain plans of care on case loads of 10 to 20 or more clients.

Certainly, input of data from multiple sources is necessary. The brainstorming can be helpful, particularly if the diagnosis is elusive or the plan for nursing treatment difficult, and particularly if the difficulties relate to staff problems with the client or his family. But from what we have observed, often this practice of planning by committee is just a means of distributing responsibility. When used this way it does not seem to be a particularly economic or efficient strategy.

We also hear, "But we learn so much from those care conferences!" Fine! If they are teaching-learning sessions, label them as such and charge them to staff development where they properly belong, not to the cost of giving client care.

By all means, use whatever data on the client that any personnel—nursing or otherwise—are willing to share that has relevance to the planning for staff development. But do not allow misuse of beliefs about democracy, self-actualization, group spirit or learning needs to diffuse the accountability for decision making to all persons. It will be the quickest route to fostering fragmentation with no personal sense of responsibility and no overall accountability for cohesive planning. Random planning may have been an appropriate model when health care was equated with medical care and the physician was ultimately responsible for it all, but it is outmoded when nurses assume accountability for management of nursing care. A nurse is responsible for decisions on nursing care just as a physician assumes legal responsibility for decisions on medical care. Each one may consult with persons in and outside of his own field, but in the end, the decisions and accompanying legal responsibilities rest, not with a team, not with contributing colleagues or nonprofessionals, but with the one assigned to the case.

THE INTERPERSONAL DIMENSION OF NURSING ORDERS

Nurses are beginning to find that nursing care plans impede individual freedom to relate to patients in a spontaneous, untrammelled fashion. Palison cited this as one of the reasons why nursing care plans were " . . . a Snare and a Delusion" (Palison, 1971).

Nurses learn early and well to accept medical orders. Research has shown that they do it so well that they may even accept orders by phone from an un-known "physician" for a nonexistent drug, or a dosage that is questionable. By contrast, the dynamics of having one's nursing behavior modified by another nurse, other than one above us in the hierarchy, has not been taught. But to be fair, to date not that many nursing orders have been written that put this behavior to the test either.

However, with the concept of accountability for decisions and the shift from the philosophy of "Suggested Approaches" to "Nursing Orders", there is a defi-nite change in the obligation of one nurse to carry out the activity and the style of responding prescribed by a colleague. This has raised some interpersonal problems.

If the concept of accountability is accepted and implemented, it means that the prescriber is charged with the results of his/her decisions and it means that the implementor is charged with the obligation to carry out the activity as ordered, negotiate for change or face the consequences of failure to carry it out as ordered. Accountability means that responsibilities for behaviors are fixed—attached to spe-cific people who then are held liable for the quality of their judgments and ac-tions—commissions and omissions.

Somehow a climate to accommodate to this concept of accountability needs to be worked through in our care systems, particularly in institutional settings. Its ramifications and its implications for day-to-day nursing behavior and nurse to nurse role relationships needs to be explored, tested, and systematized. Other-wise we will be in the same position we have been in before when we equated the *saying* with the doing. We said *team leading* and it became a euphemism for functional assignment. We said *patient centered care* and continued with stand-ardized routines. We said *total* and *comprehensive care* and continued to give high priority care. Now we may say *accountability* and continue with everyone assum-ing responsibility and no one assuming it.

We have seen a variety of strategies used to quietly but effectively subvert nursing plans that were not acceptable, or whose authors were not respected. These "games" are counter-productive. They are not compatible with accountability.

Every nurse has an obligation to be judicious about obeying an appropriate order from a doctor or a nurse. It is part of the law that governs our practice. No one in operationalizing this concept of accountability for nursing decisions is speaking of blind obedience. What is being structured is the development of ac-cepted policies of behavior when an order is seen as inappropriate or inadequate. What do you do at that time? What are you obliged to do in giving feedback to the author of the order?

Certainly an accepted protocol for action to be taken when one disagrees with an order should be fully explored and the acceptable options spelled out. In addition, these options should be tested by means of role playing with nurses taking roles of both the prescriber and the dissatisfied implementor to gain in-

225

sight into the feelings that can be generated in using these options. We know differences of opinion in nursing management occur regularly and will undoubtedly continue to occur. We handle many of them now by ignoring a diagnosis or order. If in the future that option is no longer available, then other normalized, productive means must be found to deal with these differences.

We would suggest as an early activity, designed to create a climate for genuine accountability, that rap sessions be undertaken in which accountability as applied to nursing management for clients (and particularly nursing orders) be openly explored. The discussion should deal with the disadvantages, the advantages, the attendant problems and the ways of preventing or dealing with them in a productive fashion. This may take one or more meetings, but they should be open, initially unstructured—no holds barred—ventilating, think sessions. When most of the ideas and feelings seem to be out in the open, the next goal should be to reach some kinds of agreement for formalizing some role relationships between nurses in the areas of prescribing-implementing planned care. These can be tried out on one or more units on an experimental basis for a designated period of time. Then they should be evaluated and revised as needed before they are further formalized into policies and expected behavior.

Also important in the development of a climate for accountability and growth in the skills of nursing prescription is the establishment of a climate where perfection is not the established norm. Nurses, like doctors, lawyers, social workers, and others are dealing with difficult, elusive, fluid situations where the total picture is never fully seen. We are obliged to do our best and to get better. We are obliged to learn from orders that didn't work. But we are not obliged to write infallible orders. Feedback on less-than-perfect orders should be an expected, ongoing, professional development, not an ego-shattering experience. And the styles for giving feedback to assist in upgrading nursing prescription skill need to have this positive quality. Critiques of nursing orders should include analysis of strengths and limitations. They should not be exercises in one-upsmanship.

Gaining skill in giving feedback that is helpful to the nurse prescriber can be learned. Inservice classes followed by role playing can be very helpful in this aspect of staff development.

THE CLIENT'S ROLE IN NURSING PRESCRIPTION

It is a rare occasion when the client manages his medical care—at least as long as he is under a physician's care. The client gives his data to the physician and the physician from his point of expertise decides on the diagnosis and the course of management. Sometimes there is consultation and options may be offered. Sometimes informed participation is sought (Scheff, 1965). But at other times the decisions seem quite unilateral with a minimum of truly informed consent.

Nursing management, concerned as it is with the client's living moment by moment, day by day with his health problems, must of necessity involve the client in the decision making early and regularly, if it is to succeed. In fact, the most successful nursing management results in the client's taking over entirely and being happy and successful in doing so if he has the prognosis and capability of doing so. This can be true whether he is "cured" or continues to deal with chronic illness. When he cannot take over entirely, success in nursing management can be gauged by his being a satisfied participant at whatever level. The surgeon may take out the patient's gall bladder for him, but he cannot make the decisions that will regulate his diet or other aspects of living once the individual is out of the hospital (Stimson, 1974).

Given the goal of informed participation and maximum independence, the degree of involvement of clients in the plans of care begins early and continues consistently. In acute intensive stages and in terminal stages the nurse may well have to assume the dominant planning and implementing role, with the client in a consulting role. And, where the client does not have the knowledge, the skill or the desire, the nurse may also temporarily assume a dominant role. However, successful prevention, maintenance and rehabilitation result only when the client assumes the dominant role in the planning and implementation and when the nurse becomes the consultant—giving expertise and support when needed. The nurse is more often a facilitator of client potential than a substitute for it, unless the deficits are too great and the resources too small.

The translation of these beliefs into actions in the area of planning for nursing orders means that when the client is capable of participating, and in whatever ways he is capable of participating, the plan of action with its rationale is discussed with him in terms of its usefulness to him. Where nursing actions must take place that are seen as undesirable to him, the rationale for them and for overriding his desires temporarily, or even on a long-term basis, are a necessary preliminary step.

Nurses who have been accustomed to carrying out doctor's orders routinely without informing clients or consulting them, may find the activities of validation and consultation with clients uncomfortable and strange. In fact, we may well be programming in a known role conflict if physicians are adamant that clients not be given information about their body responses and the effects of medications or treatments. In other words, if the physicians do not believe in an informed clientele or informed consent for participation in medical care, and particularly if they see nursing and medical care as synonymous, our suggestions here are sure to open up a wasp's nest. It is helpful to know what one is inviting before rushing in. There are no recipes for quick handling of these differences in philosophies between health care disciplines. It takes astuteness, courage, and often support from one's professional association where there are strength in numbers and the resources of skilled experts.

SUMMARY

Nursing orders are the means of communicating the behavior to be undertaken by the nurse or the nursing staff. Verbalization and particularly, precision in verbalization, are important whether the orders are in the form of prescriptive thoughts for oneself or written orders to others. Sound scientific rationale rather than intuition or ritual is the basis for effective prescription of nursing care as it is for medical care. Although complementary to delegated medical care and standard plans of care, nursing orders are not identical with them. Nursing orders carry with them accountability both for the prescriber in terms of the nature of the decisions and for the implementor in terms of carrying them out. Whenever possible, the client is an early ongoing participant in decisions of nursing management to the extent of his expertise, since the focus of nursing management is so intimately entwined with his everyday living and lifestyle. Interpersonal problems related to nursing orders need to be dealt with in group process on a predictive and ongoing basis. In the end, working with prescriptive skills as with each of the other aspects of the nursing process and nursing planning becomes another area for the nurse's balanced professional growth.

REFERENCES

Alexander, Ardyth. "*A Study of Nursing Measures for Improved Ventilation Following Surgery.*" Unpublished Master's Thesis, University of Washington, 1969.

Cahill, Cheryl. "*Comparison of the Yawn Maneuver to a Deep Breath.*" Seattle: Unpublished Master's Thesis, University of Washington, 1973.

Ciuca, Rudy. "Over the Years with the Nursing Care Plan." *Nursing Outlook* 20:706-711, November, 1972.

Copp, L. A. "Improvement of Care Through Evaluation—Change of Shift Report." *Bedside Nursing* 5:19-23, February, 1972.

Cullinane, M. "The Blossoming of Ruthie," *American Journal of Nursing* 68:122-124, January, 1968.

Hood, Phyllis. "*Perceived Loneliness Among the Aged and Associated Factors.*" Unpublished Master's Thesis, University of Washington, 1974.

Little, D., et al. *Nurse Specialist Effect on Tuberculosis.* Seattle: University of Washington School of Nursing, November, 1965. Mimeographed.

Manthey, M. "Primary Care is Alive and Well in the Hospital," *American Journal of Nursing* 73:83-87, January, 1973.

Manthey, M., and M. Kramer. "A Dialogue on Primary Nursing," *Nursing Forum* 9:356-379, No. 4, 1970.

Palison, H. "Nursing Care Plans are a Snare and a Delusion," *American Journal of Nursing* 71:63-66, January, 1971.

Pankratz, Deanne and Loren Pankratz, "The Nursing Care Plan: Theory and Reality," *Supervisor Nurse,* 3:51-55, April 1973.

Peplau, H. "Professional Closeness," *Nursing Forum* 8:343-358, No. 4, 1969.

Rogers, C. "Persons or Science, A Philosophical Question," *The American Psychologist* 10:267-278, July, 1955.

Scheff, T. "Typification in the Diagnostic Practices of Rehabilitation," in Marvin B. Sussman, ed., *Sociology and Rehabilitation*. Washington, D.C.: American Sociological Society, 1965, pp. 132-147.

Stimson, Gerry V. "Obeying Doctor's Orders: A View from the Other Side," *Social Science and Medicine* 8:97-103, 1974.

Trasker, R. "What is Health Planning." *Nursing Outlook* 18:33-35, January, 1970.

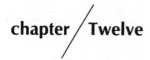

chapter Twelve

The Nurse and the Evaluation Process

How do you know when the client is moving toward the goals set? How will you recognize when a goal has been achieved? How do clients recognize when they are making progress toward a goal? How do you or they know whether or not the prescribed nursing actions being carried out are productive in terms of the client response?

When you begin to ask these questions you're ready to think about evaluation. If you are not asking these questions, or if you are not helping your client to ask these questions, you should be. Evaluation is a necessary and integral component of ongoing nursing care.

EVALUATION AS A PROCESS

Evaluation consists of three sequential steps:

1. selecting criteria or standards that will guide observation to specified areas of client response logically related to the diagnosis and goals.
2. collecting data in the currently presenting situation as prescribed by the observational guide.
3. comparing the evidence collected to the criterion standards and the baseline (if available) then making judgments about the nature of the response (such as direction, stability, achievement).

Evaluation, unlike assessment, is undertaken only *after* explicit or implicit goals have been set and some client-nurse activities have been undertaken in relationship to those goals. Thus it can never be an initial step in the nursing process. Where assessment is always concerned with arriving at a diagnosis of client status, evaluation is concerned with the client's status or movement within a specified goal area.

In both assessment and evaluation, data are collected and inferences are made; however, the sequence differs. In assessment the data collection takes place first.

The data are used as a basis for selecting which diagnostic concept best explains and organizes the findings in the presenting situation. At least initially, the diagnostician is an open, neutral, receptive surface—ready to receive any input from the client and his situation. The focusing begins only as initial tentative diagnoses are selected and branching logic exerts a directional force on the observation. In evaluation this initial, open type of observation is not present. Here the goal related criteria and their observational guides focus the data collection, so the observation is, even initially, controlled by them. Thus, while assessment and evaluation are similar in the activities involved, the sequence of steps and the purpose of the activities differ.

Now, having looked at the evaluation process in overview and in contrast to assessment, let's look at each of the steps of evaluation in more detail.

Selecting Evaluation Criteria

Obviously one cannot say that a goal has been achieved or not achieved without some supporting evidence. And equally obviously, evidence must be specifically and logically related to phenomena within both the diagnostic and goal areas. Thus, the first step in evaluation is to review the diagnostic concept that has been used and the goals that have been set, and from them either recall or develop the associated criteria for observing and measuring change. These criteria will serve two purposes:

an observational guide for collecting data from the presenting situation, and
a measuring standard for judging the data collected.

Evaluation must be related to both the diagnostic concept and the goals set. For example, the diagnostic concept in one situation may be obesity. Suppose the goal within that diagnostic area were: to achieve a normal weight for age, height, and build. The logical observational guideline would be to collect data on the weight of the individual at regular intervals and under comparable conditions (time of day, clothing, similar scale). The measuring standards would be a table of normal weight ranges for height, age, and build. But now suppose instead that the goal were to be: Satisfied with the food and eating patterns while reducing weight to that normal for age, height, and build. Then one would need additional data, subjective data, related to satisfaction with food and eating patterns and objective data on manifestations of that satisfaction. In both situations the diagnostic concept was obesity, but the goals were different and therefore the criteria and data base for evaluating client response had to vary in accordance with the goal.

Evaluation criteria are much more operationalized and specific in style than is the usual pattern in stating goals, even when those goals are behaviorally stated. The criteria, whether in one's head or on printed guidelines, should indicate what is to be collected, how it is to be collected, and the terms of description.

It does not seem realistic to believe that goal statements should fully spell out all the observations and measurements to be undertaken in the measurement of achievement. In most places one is lucky to have an explicit goal statement at all, so it would be impractical to suggest that the evaluation criteria be included. In some instances, what we are speaking of here must of necessity involve the thinking that goes on in the nurse's head as she drafts the goal and considers the data which she will collect or ask others to collect. (See also the flow sheets which appear on pages 258-262.)

Observing the Situation for Evidence

The second step in the evaluation process involves collecting data as prescribed by the criteria. (We are now back to the skills of cue collection, so all of the skills acquired in association with Chapter Four can now be put to work in another context.)

Collection of evidence for evaluation is controlled as to the kind of data gathered, how it is collected, and how it is described. This is not to say that additional data encountered in the situation that were not initially considered in the criteria may not also be used. What it does say is that evaluation requires the nurse to collect and report the required data in a prescribed, consistent way that lends itself to quantitative or qualitative measurement with some degree of reliability. The units of measurement or qualifying terms need to have been indicated in the criteria so that each observer will collect data in the same way and reports will be comparable.

Making Judgments in Terms of the Evaluation Standards

The final step in the evaluation procedure requires the nurse to place the description of the evidence against the "ruler" of the standard and make a judgment as to movement within the goal area. That achievement may mean change or stability. It may mean gains or slowing of losses. Some may be measured quantitatively in terms of numbers, amount, frequency, consistency, pounds/kilos, cc's, degrees, distance units, duration units (such as minutes, hours, days, weeks), work units, and so forth. Other aspects will be qualitatively described with whatever precision can be achieved, but using terms having a definition shared by all observers.

The idea of using terms with shared meaning is worth exploring in a little more detail. It is an area in which nurses currently experience difficulty, if the authors' experience is a usual one. As nurses we seem to be more interested in getting the work done than in determining whether what we did was actually achieving the desired nursing goals set. Thus effort is not frequently spent in operationally defining our terms in evaluation. Just look at the charts and nursing records. Listen to the change of shift report. Do you see and hear measurement terms such as:

> Good day/pm/noc.
>
> Procedure tolerated well
>
> Slept fairly well
>
> Ate poorly
>
> Voided/drank/ ate q̄ s. (quantity sufficient)?

Here is measurement with an accordion-pleated tape measure.

What does "well" or "fairly well" really mean? Does it mean the same to all nurses? One student nurse decided to find out just what the term "slept well" meant to all the nurses on one unit who were regularly using the term. Not only did each nurse use a different measurement guide for interpreting; all used different data on which to make the measurement. Some said they measured sleep by whether the signal light went on or not. And the "ruler" they used was variable, ranging from 4, 6 or 8 hours without the light going on as being the criterion for reporting, "slept well." Another group of the nurses used a different data base; they made rounds. If the mound on the bed did not stir or verbally respond to the nurse's presence, the person was judged to be sleeping. Again, 2, 4, 6 or 7 of these nonresponding contacts constituted the measurement for "slept well"; of course, the interval between rounds varied as well as the number of contacts chosen. If they only made rounds twice during the shift and the mounds did not move, then 2 might be the number used. Still others reportedly added subjective data by asking the clients how they had slept, thus broadening the data base somewhat. Any time you use both objective and subjective data you have increased the possibility of disagreement. Then how do you measure? These nurses said that if the client said, "Terrible" or "fine" and it agreed with the other measures (lights and rounds), they were evaluated as having slept well or poorly as reported. On the other hand, if the client said, "Terrible," but did not turn on his signal or had not talked to the nurse when she came on rounds, there was a reported tendency to trust the objective data over the subjective, and report, "Slept well but denies it."

Now 2-4-6-8 offer quite a range of data units on which to make the judgment "slept well," particularly when sometimes the data were based on signal lights being turned on and other times on direct observation; also, intervals of time were so variable. Would you care to buy bananas on a scale of such unpredictable weights?

Of course, sleep is an elusive phenomenon to measure and can be disturbed by the activity of observation itself. So let's take another slightly larger study in which nurses were measuring a client response that is accessible to objective data gathering—respiratory rate. Here, skillfully done, the nurse's activities in measuring do not tend to disrupt the responses as they may have done in sleep. A graduate student did a study of techniques of practicing nurses in evaluating respiratory rate (Eisman, 1970). Of the 48 nurses interviewed in three hospitals, 19 reported that they estimated rather than counted respirations. Both counters and guessers recorded numbers and neither designated whether an actual count was made. Those who estimated were asked how they decided what number to record. Seventeen of the 19 estimators decided on a number based on the "patient's appearance." When invited to share the criteria they used, however, they did not describe how appearance was associated with each number they had chosen. Two reported they had no basis for the number they chose. Even here, where access to data is quite uncomplicated and only 15 to 30 seconds of time is involved, the nurses' rulers seemed to be quite elastic.

How Changes in the Nurse's Values May Effect Changes in Nursing Evaluation

Given the busy routine of everyday activities of nurses, how could evaluation be done any differently? First, it would seem that there must be some changes in the nurse's values. As nurses we must value client responses in the area of nursing management as much as we do those responses related to medical management. If we do not, we will continue to occupy ourselves collecting data for physicians and ignore evaluation of the effectiveness of nursing care, even when nursing's goals could well have greater impact on the management of effective living. Setting priorities in any single direction (such as evaluating only medical management) can become a habit that is very difficult to change. Second, from our perspective, we in nursing could begin to value a greater degree of appropriate accuracy and precision in our evaluations. Out of these two values could then emerge changes in behavior leading to a sense of proportionate importance and higher degree of skill in the evaluation of nursing management to clients.

Let's take a very common, everyday example. Individuals who are hospitalized often undergo experiences or illnesses that make them weak. Part of the challenge of coping with living at home again is related to being able to ambulate securely enough to participate in needed self-care activities. How many of us have either thought or charted, "Tolerated ambulation well"? Let's look at the data that must have gone into the making of that judgment and see how a nurse might view the same data and consciously seek evidence and label it more precisely. She may or may not record the variables and the data, depending on how high a priority there is for the goal and what evidence of achievement of it exists. However the criteria for evaluating toleration of activity need to be just as sharp, in one's thinking, whether they are recorded or not. So pretend that you are going to observe ambulation behavior in a client and that these are the criteria that flash *into your thoughts* as a basis for observation.

234

Goal: Demonstrates endurance for ambulatory activities
needed for self care ADL at home prior to discharge
4/19

Criteria	Data		
	4/16	4/17	4/18
Dangles s̄ sx orthostatic hypotension			
Pallor?	+, +, 0	0 ———	0 ———
Cx dizziness?	+, +, +	+, 0 ———	
Knows rationale for gradual staging of movement to upright position?	given information asked ?	paced movement to sx	no need to pace self today
Sits in chair for ↗ periods s̄ discomfort	5 min x3 ex fatigue	30 min x3 < fatigue	45 min x4 no cx
Ambulates			
Longer distances?	to chair & B.R.	2x to corridor & around rm	walked 200 ft down corridor 3x
Diaphoretic?	+	0	0
P & R?	↗ 16/3	↗ 10/0	↗ 8/0
Pallor?	+	0	0
Gait?	shuffles	walks steadily	walks alone pace ↗
Rest req. p̄ activities?	lays quietly eyes closed	lay /reading	sat in chair
Initiative in self care and ambulation?	reluctant	up when asked	up s̄ reminding

Interpretation

Walks steadily s̄ untoward sx the distances to bathroom and kitchen at home. Able to stay up long enough for meals and self-care as needed.

THE FOCUS OF NURSING EVALUATION IN NURSING CARE PLANNING

Just as there are blurred areas of responsibility for assessment and diagnosis among the core health disciplines, so evaluation will involve shared territory of the involved disciplines for any client. However, just as there was an argument for a primary focus to nursing assessment, so there is a valid basis to offering a primary, but nonrestrictive, focus to nursing evaluation. It will of course be contingent on one's definition of nursing. So, while we believe that nursing will continue to evaluate client response to pathology and medical management as a delegated medical function, we also believe that it is in the client's best interest that the nurse give regular attention to, and be primarily accountable for, evaluation in the territory of nursing. In terms of individual care planning, this means making judgments about how the client and those close to him are managing the demands and goals of daily living as influenced by their health status and health-related activities and issues.

MAJOR COPING CATEGORIES AND NURSING EVALUATION CRITERIA

The major coping areas cited in the chapters on diagnosis and goal setting can offer a basis for development of general areas of evaluation criteria which can then be tailored to any given client's specific situation and goals. This would be similar to the protocols used by physicians whereby healing or cure is judged on the basis of standard indices of response to specific pathologic phenomena. For example, there are certain general indicators that inflammation is subsiding, or that tumor spread is being held in check. From these, more specific indicators are drawn for individual cases.

Let us look then at how general areas of criterion measures associated with categories of coping abilities and resources could be used similarly. We give examples associated with each of the coping ability categories on pp. 236 through 251.[1]

Strength

Strength can be measured in two ways:

1. the physical/mental work or stress undertaken at a point in time;
2. the ease with which the work or stress load is accomplished or tolerated.

When a localized or specific area of loss of strength has been observed, the observations would focus on the change in deficit in this specific area. Thus if it is only the fingers of the right hand that are weak and the person is right-handed, one would observe the amount and kind of work undertaken and the success the individual has in meeting the demands for right-handed work. If there is generalized loss of strength, as in malnutrition, and the task is to get up and walk to the bathroom, the symptoms indicating tolerance of this activity would be noted.

Accommodation to Decreased Strength.   Since coping with daily living is nurs-

---

[1] You may wish to read them all or merely to sample one or two as a basis for gaining perspective. For the reader who wishes to move directly to the implications evaluation has in terms of nursing practice we suggest turning to p. 251. The intervening pages can always be consulted at the time criteria for evaluation for a particular coping area are desired.

ing's focus, and since maintenance or accommodation to inevitable losses are as much the nurse's concern as is cure, another area for criteria setting and data gathering would be with compensatory activities or arrangements made to adjust to decreased or decreasing strength. Nurses are also concerned with *effective* living and this implies some degree of satisfaction with one's lifestyle. Therefore another essential area of evidence would concern the individual's satisfaction with any compromises or adjustments being made.

For example, when an individual does not have the muscle strength in his jaws to chew tough, fibrous meat such as steaks or some roasts, a switch can be made to meats that are made softer in cooking such as stews, braised dishes, ground meat recipes, and soups. Or perhaps fish, chicken, or meat substitutes would be used. If this diet is within the budget and the cooking facilities of the individual, and if the meals are still enjoyed, then the compensation for lost strength may be judged to be effective.

When a person's emotional strength does not allow him to deal with one more major (or even minor) family crisis, he may be able to take steps to at least temporarily "cool" the situation, putting conflict issues on a back burner until there is enough strength to take them on again.

Effectiveness in Using Support Systems. Clients with or without nurses' help may seek support systems to supplement their failed or failing strength. These might be physical, such as crutches, trusses, wheelchairs, electric typewriters or other equipment, ace bandages for weakened joints or blood vessel walls, intercoms to save walking, commodes, meals on wheels, and so forth. Clients may also seek external supports for their emotional weaknesses from organizations such as Alcoholics Anonymous or Alanons, or Weight Watchers, or from a minister, a confidant, a book, a distractor, a crisis clinic, a friend, or a family member. This support-seeking behavior may be viewed as an attempt to cope with the demands of daily living in the face of decreased strength in some area.

Summary. Thus, strength can be observed in what is done to handle physically and emotionally weighty demands. It can also be measured in: 1) the activities used to decrease demands for strength, making them commensurate with ability and resources and 2) experiences of satisfaction with the efforts and/or the outcome. The cues of satisfaction may be reported verbally or objectively observed in positive affect, relaxed demeanor, lack of nonproductive motions, and continuation of activities.

To summarize, an observer evaluating activities related to management of loss of strength in coping might seek data in:

activities to minimize loss of strength and/or to maintain or regain losses

the pattern/nature of physical or emotional work load undertaken by the client at a given time involving the area of deficit

the ease/speed/physiologic or psychological tolerance with which the "work" is accomplished the skill in locating support systems to supplement personal strength or compensate for lost strength

the deferment of "work" demands until strength is available

the lowering of goals to accomplishable work demands

satisfaction with the coping style chosen to adapt to change in strength.

Endurance

The endurance, stamina, or staying power to carry out the required tasks of the day or to maintain a desired lifestyle with zest and vigor represent one end of the endurance continuum. Fatigue, weariness, lassitude, or exhaustion before tasks are done or preventing participation in a desired way of life is seen as the other end. Again, as in the coping area of strength, a task and work are involved. But differentiated from strength, endurance is related to time. How long can work on the physical or emotional task be sustained?

A data base to evaluate endurance should consider the following areas:

the amount of activity absolutely *necessary* in a time period (e.g., tasks in a morning or a day)

the amount and kind of activity *desired* in a time period (e.g., the woman who has always done her washing and ironing on the same day, or who feels clothes aren't clean unless they've been hung on a line)

the pace either *required or desired* in activities

the observed pace and reported/observed comfort with the pace as work progresses

the duration of observed or requested recovery time after an episode of work

behavior indicating desire for or seeking of additional physical demands and/or intellectual or emotional challenges

efforts to reduce demands or delay them

behavior during rest periods (e.g., standing, sitting, lying down, talking/silent)

changes in breathing and pulse rate associated with activity; time it takes for elevations to return to baseline

observed or reported satisfaction/dissatisfaction with the amount, kind, and pace of activities in given time spans

> An example one of the authors encountered in this variable vividly illustrates this. An elderly lady who had been recovering from a severe bout of coronary ischemia was finally able to go downtown and pay her bills (she didn't believe in checking accounts). The daughter that night congratulated her on her progress in being able to expend all the effort of the bus rides and the walking that was involved. To her surprise, the mother rather than being delighted with herself, got ruffled and snapped, "It wasn't all that good. Everyone else walked *faster* than I did." Here was evident dissatisfaction with the pace of activities.

Accommodation to Decreased or Decreasing Endurance. Where endurance has decreased or is declining, the coping behavior, as in strength, may be evaluated in the following areas:

lowering of goals as to how much will be done, or how quickly it will be accomplished

success in search for compensatory equipment or persons to supplement personal resources of energy

reduction in demands

setting up of slower pace or more frequent rest periods

reported or observed satisfaction with the resultant change in lifestyle, or at least somewhat neutral toleration of it.

Knowledge

In the coping area of knowledge, the behavior being evaluated is the *acquisition* and *use* of facts, ideas, insights, or relationships between ideas and events to manage health-related aspects of living. Here, as in other areas, baseline data on initial command of the material and skills in use form the point of departure.

The evaluation of change from the baseline will have two dimensions. One will be related to the content area involved and learned. The second dimension will be concerned with the level of skill in using the content. Bloom et al. have delineated a taxonomy of six levels of thinking that suggest progressive levels in use of knowledge. Some of these lend themselves well as a frame of reference to evaluation of knowledge acquired by the client (Bloom et al, 1956).

Content. Content may well be the simpler aspect to measure. The goal statement should have identified what is to be learned (e.g., effects and side effects of a drug to be noted, the relationships of behaviors to symptoms, the responses one might expect from others when one behaves in a particular fashion, the steps in decision making, the idea of territoriality and its protection, the community resources available to assist in coping with certain deficits, steps in entering a particular system, criteria for judging a "normal family," symptoms of a heart attack, and so forth). Once the content area has been spelled out in the goal, particularly if the extent of knowledge is made explicit, evaluation of this dimension is not difficult. It can be made evident in oral or written communication.

Levels of Cognitive Learning. A more complex evaluative aspect is concerned with the level at which that content is to be learned—the skill of using the knowledge. Using Bloom's taxonomy, let's see if we can develop some observational guides for areas of data collection.

Recall

This level of learning involves remembering specifics, universals, methods, processes, and patterns. Achievement here means being able to bring to mind information when it is needed.

Examples

Remembering the local emergency phone number—how to perform a treatment or procedure, what the colors are on a urine test and what each one signifies, which symptoms mean that labor has begun or a heart attack has occurred, what to do if one wakens with paroxysmal nocturnal dyspnea.

Comprehension

At this level the learner has done something more than just memorize material as it was given to him. He can put it in his own words, offer illustrations, interpret what it means—explain it, compare it with other ideas, predict consequences and implications.

Examples

A physician had explained to an older man on diuretics that along with the extra fluid he would be urinating he would be losing potassium . . . that the loss of this substance from his body could cause his muscles to feel flabby and give him a feeling of weakness. It was therefore important for him to take the prescription that was being given to him as replacement.

Later the nurse asked if he understood what the doctor had told him. "Oh sure," he replied, "the doc said I'd be peein' out my potassium so not to forget to take that stuff every day or I might get to feeling as floppy as a half-filled hot water bottle. I don't want that!"

Application

As the label suggests, at this level the learner is able to take facts and abstract ideas and apply them to a concrete situation.

Example

If a nurse gives the client a list of foods high and low in sodium content, the client is able to indicate how the current family diet either accommodates to the amount of sodium permitted or does not.

The cardiac sets up his multiple pillows securely at night to counteract the displacement of fluid from the peripheral to the central vascular system and minimize the fluid that will tend to collect in his lungs and cause paroxysmal nocturnal dyspnea.

Undoubtedly, the three other kinds of cognition—analysis, synthesis, and evaluation—will also be used by some clients, at least part of the time.

Analysis

This type of thinking will be recognized if a client is observed or reports taking ideas or communications and breaking them down into component parts, categorizing, or organizing them in a particular way for himself.

Example

A person who is familiar with the steps of grieving may use the pattern and the behavior associated with each of them to recognize, understand, and predict his own personal behavior or that of others in situations where a significant loss has occurred.

Synthesis

Synthesis will be marked by taking ideas and creating something different or new from them.

Examples

One takes in a diagnosis of chronic or terminal illness and reorganizes one's body image to incorporate it, e.g., diabetes, blindness.

Modification of procedures, diets, recipes, schedules, or equipment for more acceptability, efficiency or convenience.

Evaluation

For the client, as for the reader, evaluation involves the use of knowledge to determine criteria, collection of data, and measurement of the data against the standard to make judgments about it.

Examples

A client reports progress toward a goal and gives supporting evidence. "I've been walking each day and now I am able to walk 4 blocks and back, instead of the 2 last week, and one of them was uphill. My heart wasn't going nearly as fast and I didn't even have to lie down when I got back. It's getting easier and I'm even beginning to enjoy it."

Each of these levels of learning will be evaluated in a different way and each content area of knowledge will also modify what kind of data is collected. In *any* instance, evaluation of this area of coping will concern itself with content to be acquired and the appropriate level of learning desired or achieved.

The data base associated with achievement of knowledge is both subjective and objective. Learning is a "black box" phenomenon; we cannot actually view the internal process of learning. We can see what we think goes in. We can listen to what the person reports is happening and what is changing within him. We can observe how the individual behaves on assigned tasks (e.g., answering specific questions, using knowledge in structured situations) and in incidental, unstructured situations. We can notice the words used, the relationships drawn between ideas or events, the discoveries made (sometimes known as the "aha!" syndrome). We can observe when new goals are set by the client, when different problem solving approaches are tried, when new relationships with others are attempted, or when new perceptions of himself seem to grow out of the input that has been prescribed and implemented.

Whole volumes have been written, whole curricula developed, whole research projects undertaken to identify and measure learning. As practicing nurses each of us will evaluate to the extent of our sophistication in this area. But let's not let our limitations in this area keep us from using our senses and our creativity to deal with the day-to-day knowledge and cognitive skill changes in our clientele that are so important to their effective living.

Skills

Skills may be easier to evaluate than knowledge, particularly if the observable behavior and the context have been spelled out sufficiently in the goal. The evaluation then consists in either observing the performance in the prerequisite settings or receiving reports from the client or those who have opportunity to observe, and then comparing the data with the behavior indicating achievement of the goal. One can observe a client:

walk up and down all types of stairs on his crutches, using the correct gait without waivering or interrupting his stride

draw the correct amount of injectable substance from the vial without contaminating sterile surfaces, inject it at the angle of x° to the depth of x cm. in the correct site for this occasion, check for its entering a blood vessel and do all this at the appropriate time for administering the medication

work for greater joint flexibility by increasing the range of motion achieved

work on a task against the clock and achieve greater speed.

There are many concrete cues, readily observable and logically tied to the skill being evaluated.

Even with intra- and interpersonal skills, such as confrontation, showing affection, conflict resolution, role negotiation, and so forth, there are reportable and observable cues that are identified in the literature and reported research with each concept. If the nurse learns and stores the concept with these evaluation criteria grouped together in a retrievable cue syndrome, then evaluation of these phenomena is quite possible.

Desire

Most of us know of people who seemed to have many resources, but have a low level of achievement. We also know of others who, with modest resources or even deficits, were able to achieve at a high level. The difference seemed to lie in the elusive quality of desire for the goal. In health care problems also, outcomes are related to how much people want to participate, to try, to endure, to achieve, to live.

Wanting, like learning, cannot be viewed; we hear only the subjective reports of it and see behavior in the related area that indicates it. The subjective data on desire will emerge from verbal reports about this internal state, either in response to questions or in spontaneous expressions. A continuum of wanting to not wanting can be expected. Non-wanting may take the form of explosive, vehement rejection of ideas, goals, or approaches if the client is of this temperament and feels safe to respond in this way. Equally negative responses may take the form of quiet, polite refusal, lack of interest or nonverbal expressions of rejection. Covert activities to undermine or prevent goal-related activities would also reflect lack of desire. These may be expected where an individual has either been socialized into these behaviors with health care workers, is afraid to express the true degree of his aversion to ideas or may be a normally less aggressive person. In the midpoint of the continuum, one might find a degree of neutrality or tolerance in the expression of desire—not against the idea, but not really wanting it much either, a verbal, "It's OK," with a downward inflection. At a positive extreme, expressions and behaviors reflecting eagerness, initiative, excitement, creative ideas for incorporation of the goal or plan into one's lifestyle, and enthusiasm for the outcomes may be heard and seen. Between these extremes one should be able to place any subjective expressions of desire for the goal or the nurse's plan of action.

Desire can also be evaluated by objective data. The expression, "your actions speak so loudly I can't hear what you're saying," applies well to the nonverbal data on desire. Objective data may either support or negate the subjective expressions of the individual. Mager suggests the behavior ranges between aversion and approach (Mager, 1968, 21-30).

With aversion, the behavior will indicate varying degrees of avoidance or participation with distaste.

A baby gulps down ice cream or mashed peaches but clamps down his lips or spits out puréed spinach.

The person on a low-calorie diet sneaks candy or goes on eating binges.

The person forcing fluids "forgets" to drink.

The person on restricted activity "forgets" he shouldn't turn himself.

The one who is to exercise has so many other things that must be done that there just isn't any time for exercises.

In general, the person who does not desire a goal or activity finds a way to avoid it, minimize contact with it, or engage in lapses from it. When engaged in it, the expression is anything but happy. No effort is observed where the person tries to find ways of engaging in the activity or moving toward the goal. Activities of the nurse to try to get the attention or interest of the client in this area may be met with avoidance, business, changing of the subject, lack of questions, avoidance of eye contact, or even a request to leave.

By contrast, desire to engage in the goal and activities will be evidenced by approach behavior. The observer should see the client not only *not* forgetting, but actually taking or making opportunities to participate in related activities. Related ideas from the media or reading may be brought up. There are questions that go beyond the material given, or give evidence of thoughtful consideration of content covered. Sometimes the client will show initiative in incorporating the ideas or equipment into his lifestyle, or will change the lifestyle to accommodate to the goal. There are cues indicating excitement, enthusiasm, and eagerness.

Pleasure is seen or expressed as the individual engages in activities. There is pride in accomplishment. The individual may go so far as to try to share his own positive experience and expertise with others who are encountering comparable health care situations.

In this continuum, as in so many others, the extremes are easy to document, it is the grey areas in between that are difficult. Still, variations and degrees of approach and aversion can be identified and verified in so many ways even as one interacts with the clientele. These are important variables to evaluate in ongoing contacts.

Courage

Since a deficit of courage is identified in terms of self-perceived personal risk or threat, rather than lack of understanding or desire, the changes will be evaluated in terms of risk-taking behavior and degree of comfort in both vulnerability and the decisions and actions. In the area of objective criteria one may see the client engage in the behavior that has been perceived as threatening. This may be in several areas such as:

> performing activities that cause physical pain (burn dressings, injections)
>
> risking exposure of inadequacies of performance (mothering, carrying out skills, indicating one's area of knowledge in a subject, ability to carry out an activity such as intercourse for a male concerned about impotence, and so forth)
>
> agreeing to accept a changed and unwanted body image (as in a surgical procedure)
>
> risking loss of life in a choice or an activity
>
> choosing to give up a desired or needed goal
>
> participating more openly in an encounter group or with a psychiatric health worker with the risk of increased disclosure with or without awareness.

It may also be seen in behavior aimed at reducing the feeling of vulnerability.

> rehearsing or roleplaying the threatening situation (Parents and children often do this in terms of hospitalization. It can also be done when a client has a difficult disclosure to make to a doctor, for example, and practices on himself or others what he will say, what words he will use.)
>
> discussing the range of risk (What's the worst that can happen? What's the least?)
>
> testing the fringes of the threatening situations (injecting the orange, pulling the tape off the skin, but not cleaning the wound, looking at the colostomy or the wound but not dressing it.)

All of these activities may be observed as indicators of behavior to reduce the risks in the situation and thus bring them within the range of courage which the client perceives he has available—certainly this is evidence of coping.

Courage is a subjective experience and, therefore, it must be measured in terms of the client's version of the degree of risk. A nurse may see a procedure such as injecting a drug or giving data on a history as being routine. To measure the deficit of courage on that scale would be inappropriate. Data on the client's perception of risk is the yardstick on this variable.

The subjective data can include data from several areas of personal insight. Among these the client may report:

identification of the nature of vulnerability/risk he perceives in the presenting situation

plans to engage in behaviors that gradually escalate the risk-taking behavior in a tolerable manner

creation of test situations to rehearse the threatening situation

decrease in discomfort of symptoms associated with the risk-taking

decreased perception of risk in the situation.

You can no doubt think of many other aspects to evaluate in the area of courage. Get them together in your concept of courage and risk-taking so that they are readily retrievable when you need to evaluate them in terms of this diagnosis.

The following is a situation in which a man was experiencing paroxysmal atrial tachycardia (PAT).

Mr. Dominick's symptoms would seem to fit the diagnosis of a demand for courage in order to achieve effective living with a condition that was expected to persist. Mr. Dominick experiences paroxysmal tachycardia, a condition that has been present for years. During the last few months, these episodes seem to exhaust him physically. His behavior indicates that he is very apprehensive during them (he seeks out a nurse and breathlessly asks to have his pulse counted.) Currently, the attacks occur four to six times a month, last 2 to 10 minutes with heart rates in excess of 160 beats per minute.

The doctor indicated that this condition is unlikely to disappear so the nurse sets as a nursing care objective the client's coping with the episodes with a minimal amount of emotional distress. She planned to have the staff alert to his signal so that they could go to the bedside as soon as it was known that an episode was occurring (rather than have him expend energy at this time in seeking the nurse) and then remain with him after the symptoms subsided to allow him to verbalize as needed.

The anecdotal notes and monthly summary notes on this aspect of nursing care and client response were:

November 3

Client had an episode of tachycardia. Stayed with him. Unable to count pulse, neck veins virtually fluttering. He seemed relieved by my presence. Asked client to inhale deeply and hold breath, then to exhale. Client surprised, said "It worked." He could feel his pulse slowing down. Procedure repeated. Pulse 86. Spent few minutes talking with him.

November 14

Client told me he had a short episode of tachycardia, 2 to 3 minutes. Said it ceased when he belched. Pulse now 68, weak. (Evidence of willingness to face episode alone. Presence of mind enough during the attack to notice change in heart rate following release of trapped gas.)

November 24

Client's attitude toward work seems to be changing. Previously he has indicated that he shouldn't participate in the work program because he is here to get well. In the client group meeting today he talked about the therapeutic value of working. No reported increase in episodes of tachycardia related to increased activity. (Evidence of willingness to risk work despite his perception that it might trigger another attack.)

Summary of November

We know of a least four or five episodes of tachycardia, 3 to 7 minutes in length. (Faces episodes with minimal reporting within the hospital setting.)

December 13

Out for ride with wife. Had short episode of tachycardia. It didn't interfere with his activities. (Faced episode outside of the support system of the hospital.)

Summary of December

The short episodes of tachycardia professed have not been confirmed by observation, since the client only casually mentions them at the present time. In December he never rang the bell for nursing care in regard to an episode of tachycardia. (Handled as a relatively routine phenomenon, not requiring unusual courage.)

This example serves to illustrate progress toward coping with a self-perceived recurring, life-threatening experience. The client's progress reached the point where it was no longer seen as requiring unusual courage.

Courage is not a diagnostic area that nurses have dealt with in an explicit way very often. For this reason, our criterion package for evaluation may be quite skeletal. Hopefully, over time, everyday observations and more formal research regarding risk-taking and vulnerability will enable us to make more discriminating observations and finer judgments based on increasingly refined criteria.

Support System

In earlier sections we alluded to a client's willingness to accept, use, seek, and maintain support systems to supplement inadequate resources on his part. Evaluation of the use of support systems would seem to fall into the following areas:

Were needed or prescribed resources available?

Were they accessible—geographically, financially?

Were they acceptable to the client and his lifestyle?

Were they appropriate to the diagnosed deficit?

Have they made a productive difference in the client's (person/family) coping with the demands of daily living involved in the presenting situation?

Have they reduced the functional deficit? The demands to be met? Have they increased the satisfaction with daily living?

Is the client able to maintain them in a satsifactory working state or relationship? Is the equipment intact, running smoothly? Do persons involved feel satisfied/gratified/sufficiently rewarded to continue to function in a support relationship?

Obviously, the specific criteria and cues will be related to the exact nature of the support system. Let's look at some examples.

If the relative of a dying person or mother of a severely handicapped child needs time off to regroup once or twice a week, is this being provided in such a way that she doesn't worry about the adequacy of the care while she is "off duty"? Is it dependable? Is it financially feasible? Is the time off sufficient to enable the mother or relative to regroup—sleep—be away from the stresses? Is the person providing the surrogate care feeling good about the service?

If Alanon is being used by relatives of the alcoholic, are they gaining perspective on the problem? Do they feel less alone? Are they finding new approaches to try in their problem solving with the alcoholic? Are buddies in the system available when crises come?

If the person with cancer needs dressings, supplies, transportation for therapy, is the local unit of the Cancer Society available for this?

If the beige walls and steps in the hallway of the older person's home are causing a safety hazard due to resident's visual changes, is there someone to supply the paint and provide the labor to get more contrasting colors applied to one of the surfaces?

Is the hearing aid available? Can the batteries be afforded? Will the device be accepted in terms of appearance? Will there be someone who has been through the adjustment period or who knows of its stresses to be there as a sounding board when the distortion of sound and inability to screen out some noises gets too stressful?

In each instance the shopping list of cues are very much related to the deficit and the particular support being used. However, in all kinds, the basic questions still apply.

Sensory Input

Usable sensory input is a subjective experience, so it is the client's (not the nurse's or the institution's) norms and perceptions that must form the baseline and evidence of change. There are, of course, objective data on stimuli *available* in the environment (sounds, light, monotony of view, some knowledge of meaningfulness of stimuli such as when the client only speaks another language or a different version of English, casts or other factors known to change tactile or kinesthetic input, and so forth). We also know that when the overload or underload are extreme there can be observable physiologic and psychological manifestations. So, both subjective reporting and objective data are available in criteria setting and data gathering.

There are several major areas for evaluation of sensory input. These include changes in:

> the nature of the stimuli in the environment
>
> the status of the sensory receptors
>
> the status of the central nervous system as a mediating system
>
> the drugs being ingested which affect receptors or central nervous system
>
> the response to the sensory environment, including not only the observed responses to the sensory input, but the initiative taken in changing the environment to make it more compatible with sensory needs and desires.

Stimuli. Evaluation of stimuli consists of a comparison of the stimuli in the present living environment (long- or short-term) with the goal of usual/needed or desired input. For example:

> An elderly man in his eighties had been living with his wife in their large home in a quiet neighborhood. An introspective person, he had become accustomed to a very quiet environment. Admission to the coronary unit and, later, transfer to a private room with just the normal flow of hospital traffic was seen as an uncomfortable sensory overload.
>
> On the other hand, his 13-year-old grandson was admitted to the same hospital He was placed in a four-bed unit and was delighted with all the activity, even when he was quite uncomfortable in the immediate postoperative period.

These two related persons had different norms of environmental stimuli. Evaluation had to take these differences into account.

Using the baseline and the goal, one may collect data in terms of:

Amplitude
> Volume of sound
> Brightness of color
> Vigor of tactile contacts

Amount of illumination

Amount of movement yielding kinesthetic input

Intensity of tastes and odors.

Variety (or monotony)

Sounds

Color

Movement

Tastes and food texture.

Clarity (or distortion)

Blurring of vision

Diploplia

Loss of high pitch

Blurring of sounds

Decrease in sweet and sour tastes

Tactile hyperesthesia or numbness.

Availability

Presence of stimuli in the environment

Accessibility within control of the client.

Receptors. In this subcategory, one notes changes of any direction in the effectiveness of sense organs. The direction of change may be toward more effectiveness, as in surgery to remove cataracts or transplant the cornea; removal of ear wax; restoration of tactile, kinesthetic sense in recovery from nerve damage; and being fitted with corrective glasses or a hearing aid. Or it may be the reverse, with decreased effectiveness or barriers between the stimuli and the receptors (as in a body cast).

Central Nervous System Change. Changes in the central nervous system can enhance perception of stimuli, as in mild anxiety, certain drugs (e.g., mind expanders), and pathology. On the other hand, depressant drugs, disease, and sensory deprivation can also depress the central nervous system, raising the threshold for entry of stimuli to the brain so that stimuli once perceived now no longer can reach the threshold level to become usable to the individual.

Response to Sensory Environment. Research in sensory underload and overload has demonstrated both physiologic and psychological responses to sensory input that goes beyond the comfort range of the individual at any given point in time. The criteria for sensory *underload* include:

Physiologic response

Progressive slowing of alpha brain waves

Decreased cortical arousal leading to reduced amplitude of received stimuli and minimal stimulation resulting in "no information" being received

249

Increase in cutaneous and pain sensitivities

Decreased galvanic skin reaction

Suggested increase in visual and auditory sensitivity as the deprived person attunes to any and all S.

Cognitive

Increased difficulty in directed thinking and concentration.

Other difficulties reported have not been substantiated by objective tests.

Affective

Sx of anxiety that may approach panic, claustrophobia

Increased reports of somatic complaints

> Explanation: emotionally aroused state may compound the normal discomfort.

There is minimal competition between external and internal S for attention

Delusions and hallucinations—present more with diminished sensory input or distorted input, as it is thought that some stimuli are needed as a basis for them

There may be attention paid to background "noise" as opposed to external stimuli present in the environment, leading to behavior described as confusion (marching to a different drummer).

For *overload*, the signs and symptoms have been reported as:

Physiologic

Increased sweating, blood pressure, heart rate, and activity of voluntary muscles

Firing of nerve cells of high rate and low amplitude

May interfere with delicate behavior involved in cue or guiding functions.

Cognitive or musculo-cognitive

May interfere with responses already in repertoire

May prevent acquisition of new responses of adaptation.

Affective

Distracted, "wild with pain."

In addition, the individual may act in a manner to create a more suitable and comfortable sensory environment. This behavior can be observed. For example, he may tune out stimuli, place barriers (close a door), request a change in the behavior of others—all these in the interest of reducing the stimuli. Or he may create stimuli in terms of singing to himself, rocking, getting a book and reading, turning on the radio or TV, moving to a more active area in the environment, pulling up the blinds, opening the door, talking to others, listening to others, talking to himself, moving to a more stimulating environment, e.g., from private home to retirement center. All of these could be observed as a means of increasing the available stimuli.

Specific Phenomena Creating Coping Deficits

Physicians may diagnose and treat diseases, or they may diagnose and treat only symptoms. In *either* instance the client's response is evaluated. In nursing also, there are times when specific phenomena affect the coping ability. These, too, are diagnosed as complaints requiring medical and/or nursing management. They are treated and evaluated. Their evaluation, however, should probably be done as a *subproblem* of the coping deficit to which they contribute. For example: anorexia, insomnia, contractures, corns, pain, dehydration, confusion, angina, all create coping difficulties. Yet they, as well as the coping difficulties they create, are amenable to nursing actions.

When nursing activity is addressed to any of these conditions, evaluation should take place at this level as well as at the level of the coping problem. The criteria for evaluating these conditions may be quite obvious—the individual reports or is observed to: sleep more, eat more, and enjoy it more, have greater range of motion in the affected joint, have smooth unthickened skin where the corn had been, report relief of pain for longer periods, find control of the angina with pacing of activities and/or use of nitroglycerine, and so forth. On the other hand, there may be no change, or the observed and reported status may become worse. In any instance, the cue syndromes that indicate change in status relative to the complaint would be used as the guide to collect data and measure change.

Summary

There is no reason of course, why cue syndromes of reportable (subjective) and/or observable (objective) data needed to evaluate responses in areas of nursing diagnosis should not be collated and standardized into algorithms, just as medicine is doing. We, as they, must take into account individual differences for both the baseline and potential range of changes, but there are norms and ranges associated with clients in general or subgroups according to age, sex, or any other group characteristic. Human variation should not deter us from our endeavor. We need comparable criteria and comparable data as a basis for measurement. Hopefully, nursing research and nursing practice will join forces to address this need and in the forseeable future, some standardization of criteria for evaluating common nursing diagnoses will be forthcoming.

EVALUATING RESPONSE TO NURSING BEHAVIOR

In the previous section, we delineated criteria related to evaluating coping deficits and goals. A concurrent kind of evaluation by the nurse needs to go on. This is the observation of client response to nurse behavior, the immediate feedback that signals a need to continue the activity unchanged or to adjust it in terms of client response.

Let's take an example in our own lives with which any of you who have ever taken or taught a class can identify. In our nursing care planning workshops and classes we try to watch what is happening with the participants. We watch to see if they are:

> getting restless
> going to sleep
> asking relevant questions
> asking no questions
> not participating in the "games"
> talking about the weather or nonrelated topics during a small group activity or class
> decreasing the amount of eye contact
> generating a lower level of noise during activities.

We have found that there are a host of audience responses that let us know whether a workshop is "bombing" or really soaring—or someplace in between. Similarly a nurse who takes the trouble can ascertain whether she is functioning effectively with the client, the family, the support persons, or whoever is the object of her ministrations. Does their behavior indicate that the help you are offering is really being seen as usable to them? Are they participating in the thinking/feeling activity with you? Are they tuning you out? Are they turned off and trying to turn you off?

Of course, there will be many times when the activities being offered or given by the nurse are not immediately wanted or enjoyed by the clientele. Still, this too can be acknowledged by both, and a sense of partnership or sharing in misery can evolve. At other times, a nurse may deliberately behave in such a way as to invite nonacceptance/anger/self-sufficiency. When the client response occurs as predicted/desired, this too can be evaluated. The point is that, regardless of what the nurse does, whether it be a backrub for relaxation, a preoperative orientation to postoperative role expectations or whatever, the client response during the intervention is a part of the movement toward the goal. There should be an element somewhere in the nurse's consciousness that is noticing the nurse behavior, the client response *and, as importantly,* the reverse situation of client behavior and the nurse's response.

NURSING ACTIVITIES AND COLLECTION OF DATA FOR EVALUATION

If, as we advocate, buck-passing in care planning stops with the registered nurse (or where there is no registered nurse, with the best prepared licensed practical nurse), then the nurse has accountability for the collection of data on which to base evaluation of client response and the effectiveness of the nursing care planned and implemented. This is not to say that the data will always be collected by the nurse, but she does have *the ultimate responsibility* for designating what data are to be collected and for seeing that the client, his family, the nursing nonprofessionals, or other health care workers know:

what to watch for

how to collect the data

how to describe or report what is experienced or observed

when and how to report (verbal, written, to whom, when).

These responsibilities and activities or delegated activities have implications for the nurses' activities and roles in a variety of ways.

Managing Client Input to Evaluation

In addition to facilitating self-evaluation by the client, the nurse is often interested in maintaining updated information on situations under nursing management. In order to receive the kind of data needed for nursing evaluation, the nurse has responsibility to make the client or those who report on and for him aware of what information is needed, why it is needed and how it will be used.

The nursing situations in which client or family feedback is needed are usually related to ambulatory or home care settings. The nurse may be in an office, clinic, school, industry, retirement, recreational, or community setting. The contact for pre-data gathering instructions as well as feedback could occur in face to face contacts during an appointment or visit or in phone contacts. (Increasing numbers of clinics, offices and HMOs are using nurses' skills as screening diagnosticians and evaluators via phone contacts) and good office nurses have been doing it for years.

In the initial contact, the nurse would indicate why observations need to be made, what to look, listen, and feel for, and how data are to be collected if any special techniques are involved. If the observer needs any special equipment, this would be discussed as would the skills for using it. If the observer needs new words to describe what is seen to communicate accurately, these terms should be operationalized. And, of course, paraphrasing should be requested, to be certain the client or non-client observer feels secure in the activities. If the situation to be observed is a recurring one in the nurse's practice, then written observation guides may be cost effective. Finally, expectations should be set as to when or under what circumstances the observer is to contact the nurse with the information.

Let's look at some examples.

Nurses in obstetricians' offices, prenatal clinics, and classes are familiar with preparing expectant mothers and fathers to collect information regarding onset of labor as a basis for making decisions on when to contact the health care worker. They learn what to look for, how to time contractions, what to be concerned about, what to report and when, and whom to call.

Nurses in diabetic clinics routinely teach parents of young diabetic children how to regularly monitor data on eating, illness, activity, stress, and diabetic symptoms. They learn urine testing. They learn what data to collect, when they should contact a health worker, and whom they should call with various problems.

In a specific situation, we were caring for a wife and husband during the husband's terminal illness. He had a malignancy of the stomach and wanted to die in the retirement apartment where they were living. The wife was taught the symptoms that would indicate that death was imminent, and was given the phone numbers where the retirement residence nurse could be reached at particular hours of the day, so that she could support her during this traumatic time. Other residents who were serving as a support system were also oriented to the situation and made aware that the nurse wished to be phoned.

In recent times, more and more clients expect, want, and are able to actively and effectively participate in monitoring and evaluating their health care situations. The skyrocketing costs of health care make it almost mandatory—if there were no better reason. Thus, where nurses were once protective of the mysterious knowledge of numbers on thermometers, sphygmomanometers, laboratory values, findings, and diagnoses, there is now an increasing openness. Nurses have a major role in facilitating client's and client families' participation in effective evaluation.

Managing Input from Nursing Personnel for Evaluation

Where, in ambulatory care settings the clientele assume major responsibility for observation and often for evaluation with guidance from the nursing and medical staff, in institutional care it is the nursing personnel who are more involved. Obviously, the nurse who plans care must see the person for whom nursing care is planned, even though some observations are delegated to others.

The nurse who is assigned to the clients in a planning case load for a shift, a day, or hopefully, a more prolonged period (like the duration of client stay), has to incorporate two distinct kinds of activities related to data collection for evaluation. One is concerned with effective delegation of observation to others. The other is personal ongoing data collection. Both of these activities and skills are part of the role.

Planning Rounds.   There are rounds and rounds—teaching rounds, change of shift rounds, grand rounds, medical rounds, student evaluation rounds. In some settings one might expect clients to be rounded into exhaustion. For the purposes of this chapter we are not going to concern ourselves with these other uses of nursing rounds, but will limit ourselves to evaluation/planning rounds.

The purpose of planning rounds is for the nurse planner to validate with first-hand data the client's current status and to involve him in the plans for nursing care to the extent that it is appropriate, given his presenting situation. The degree of participation may vary from the unconscious person's sharing of only objective data to the other extreme of objective data plus verbal involvement in validating findings, goals, prescription of nursing activities for the future, and evaluation of activities in the past.

In some places teams, not individuals, plan care. Presumably, there is team accountability for care planning decisions. If this system is used, then the planning team needs to make rounds. *Team rounds* have the advantage of having all members of the team see each of the clients assigned to the team and gain some familiarity with the presenting situation as well as with the planning. The disadvantages are related to the cost of occupying so many individuals in the activity, the delay of care they might have been giving while on rounds, and the nature of the data sharing in which the client may not feel "I-Thou" but "I-Youall." If the latter perception is present, the client may be reluctant to share particularly sensitive data, or may feel outnumbered.

In most places, and with increasing frequency, individual nurses have planning accountability for a client case load for a specified period of time. Here, individual rounds may be used. *Individual rounds* will have the advantage of being less costly of personnel and time and can enhance a one-to-one sharing. Its disadvantages are that not all who give care participate in the data gathering, and therefore they will see the data only through the screen of the nurse who made the contact.

Let's take a look at how a nurse making rounds might function. We see the RN entering Ms. Liston's room with the Kardex or chart (whatever place the nursing care plan is located). This client has been admitted for observation and care following an automobile accident in which she suffered a concussion and generalized bruising. The client is responsive, verbal, and physically able to participate in a dialogue with the nurse on her planning rounds. The scenario might go something like this:

RN   Hello, Ms. Liston. How are things going for you today?
     (the open enedeness and general nature of the question leaves the choice
     of subjects and priorities wide open.)

RN   Mmm. Well that sounds as if last night wasn't much better than the night
     before. Those two hour checks on your vital and neurologic signs must
     make sleeping almost impossible. . . .

RN   Were you able to nap any today?

RN   Uh huh. Feeling a bit more rested. Well, everything has been showing up
     very normal on all these checks we've made and the critical time for close
     watching has passed as of noon today—so we won't need to waken you as

255

often. You told me you usually sleep best the first part of the night, starting about 1 a.m. Right? . . . If we get you settled down by then, we won't need to waken you for any medicine or checking for four hours. Do you think that will help?

RN Is there anything that helps you to sleep at home?

RN I'll note that here and call the next shift nurse's attention to it. If you have trouble sleeping, the night nurse wants you to be sure to let her know so you won't have to spend another sleepless night. As of tonight, we do have a medication for you to help you sleep if you need it.

Anything else you feel we should be considering for your nursing care during the next 24 hours?

RN Fine. Ms. Ferris, who cared for you this morning, said you were doing very well on keeping up with your muscle setting exercises and deep breathing and that food was beginning to taste better to you. Things seem to be looking up. . . . If anything comes up that concerns you, be sure to let one of us know.

Either during or following the encounter, notations are made on the nursing orders sheet or care plan, updating the plan of care. If appropriate, a summary note may also be made on the nurses notes or progress sheet (depending on the recording system being used).

Now what about the *timing of planning rounds?* Probably rounds will occur in most instances on the day or evening shift at an hour after at least some of the care has been given and the pace of activities in and out of the clients' rooms permits some uninterrupted conversation and thought.

Some nurses have told us that clients seem to prefer a regular time for these rounds so that they can anticipate them and be prepared. They know someone is coming who is interested in the nursing management and the client's input on how well it is working for him. Then he can judge whether he wishes to hold questions and data in abeyance until that time or share it with another worker immediately. One group of nurses told us that they were making an announcement concerning the time and nature of nursing rounds in the orientation letter each client found on his bedside table on admission—it alerted the patient and made a binding commitment on the nursing staff. They felt both were needed.

There is one other pragmatic consideration about planning rounds that has nothing to do with evaluation but is a point that many nurses have brought up in workshops. We have suggested that when the individual nurse is making planning rounds, the activity be limited to just that. This always brings some flak about giving the client the impression that, as a nurse, you see yourself as "being too good" to give a bedpan. Actually, the nurse is no more snobbish about giving any aspect of care at this time than at any other. It is a matter of cost effectiveness. For the few minutes to half hour it takes to make planning rounds, the planning nurse (team leader, primary nurse, head nurse, clinical coordinator, staff nurse) should be free to concentrate on just this. Another person could be designated to answer lights (if there is more than one person on the unit). It is a matter of giving cost effective care and being able to focus for a precious few minutes; and it is harder work any day in the week than answering the majority of the lights. If there is any need to prove to clients and others that one is not too good for other aspects of nursing care, certainly there will be opportunity to take over the lights while other nurses make their planning rounds at another time. But do look to what you as a nurse can do best and see to it that the client gets the benefit of these services.

Assignment Conferences. In addition to the personal observations made by the nurse, she undoubtedly will delegate observations to others as well. Often the occasion for structuring data gathering activities along with other nursing actions is the assignment conference. Here the person accountable for the planning of client care updates the current nursing diagnosis, reviews the goals, integrates the nursing orders and the delegated medical activities. In addition, *she identifies the evaluation criteria and data to be collected* as care is given. (See p. 276 for example.)

While assignment conferences are not set up as teaching sessions, there is no question that they can be a source of ongoing staff development—if they are well done. With thoughtful preparation, they need not be time consuming, either. But it does mean that the nurse must invest some time and effort in preparing a compact experience that relates defined staff growth needs to the presentation of the client's situation of the day and his care. Skill in this area separates outstanding nurses from the run-of-the-mill in roles of nursing leadership.

The finale of the assignment conference structures the time and expectations for feedback which the associate or team member will offer orally and/or in writing.

Feedback Conferences. Expectations, mechanisms, and occasions are needed for regular feedback sessions from those who have been delegated to make observations. Charted notations are of necessity somewhat cryptic, and often writing skills and time are lacking among many nonprofessionals. An oral interaction where the nurse can probe, validate, and test her own impressions and expand her ideas becomes a much more effective and sensitive means of achieving continuity in the data chain. Again, as in the assignment conference, the thinking, caring nurse will make it an occasion for staff development. This includes giving recognition for effective data collection, precise description, and logical creative thinking. It also includes sharing perspectives for new vistas in observing and giving care, and more precise techniques or more descriptive vocabulary where these are seen to be needed. It is an efficient way of combining data exchange with staff growth. Ask any student, LPN, or aide who has been fortunate enough to encounter a nurse who was really good in utilizing assignment conferences and feedback sessions. They will tell you it is worth full tuition any day.

RECORDING EVALUATIONS

Nurses have always been taught that it is important to chart action taken and client response. In practice, more emphasis seems to have been placed on what is done, than on how the client responds, unless the response is both dramatic and untoward. Most responses to nursing care are anything but dramatic, and, hopefully, they are not untoward. The result has been that nurses' charting about nursing care is frequently not worth reading.

The movement toward problem-oriented recording bids to change that. At least it will if nurses become conscious of clients' nursing problems and the significance of nursing care. In the trend, we are seeing greater use of flow sheets and progress records. These can be very useful (although difficult) in highlighting client responses to nursing care.

Flow Sheets for Data

One of the features of problem-oriented records that can easily be adapted to any client record (even those not on problem-oriented systems) is the use of the flow sheet. We are all familiar with the graphics used for recording data on vital signs, with intake and output sheets, and, more recently, with other printouts for recording client response over time. Some specialized nursing units such

			TIME	A.M.	8			9
			Temperature					
HEMODYNAMIC STATUS		Heart Rate	EKG					
			Apex					
			Radial					
	Pressure	Systemic	Cuff					
			Gage S/D					
			Gage mean					
		LA	cm H$_2$O mm Hg					
		Venous	cm H$_2$O mm Hg					
		PA	S/D					
			Mean					

as coronary care units, neurologic intensive care units, and other intensive care settings have developed flow sheets incorporating essential physiologic variables so that one can see patterns in one or more variables at one time or over time. This flow sheet, allowing three recordings on hemodynamic status per hour, illustrates pre-set variables.

The following segment of a flow sheet illustrates spaces for numerical data in unstructured time intervals and a graphic option for half-hourly observations of respiratory rate.

Time			
Control/Assist			
Resp. Rate			
Tidal Vol.			
Max. Pressure			
Flow Rate			
O$_2$ %			
B.B./min.			
B.B. Vt.			

Time	0800	0900	1000	1100	1200	1300	1400
50							
40							
30							
20							
10							

RESPIRATORY RATE ○ ● PATIENTS RESPIRATORY RATE (IN RED)

Nurses in labor and delivery rooms are also using two-dimensional graphics to visually plot the relationships of contractions to rate of cervical dilation.

In some conditions where there are predictable learning needs, flow sheets with pre-set variables have been developed. You will note on the following partial sample that the dates are left open depending on the rate at which the topics are handled.

Date/time			
Understanding of physiology of colostomy			

Irrigations:
  Importance of routine
  Has appropriate equipment
  Demonstrates irr. procedure
  Discusses adaptation to
     environment and life
     style			

Diet:
  Identifies foods that cause
     gas, diarrhea, constipation
  Applies to his usual diet
  Explores potential difficulties
     and techniques of coping			

Organization:
  Knows about local and national
     colostomy clubs
  Has a local contact			

Lifestyle:
  Has explored ways in which col-
     ostomy may require adaptation in
     dress, routine, work, sexuality,
     social engagements, recreation			

With some clients progess in activities of daily living becomes important in evaluating coping with a disability. The segment of this flow sheet indicates gradations in self care.

HOUSE-HOLD TASKS	Prepared Meals							
	Dishwashing							
	Shopping							
	Laundry							
	House Cleaning							

Key: I = independent   SI = semi-independent   D = dependent

Beyond these structured forms however, there is the concept of open-ended flow sheets or a combination of the two. Here the nurse and/or the physician determine the variables to be observed, kinds of data to be plotted, and the interval at which data should be collected. Nurse practitioners are using these in ambulatory care settings. Other nurses are using them wherever they happen to be working.

DATE →

	WEIGHT								
VITAL	Syst. / Diast.								
SIGNS	PULSE								
	RATE								
	RESP.								
	TEMP.								

Open-ended flow sheets do present a challenge however, in that the nurse or the physician must decide the critical variables on which data are to be gathered and the intervals of data collection. This is quite a different skill from just collecting and recording the data in predetermined areas. Criteria associated with nursing diagnosis (see pp. 143-146), the presenting complaint, and/or the medical plan could all be considered as a basis for setting priorities of attention.

Let's look at an open-ended flow sheet as it might be completed by a nurse on a unit where a structured flow sheet has not been developed. In this situation the nurse having major responsibility for the management of the nursing care of Lisa Porter, a new 11-year-old diabetic, creates a flow sheet addressing some of the daily problems of living associated with being a new diabetic. The mother, Joan Porter, is also involved. It summarizes responses and activities for a 24-hour period so that it is possible to view a day at a time across all variables or a single variable over several days.

FLOW SHEET

Lisa Porter (and Joan Porter, mother)   *Diabetics* (Dx 4/9/75)

Variables	Time					
	4/10	4/11	4/12	4/13	4/14	4/15
Hypoglycemic Episodes	X2	X1	0	0	0	0
Weight	115	112	111	111	111	110
Insulin techniques	by RN	LP & gf watching steps	LP meas. RN inj	LP meas accurately & inj. JP watch	JP meas LP inj.	JP meas. & inj 1x / LP meas. & inj 1x
Urine testing	RN	RN explain (+ written info) & show LP/JP	LP explaining & demon. to RN	LP explaining to JP & testing	JP explaining & testing	LP Testing on own
Urine Sug/Kit	4+/4+	2+/0	0/0	tr/0	tr/0	0/0
Ambulation	0	5'x2	30'x2	30'x3	ad lib	ad lib
Diet — Food Composition	/	Explored: Understanding	RN identifies Hi COH, Fat & Prot. food on tray	Lack of interest	List of food composition given	Identified COH Fat Prot Comp. of food on tray x3
Rx diet	/	/	/	Explored implications LP angry JP worried	Cont. discussion of implications for	Showed MD Rx diet
Exchange diet	/	/	/	/	How to get control by knowing exchange system	Planned menus x3 days built on family patterns & lists. LP/JP
Relationship of blood sugar to life events	0 Understanding	LP Angry JP interested	Explored that understanding → control c̄ LP	Asked LP to relate usual ↗↓ phys act to BS	LP Emot. stresses & B sugar	Illness & B sugar

These flow sheets may present a challenge since nurses have been less accustomed to making explicit the variables on which they make judgments for arriving at the statement or sense of progress. However, there is no reason why practicing nurses and nurse researchers cannot develop these criteria and why nursing educators and continuing education programs cannot teach both future nurses and currently practicing nurses so that each of us is sufficiently capable of carrying out this function and building valid, reliable flow sheets.

Progress Reports

There has been a growing tendency in recent years to move away from ritualistic charting on nurses "notes."

E.g., "Gen A.M. care c̄ backrub. Pt. comf," or "Good day. No cx." Instead, there is a movement toward problem-oriented charting, whether the charts are structured for this or not. Problem-oriented charting merely implies that the statements regarding the client are organized and labeled according to the problem rather than some other organizing system. It can be done on any open-ended recording system. Of course, the current emphasis is on problem-oriented medical records. In fact, many are so labeled Problem-Oriented Medical Records (POMR), rather than Problem-Oriented Health Records, that would incorporate dimensions of health care other than medical. The notion of problem-oriented organization of recordings is catching on for many disciplines, and so it has implications for nursing. It means that nurses will be expected to deal with findings and care in terms of problems rather than only recording tasks done for the client. The latter are still recorded, but more often than not, on a check-off sheet —as medicines and treatments are, leaving other descriptions of the client's presenting or changing situation to be recorded on a progress record or in a progress type of recording. In some situations the progress records are integrated with all health professionals noting progress on one form. In more, the form labeled "Progress Notes" is restricted to physician recordings, with others making notes elsewhere, or through the physician.

For nurses, the usual expectations are that they will write progress notes in terms of diagnosed problems, interventions, and goals. Subjective and objective data are summarized as a basis for evaluation of the client status, goal achievement, and effectiveness of nursing prescription.

The progress notes which appear on p. 264 written by a nurse practitioner reflect the recording about a client's problem of managing to live effectively with diabetes and arteriosclerotic heart disease.

The interval between progress notations (given daily nursing charting on routines and observations on other forms for legal obligations and a data base of therapy) will be determined by the pace of response and the nature of the problem. There should, however, be a *maximum time period* within which the problems, goals, prescribed regimen, and responses must be reviewed, evaluated, and updated. This interval may be by shift in acute care settings, by day or week in less acute situations, and monthly in maintenance situations. Ambulatory care settings often make a progress note per visit, again depending on frequency. There is, of course, no reason not to make a progress notation more

Progress Notes

DATE

12/1

Sx: Felt "better" until 3 days ago—"unbalanced" p̄ standing. Thirsty ↑ fatigue ↑, intermittent diarrhea (6x/day) ↓ amts of urine, sweats on exertion & during meals. Ex-wife states appetite better and urine testapes 4+ 3x/day q.d. since going home.

Ox: rash appears improved c̄ less itching. Neck veins not distended. Edema 1+ pretibial.

Nsg. Assessment: Ex-wife has been giving insulin & testing urines c̄ fair degree of confidence. Trying to observe Na restriction and diabetic diet. Pt. appears less depressed & is enjoying tapes for ham radio instruction.

Plan: Referred to Soc. Serv. for financial matters.
Diet reviewed—insulin technique with sliding scale coverage discussed—began discussion of rotation of sites
Nail care and foot care briefly discussed
Per consultation c̄ Dr. Roger. Dc. Lasix. ↓ Digoxin 0.125 mgm q̄od
Lente Insulin U-40 25 U q̄ a.m. and Reg Insulin 10 U if 4+ testape beginning 12/3/ Cont. other meds.

N. Nebor R.N.N.P.

Telephone Tues. p.m. Ret. appt. 1 week.

12/5

Tel. call: managing well. Urine testapes 2-3+ c̄ ↑ Lente. ↓ thirst and ↑ equilibrium on standing.

N.N.

12/8

Sx: Feels "better & stronger" Activities ↑ outside apt. Balance improved. Notes ↑ swelling in extremities as day progresses. No PND or orthopnea. Urine testapes 2-3+ Required Reg. 10 U 1 day for 4+. Planning remarriage.

Ox: Rash improving s̄ Vistaril past week.

Nsg. Assessment: ↓ depression. Following treatment plan easily and confidently.

Plan: Referred to Soc Serv. re diabetic son needing care @ the County Mental Health Clinic. Referred to hospital chaplain for marriage plans.
Reviewed diabetic instructional material provided.
Outlined injection rotation pattern. Taught radial pulse counting.
Per consultation with Dr. R restart Lasix 40 mgm. q̄od
Lente Insulin 30 U q̄ a.m. and reg Insulin 10 U for 4+ testape
Aldomet & digoxin q̄od as before.
Telephone Tues. p.m. Ret. app. 1/week./

Sched. M-G, CBC, EKG.   N. Nebor R.N.N.P.

frequently. All this regulation would require is that the nurse assigned the management of the client be expected to delay no longer than this in evaluating and recording the progress and then updating the rest of the plan.

Final Summaries

When a client leaves a care system, of whatever nature, a final summary note on nursing management and response should be made. This summarizes the current situations. It may be helpful to include aspects of nursing management that were attempted and not successful, as well as those which were. It certainly should include the coping challenges abilities and resources involved in the client's current situation and any predicted future challenges. To improve chances of continuity, xeroxes of such a final summary can be attached to any referral sheet or transfer materials when the individual moves to a different health care system. Following is an example of a final summary note on a client who came in for a diagnostic D. and C. with high risk of a malignancy.

> Pre- and postoperative preparation adequate. Understands care of self on discharge. Likes to identify with one nurse. To return to doctor's office in 6 weeks if diagnosis benign. Understands importance of follow-up care and periodic check-ups. Anxious to return to home and family—relationships seem warm and close. Reluctant to express fears with a variety of different nursing personnel. Enjoys talking about children and husband. Still realistically concerned about possible malignancy. Seems reassured by straightforward explanations.

Below is an example of communication of the plan of medical and nursing care on a referral from a nurse in a hospital to a community health nurse. Mrs. Clark has been referred for home care by her physician and the nursing staff at Skyline Hospital. The referral gave the following information:

Two-week hospitalization; discharged Monday, October 10.
Inoperable breast cancer, rapidly metastasizing to spine. In late stages.

PHYSICIAN'S ORDERS:

1. Testosterone 2 cc. I.M. weekly.
2. Colace 100 mgm BID.
3. ASA gr XV prn for pain.
4. Fleet's enema prn.
5. Up in chair as tolerated.
6. Bathroom privileges if tolerated.

The nurse at the Skyline Hospital had written the following information:

Current status of implementation of physician's orders: Testosterone usually given every Wednesday at 9 a.m. Rotation of sites rt and lt leg I.M. sites (little muscular tissue in arms).

Suggest to continue colace and 1 glass of water at 7 a.m. and 9 p.m. (Patient unable to give own

265

medications, and husband and 17-year-old daughter are home at these times. They have been instructed.)

Elimination

Enema has been needed every 3 days. Enema given on day of discharge. Retains fluid well when placed on left side. When on bedpan, use a small pillow in small of back. If unable to expel stool, remove manually. Usual bowel routine: place on bedpan at 7:30 a.m. Husband and daughter have been taught bedpan technique. Prefers to have bedplan placed on chair at right side of bed. Needs assistance to transfer from bed to chair. Tolerates assistance in transfer. Family has bedpan. Tolerates being up in chair for approx. 2 hrs. at a time. Enjoys being up for meals. Family has wheelchair.

Support Systems

Mrs. Clark and family are aware of diagnosis and prognosis. Husband and daughter seem very devoted. They asked that she be allowed to come home, and indicated willingness to assume responsibility for care. A neighbor, Mrs. Leary, is available to assist client during day when husband and daughter are not home. Client able to help self with some difficulty.

Nutrition

Buttermilk, fruit juices, and soups. Needs some assistance with feeding—tires easily.

Dyspnea

When dyspneic, client prefers lying on either side with head of bed elevated 30 degrees. Family has hospital bed. Has difficulty talking when dyspneic. Family aware of problem.

Pain

Client uses self-hypnosis and post-hypnotic suggestions of her physician for relief of pain. Has been very effective. ASA usually requested 7 a.m. and HS.

Hygiene

Enjoys bed bath after breakfast. Uses TV as diversion, usually in evening. Mrs. Clark is alert and pleasant. She seems to hesitate to ask for things at times.

Catherine Murdock, R.N.
Skyline Hospital

SUMMARY

Evaluation and recording of patterns of management together with client response are as essential in the nursing component of health care as in any other. The skills of determining the criteria to be used, the data to be collected and the recording system to be used are currently not well developed in many nurses, nor in nursing's body of knowledge, for that matter. We are functioning, however, in a system where responses to disease and treatment are evaluated every day both by doctors and nurses; so there is an established climate, lifestyle and protocol for this behavior in the medical dimension of health care. It should not be extraordinarily difficult, then, to add nursing's focus of evaluation to that of the other disciplines—to add variables concerned with strength, endurance, knowledge and its use, desire for participation, skills, development of support systems, and risk taking. They fit very naturally and serve to expand the total picture of the client's progress in coping with his problems of health and their impact on his daily living.

REFERENCES

Bloom, Benjamin, et al. *Taxonomy of Educational Objectives, Handbook I: Cognitive Domain.* New York: David McKay, 1956.

Eisman, Roberta. *Criteria Registered Nurses Reportedly Use in Making Decisions Regarding Observation of Respiratory Behavior of Patients.* Unpublished Thesis, University of Washington, 1970.

Mager, Robert F. *Developing Attitude Toward Learning,* "Recognizing Approach," pp. 21-30. Belmont, California: Lear Siegler Inc./Fearon Publishers, 1968.

chapter Thirteen

Communicating Nursing Care Plans

Continuity of care and systematic communication go hand in hand. Nursing care plans have a two-fold purpose in relation to communication. First, they form a written basis for communicating the nursing diagnosis, planned goals, and prescribed nursing actions that can provide for a smooth progression of the client's nursing care. Second, care plans can be used to communicate to nurses data on the nature and quality of care that they are providing for their clients.

Written care plans form the foundation for the methodical communication of important elements in each client's nursing care. This is true, whether the nurse is communicating with:

> the client
> herself
> her colleagues
> other team members
> the physician
> the family
> the nursing staff on other units or departments
> nursing staff in subsequent admissions or
> staff in other health care agencies and institutions.

COMMUNICATING THE PLAN OF CARE TO THE CLIENT

Let us look first at our communication of the plan of care to the person who probably has the greatest interest in it—the client. If we truly believe in autonomy, if we believe we are assisting the client to cope with his problems and not solving them for him, then it follows that he should have a collaborative role whenever possible. Admittedly, there are times when his physical and mental status do not permit this; however, whenever it is feasible, the client is a partner in the plan.

We have all had occasion to visit a physician for examination and treatment. We participated as he collected data and then waited in varying degrees of fear and anticipation for feedback on his interpretation of findings and his plan for our care. Suppose he failed to give us any satisfactory feedback? Then, even though we have a vested interest in our own well-being, how much motivation would we have for following through with the prescribed care? Fortunately, most of us have been informed (to the extent that the doctor considered it therapeutic) of the nature of his findings and the plan of care he is recommending, and often we are given the rationale for the treatment being instituted. Then the road back to health seems to become a mutual responsibility. There is usually no reason why the same feedback should not occur between the nurse and the client when it comes to the plan for nursing care.

Pretend for a moment that you are a client who has been interviewed for a nursing assessment. A short time later your nurse returns and says, "From what you've told me and from the doctor's orders for your therapy, these . . . seem to me to be the problems with which we nurses can help you during your illness and in your recovery. . . . We'll be trying to help you by. . . ." She then, like your doctor, is sharing with you her interpretation of the findings and the plan that has emerged in her thinking.

Suppose we look at some specific examples. This time, imagine that you are facing a gallbladder operation in the morning. You have never had surgery before. Your nurse has made a tentative decision that you need some help in preparing for the early postoperative period so that you will be able to participate effectively. So the nurse says:

> You told me that you expect to experience some discomfort after surgery. It may tempt you to lie very still, but we know that you will tend to avoid complications and have a smoother recovery if we keep you comfortable, help you to move regularly, and assist you with deep breathing. . . . We could go through a rehearsal of it now so that you may know how we will help you in moving and how you can help yourself, and also what you will be expected to do in deep breathing. . . . I will tell you how you can move most easily and help you to move as we will tomorrow—that way you can know how it feels. . . . Now, let's go through the steps of moving from a lying position to sitting on the edge of the bed. . . . This is the position where you can get your deepest breaths, so that your lungs get fresh air to the deepest parts. To deep breathe, I'll support the area where your incision will be so that you can be assured that it does keep it from moving so much. . . .

Or pretend that you have low back pain. Your doctor has ordered pain medication every four hours at your request, but you also told the nurse who took the history that backrubs of the upper back and neck help you to relax. In giving you feedback on the plan of care, she indicates that the medication has been ordered for you and that a backrub is scheduled for you during your morning care and again at bedtime, but you may have them more often if you experience discomfort.

If you were a client who received this kind of nursing attention, would you feel that:

1. The information you shared was being used?
2. Nurses cared about what you thought and wanted?
3. You could ask for changes if the plan was not agreeable to you?
4. You could remind the nurses if activities were omitted?
5. You were involved in "doing with," rather than being "done to"?

This sharing of the plan of nursing care communicates the nurse's evaluation of client information, and it also communicates her expectations for client involvement and responsibility. In addition, it serves to set the client's expectations regarding the limits of nursing activities that are possible within the realities of this health care setting, so that he too can use nursing resources more wisely.

COMMUNICATING PLANS OF CARE TO THE CLIENT'S FAMILY

Health workers as a group in institutions of the Western world have become aware that families are an important factor in the client's response to illness and recovery (some other cultures never lost sight of this resource!). In retrospect, it seems that we have only gradually found that health care may be given in the presence of families at many hours of the day and night. And, surprisingly enough, we have found that families have not lost their ability to help care for the client whether he has been placed temporarily in a health care institution or remains at home.

Families *can* be a part of the client's resources and support system when health problems occur. As such, they need to be involved *to the degree* that *primary* data from:

the client

involved family members

indicate a desire and a potential for contribution. Before doing any planning or sharing of client data, the nurse needs to collect current primary data that the client wants a family member involved in either knowledge of his status or in care activities. By the same token, the family members, as a primary source of data, need to be interviewed or nonverbal data need to be collected to determine their genuine desires and capabilities as a resource.

For example, a husband has an extreme aversion to illness in himself and, particularly, in any member of his family. He gets frightened, he worries, he gets angry, he avoids contact. The wife, knowing this response and behavior pattern, may well wish that neither the nurses nor the doctor tell the husband what her diagnosis or prognosis is, preferring to maintain their relationship on a status quo basis as long as possible. She may well have other resources she has built over the years which she prefers to use. Given this situation, what right does the nurse have to interfere in an ongoing marital relationship?

This example represents one extreme of a close family relationship where non-involvement is chosen. The other extreme is much less rare. How often have we observed situations in which the client and family each wish family involvement, but nurses fail to share information, goals, or activities with them.

It is important to communicate nursing goals in caring for the client to the family or to those important others who sometimes substitute for family. *If* they are going to help, they should know the direction his care is taking. If they should not or cannot help, or are not permitted to do so, they may have a need to know what we are attempting to do. In a time of stress and fear it may give them a sense of being cared about too.

When members of a family are to assume an active role in the client's care, they must know how they can participate appropriately. Suppose a client's daughter comes in after work and notices that her father is slowly and awkwardly feeding himself. Seeing that nurses are occupied elsewhere, she steps in and feeds him. Perhaps she even plans her schedule so as to come in and feed him the next night as well, and asks her sister to drop over to help at lunch. Now, on the other hand, suppose that the goal is for the father to develop increasing strength and endurance by feeding himself. Then the nurse and the daughter are working at cross purposes. How much better to share the goals of nursing care with a responsible member of the family who, in turn, can alert the others to the goals and current approaches! Then they may come—at mealtimes, if they wish—and talk with him or help in small ways that do not interfere with his needed activity. They may notice and help him to see the steps he is making in gaining strength through his laborious efforts and convey their confidence in him.

Sharing plans with families often helps them to clarify their role in the illness and therapy, thus minimizing conflicts of expectations. Does the family believe that medical costs are so high that nurses should do all the care? Are they aware that some aspects of care may be more effective when given by a member of the family? Do they want to ask questions but dare not? Do they want to help but doubt the acceptability of it? A frank discussion of their questions and desires, and of nursing goals and approaches, can attune them to client needs and give them security in their role as participants in the planned care.

Another reason for sharing aspects of the nursing care plan with the family is that many of the client's problems involve them. Therefore, a family that has been kept abreast of problems and achievements may feel less fearful about assuming more responsibility when he returns home. And, if they are not only aware but have participated in activities, they assume responsibility much more easily.

Many factors influence the degree of involvement members of the family may want or be able to accept, not the least important of which is their previous relationship with the person. The nurse should note in her data how family members affect the client. Those who have a contribution to make to the person's well-being ought to be motivated and encouraged to participate as effectively as possible. Communication of the plan of nursing care can channel that contribution toward a common goal.

CARE PLANS COMMUNICATE TO THE NURSE WHO WROTE THEM

Nursing care plans are effective in achieving orderly progression of nursing care when they are used consistently by the nurse who wrote them. Case loads, distractions, and time intervals between client contacts, as well as the normal frailty of human memory, are excellent reasons for a nurse to use the care plans she herself has written.

Nurses Who Work Alone

In some health care situations all nursing care is provided by one nurse—the public health nurse, the school nurse, the office nurse, and, in smaller industries, the occupational health nurse, or the nurse practitioner. Here the nurse finds the plans an effective means of reorienting herself to the client's situation as she saw it in her last contact, and from this she can assess changes that seem to have taken place in the time interval between contacts. A glance at the written diagnosis, goals, and nursing orders, as well as notes on client response, can quickly bring the client situation into focus. To prove it to yourself, try the care plan technique with part of your case load, and give nursing care to another segment without the care plan system, using your usual narrative nursing notes.

Not only do care plans and client progress records refresh the nurse's memory of her previous perceptions; they also help her to identify to herself and to her client the changes that take place over a period of time. We are always so sure that we are going to remember those small but critical client responses; but, if you are like most of the rest of us, you will be surprised in reviewing your plans and progress notes to see the data you would have forgotten. Sometimes the client, too, will have passed significant milestones in his progress without being aware of them. It is stimulating to the client, and to the nurse, to be able to spot progress or to see areas where the client has held his own or coped with stresses more effectively over a period of time. Data on coping ability serve well as guidelines for prediction and prescription in subsequent planning for this client.

Nurses Who Share Responsibilities for Client Care with Colleagues

The nurse who shares client care with other nurses uses care plans *to communicate to herself* as well as to her colleagues. The usual work setting in which this occurs is in the hospital or nursing home. In institutional nursing, it is distraction, perhaps, more than length of interval between contacts that tends to disrupt the nurse's ability to provide organized continuity of care within her own sphere of influence. The distractions take the form of numbers of clients, numbers of personnel, visitors, traffic, noise, and so on. However, in addition to distractions, there is also the element of time away from the work setting, when one considers days off, illnesses, vacation, holidays, educational or professional leave.

With the communication from prior plans combined with observations of present client status, the nurse is able to satisfy herself that continuity is being maintained in spite of the "Grand Central Station" nature of many nursing units or that occasional four-day weekend.

Nurses today are using *nursing rounds* to assure themselves that the care being given is moving at the client's pace. On these rounds of the clients in her case loads she carries her nursing care plans to communicate to herself the diagnoses, goals, and orders that currently guide the nursing care of her clients. As she visits, interviews, and observes each client she either validates care given or notes changes that are needed in caring for this client. She can re-date the orders she wishes to be continued, discontinue those that are now obsolete, and jot down notes regarding the changes in the care plan she wishes to make. In nursing care rounds, as in the assessment interview, she primarily collects data on client response and expectations. However, she also reinforces the client's original impressions that a registered nurse is assuming responsibility for the quality of nursing care, is interested in him, and is listening to him, on a continuing basis, and is maintaining the relationship that was begun in the first contact.

CARE PLANS ARE COMMUNICATED TO NURSING COLLEAGUES

Nursing care plans communicate the essence of care to a nurse's colleagues through their very existence in writing and through verbal communication—usually at the change-of-shift report.

On relatively rare occasions, a nursing care plan may have to speak for itself without any additional oral interpretation; for example, someone falls ill during a shift and must be replaced by a float nurse, or some other emergency measure is taken in which the time for verbal interaction is limited. If the nurse who comes on can give the client the same kind of care he has been receiving after she has read the diagnosis, goals, and nursing orders, then the author of the care plans has communicated well. Nurses who have floated to units in which care plans are conscientiously carried on have commented on the ease with which they can fit into the nursing care needed by a group of totally new clients.

The most common situation in which nursing care is transferred from one group of nurses to another is at the change of shift. Here the written care plan is supplemented with a verbal report and is more open to explanation or questions. Currently, because most Kardexes are oriented to maintaining continuity of delegated *medical care,* these are the aspects of care that receive priority of attention as nurses give change-of-shift reports. We learn when the last Demerol was given, that the pre-op enemas till clear have been completed, that the urine was sent to the lab, that a breakfast is being held, that the client is on IV #4, 5% in DW—due to complete at 10 A.M., and so on. All of these units of information are important to clients, but they are only a part of the nurse's responsibility for care—only a part of what she needs to know to function effectively in caring for her clients during the next tour of duty. Through the use of the nursing care plan system the nursing care aspects will also receive their rightful share of attention.

Let's contrast a few samples of reporting as they might occur during a change of-shift report, without and with nursing information.

Name and Status	Medical Care Information	Nursing Care Information
Mrs. Graham 80 years aphasic hemiplegic (old)	Needs to have food and fluid intake increased as tolerated.	Will open her mouth automatically if spoon is held 18" from face so she can see it. Likes hi-prot. milk shakes. Will eat most of food served, but *slowly*. Poss. volunteers in family for feeding?
Mr. Jones 73 years pneumonia, Parkinson's disease	Needs to have food & fluid increased as tolerated.	Food should be almost liquid consistency Tell him when to swallow. Does not like eggnog.
Mrs. Green 72 years recent left hemiplegic (CVA). Responsive but forgetful. In and out of reality.	Do range of motion and encourage activity. Prevent shoulder joint damage. Wheelchair. 1 hr BID.	Able and willing to do ROM and isotonics on unaffected side and on fingers and wrist of affected side. Needs help on other joints. Does on cue of "someone leaving the room." Will brush own hair. Will feed self if food cut and fixed. Use sling on arm when up in chair. Daughter-in-law helps with exercises. Good resource.
Timmy White 12 years appendectomy 1 day p.o.	Ambulate TID.	Will move self if given time. Dislikes others moving him.
Mr. Ferris 46 years Cholecystectomy 2 days p.o. Chr. resp. infection	Cough and deep breathe.	Coughs and deep breathes most effectively 30 min. post-analgesia. Sits on side of bed. Towel around waist for splinting. Willing to C and DB at other times, but less effective. Needs encouragement, but knows technique.

Name and Status	Medical Care Information	Nursing Care Information
Mrs. Lehman 76 years pneumonia and or- ganic brain disease. No verbal feedback.	Range of motion, turn.	Responsive to auditory stim. Responsive to praise and posi- tive expressions. Will open eyes and do ROM with arms when asked. Can't turn self. Needs more auditory and tac- tile stim.
Mr. Frank 53 years Myocardial infarction 2 days ago	Absolute bed rest. Feed patient.	Balks at orders but responsive to joking and to compromise or "deals." Few teeth, eats slowly.
Mrs. Keely Rt. cataract First p.o. day	Keep both eyes patched.	Identify yourself on entering room. Wants to touch person talking to her. Cooperates with instructions.

Next time you listen to or give a change-of-shift report, note what proportion of it is given over to communicating medical treatments and also to nursing care. Would it be possible to communicate both in the time allotted for report? If not, how could non-essentials be communicated in other ways to that essentials of both medical and nursing care receive attention?

COMMUNICATING CARE PLANS TO MEMBERS OF THE NURSING TEAM

Once client assignments have been made on any shift, the next step is to ac-quaint the staff with the current priority of nursing goals, the nursing actions and approaches to be tried, and the feedback on client response that is desired. This assignment conference should be a two-way dialogue, not an "I'll talk, you write" lecture. There are often honest disagreements as to the nature of the diagnosis, the current goals, and the approaches prescribed. If a team member or an "asso-ciate" of the primary nurse is giving only lip service to the plan of care, one may safely predict that its execution will be less than effective. So, it is important to achieve at least a shared understanding of the rationale, if not wholehearted agree-ment on the nature of the care to be given.

Often the nurse wants to retain responsibility for some segment of the client's care—some treatment or teaching, or the discussion of a particular problem area. She should so inform the team members or associates, to avoid conflict or duplica-tion. A mutually acceptable time schedule also needs to be worked out. The nurse may want to elicit ideas or data related to the care she intends to give: first, to become aware of her perspective of the client and, second, to stimulate the in-volvement of the others in all aspects of client care. For, while the nurse may do the writing of the care plan, the plan itself is a composite of the participants' actions and observations—a mutual responsibility and achievement.

The nurse should also explore the feedback that she needs on client response, being quite specific about the cues that should be observed and measured. This serves several purposes:

1. It forces the primary nurse or team leader to think in terms of specific, relevant cues in patient response.
2. It results in less vague, subjective, impressionistic information being returned in the feedback conference.
3. It upgrades the observational skill of the associates or team members.
4. Hopefully, it stimulates them to think of additional cues that would describe more accurately or more extensively the nature of client response.

The elements, then, of the nurse's report to the staff about the client are: a report on client status; an indication of goals that are receiving current attention; nursing approaches and actions being tried; cues on client response to be observed; and potential problems to be kept in mind.

Let's take an example of the way the nurse might talk with a practical nurse about one patient. We shall use Mrs. Green (p. 274) as our sample:

RN: Mrs. Green in Room 47, bed B, was transferred in from Midvale Hospital Tuesday. She had a CVA two weeks ago with left hemiplegia.

She's responsive and gaining strength, but she leaves the world of reality frequently. Our current goal is to help her gain strength and prevent contractures. She is able and willing to do range of motion and isotonic exercises on the unaffected side. She'll brush her own hair and feed herself if you set it up. She's embarrassed about spilling and loss of control of food in her mouth.

PN: She might enjoy brushing her own teeth and washing her face, neck, and chest if I help her with the washcloth and soap.

RN: Sounds like a good idea. She began yesterday to do ROM on her affected fingers and wrist, but couldn't manage the elbow and shoulder. Why don't you see if she'll go a bit higher today? We tried making a contract with her to do some exercises whenever someone leaves the room. We need some data on whether she is able to remember to exercise and understand what she is doing.

PN: I'll keep an eye on whether she does it and what she does, while I care for her and the other women in that room.

RN: I'll make a point of coming in myself and then leaving, so you'll be sure to have a situation to watch. If she does remember, let's compliment her to reinforce the behavior. If she forgets, remind her. Notice how she reacts to both praise and reminding. We need to find the best way to motivate her.

When you do the ROM on her affected side, let me know the amount of limitation as compared to her good side.

Incidentally, her daughter-in-law told me that she was unable to walk long before her CVA. They used a wheelchair. You'll need help getting her into the wheelchair. Mr. Gibbs is caring for the men in 49 this morning. I'll alert him that you'll need help getting Mrs. Green up and back to bed. There's a sling for her arm in the bedside stand.

PN: Fine. Do you think she's getting bored and needs something to do? I could explore with her what she has been doing before.

RN: Sounds good. So far, the pressure areas on her back look normal, but we're watching to see that she turns, and massaging them with care. Now for Mrs. Carlson in bed C. . . .

The highest quality of care can be offered by concerned nursing personnel, all of whom share a sense of concern for the well-being of the clients in their case load and who have an *esprit de corps* about their ability to give good nursing care.

COMMUNICATING BY CARE PLANS WITH NURSES ON OTHER UNITS

Clients are frequently transferred from one unit to another. Often this is routine practice, as in the case of obstetric clients who move from the delivery unit to the postpartum unit, who are also closely involved with nurses from the nursery. Similarly, clients on the medical units may move to surgical or specialty units or vice versa. In progressive care units, the clients anticipate moving from intensive to intermediate to self-care units. Since mobility is a "way of life" in our institutions, it behooves us to systematize the exchange of information about the client.

It seems unfair to the client to require him either to adjust to radically different patterns of nursing care or to have him repeat the data he has already given to the nurses. It also requires more of the staff's time to individualize care if they have no data with which to work. The smoothest and most economical transition is made when the nursing assessment, the current care plan, and the progress report accompany him as a part of his chart. A short, focused conference between the nurse who has been caring for the person and the one who will be assuming responsibility for his care on the new unit can quickly bring the latter up to date on problems (solved and unsolved), his strengths, and nursing intervention that has seemed to be successful.

Also, if the client is aware that efforts are being made to maintain the continuity of care and that his contributions toward this continuity are still welcome, it may offer a sense of security and of being well cared for.

USE OF CARE PLANS IN SUBSEQUENT ADMISSIONS

Just as data on client problems and responses are helpful when they transfer from one unit to another, so data on his experience in a previous admission can help the nurse to plan orientation, teaching, and other aspects of nursing more appropriately. For example, the previous care plan and progress notes may indi-

277

cate some of the client's experiences and responses, procedures done, and problems encountered in previous hospitalizations. On the basis of these data, the nurse can intelligently explore the client's perception of his previous experience and his expectations of the current one.

An example might highlight the way in which the previous data contribute to planning for subsequent care. Mr. Moore was being admitted for heart surgery for the second time. In the previous postoperative period he had spent several days in the intensive care unit. The nurse said:

> "Mr. Moore, I understand this will be your second visit to the intensive care unit. Are there any things that the nurses can do for you this time that would make your stay there a bit easier?" "Yes," he said, "there were a few little things I would have liked different. I know I couldn't have water to drink for a while, but my lips got so dry—it'd sure help if they'd wipe my lips with some ice chips inside a washcloth or some gauze or something. And the washcloth wrung out with cold water and put on my forehead felt good too. There were a lot of tubes to keep going, but I like a cover over me. Guess it's just what I'm used to. And oh, if I could get my teeth brushed a bit more often—my mouth tasted awful."

The nurse made notes of his requests and learned that in all other respects he recalled few problems. The nurses' notes had indicated that he had been able to participate quite effectively in postoperative exercises and had an uneventful recovery. She reviewed with him the aspects of the pre- and postoperative period that were likely to be similar to his previous experience and noted his comments and reactions. From this short interview based on prior data, she began making her own plans for his preoperative care and made notes on his requests to the nurses in intensive care.

Nurses caring for clients who have had several hospital admissions (injuries, orthopedic conditions, or chronic diseases) have found the nursing care plans from previous admissions a good starting point for planning care during the present admission. There is, however, the danger of not being alert to changes in responses. In the case of children, for example, there are developmental stages to consider. In every instance the nurse should not take previous plans at face value, but use them simply as a point of departure.

COMMUNICATING BY CARE PLANS WITH NURSES IN OTHER AGENCIES

A pattern in client care that is being seen with increasing frequency is the transferring of clients' health care management from one health care setting to another as their health needs vary. They are moved easily between clinics, offices, diagnostic centers, acute care institutions, convalescent centers, rehabilitation centers, retirement residences, and home care with or without public health nurse supervision.

Any change in the health care setting poses problems for both the client and his nurse. For the client there is the uncertainty of the new environment, questions as to how his needs and preferences will be met, and concern as to the acceptance he will receive as a person. Some of the energy he needs for healing and recovery, or perhaps even survival, is diverted into reacting to the stress of the change. In some instances, this is a dissipation of energy he can ill afford at this time. If, on the other hand, he is made aware that facts about his patterns of daily activity and living, his needs and his preferences are being communicated to receptive listeners in the new agency, some of the tension of moving may well be reduced.

For the nurse in the receiving agency, the new client represents extra demands upon her—an equation with some knowns and many unknowns that she hopes to balance. If she too is aware that some of the data on the unknowns will be passed on by colleagues who have already been working with him, she also will feel more secure in picking up the problems. She expects to have some data on problems that have been solved, the techniques that were successful, and the areas of limitation in which the client still needs help. Although the priorities of medical therapy may change with a shift in institutions (e.g., moving from an acute care setting to a rehabilitation center), the client resources and responses with which the nurse must work tend to change slowly, and represent the framework within which the new nurse must offer her assistance to him in his coping efforts.

When a client moves from one part of the health care system to another there are certain areas of nursing information that should be predictably available. These include:

> Problems that have been resolved
>
> Continuing unresolved problems—current status, prognosis
>
> Coping abilities and resources identified
>
> Deficits in abilities and resources identified
>
> Nursing prescriptions that were successful/unsuccessful
>
> Identification of referring nurse, means of contact (phone, address)
>
> Date

These may be contained in a summary of progress, in a narrative form, or in a concise outline based on predetermined headings. It also seems appropriate that these reports be signed by the nurse and that her phone number be given; sometimes a short phone call can save a great deal of time and spare the patient and nurse some unnecessary difficulty. Verbal interchanges also have the faculty of strengthening the bonds of communication and sense of responsibility for continuity between nurses in the agencies.

COMMUNICATING WITH PHYSICIANS BY CARE PLANS

Nursing care plans are predicated upon the belief that nursing care is different from medical care, but that the unique contribution that each one makes must be closely interwoven with and supportive to that of the other. Before nurses became aware of the unique contribution they had to make to client's care, doctor's rounds tended to be primarily a receiving process on the part of the nurse—one in which the doctor looked at the chart, heard any comments from the nurse, visited the client and gave the nurse the new orders that were to guide the medical therapy for the next 8 to 24 hours. This is not to say that nurses have not served as liaison or advocates for the client or that they have not reported on observed response and, in this way, contributed to the doctor's data. However, when the nurse's primary function was to carry out the assigned medical therapy, there was less sense of responsibility for, or awareness of, the need to communicate problems of nursing nature not related to medical therapy.

With a planned approach to nursing care, the physician's rounds can be used by the nurse: 1) to validate her perceptions of nursing care problems with the physician, 2) to indicate how she is individualizing the medical therapy, and 3) to discover more effective ways of dovetailing her intervention with that of the physician. There will be times when the nurse needs the medical expertise of the physician; there also will be times when he needs her expertise in the nursing area. As recognition of the unique contribution each one has to make to client well-being develops, this sharing of expertise should grow.

Written nursing care plans can be an important component of the physician's rounds, as well as nursing rounds. Again, they serve to give the nurse reminders of what she wants to communicate to the physician and of client needs that she should share.

This pattern of shared communication should not be limited to institutional settings. Nurse practitioners and nurses in traditional roles in ambulatory care settings also need to use the same approach of assuming responsibility for the nursing component of health management. They too need to make the physician as well as the client aware of their data base and plans for nursing management so that there is continuity and commonality in their approaches and the client is not caught in the middle.

In situations in which this collaborative approach to physicians' rounds has been instituted, nurses and physicians alike have reported developing a greater awareness of the contribution each has to make. The result has been more efficient and economical utilization of each one's particular skills and knowledge.

SUMMARY

We have explored the idea of utilizing written care plans to communicate the past and current status of nursing care to: the client, his family, the nurse who wrote the plans, her colleagues on the ward, her team members, nurses, physicians, and to those on other wards, in subsequent admissions, and in other agencies. Nursing care problems that have been solved, as well as those yet to be solved; unsuccessful as well as successful approaches; and reports of patterns of client response and coping ability were seen as being useful information to be shared. The well-written care plan may speak for itself without interpretation, but verbal interchange as an adjunct is helpful to both the nurse giving and the one receiving the report.

The client who knows efforts are being made to provide for continuity of care may experience less stress in adapting to the new situation. Certainly, the nurse with some foundation of knowledge of the nursing care and client activities that have preceded her care feels that she can progress in a more orderly fashion, although she expects to validate the data she has received.

chapter / **Fourteen**

Environmental Factors for Maintaining Nursing Care Plan Systems

Any nurse with a reasonable case load who is skilled in nursing process and well grounded in nursing knowledge will plan nursing care with or without supporting systems. It becomes a usual pattern of thinking, an established nursing lifestyle. But, for a *system* of care planning to survive, one that is consistent, one that involves all nurses, many factors in the work environment must be considered. These factors have their foundations in the organization's philosophy of nursing services; and from this beginning, branch out into every facet of the nursing system (small or large) to shape decisions and behavior regarding:

philosophy and objectives of nursing care
policies
budget
staffing
job descriptions and evaluation
assignments
staff development
records and recording systems
relationships with non-nursing departments and disciplines
leadership

Let's examine each of these and their relationship to the orderly development of the nursing care planning system.

NURSING DEPARTMENT'S PHILOSOPHY AND THE CARE PLAN SYSTEM

The written philosophy of care in a hospital, on a unit, in a clinic, office, or retirement home—in any nursing system—*ought to* reflect an honest, genuine belief concerning the nature of the care planning system within that setting. The reverse side of the "ought to" of a written philosophy, the *working philosophy* of any institution, is quite identifiable by observation of the behavior of the staff, often in the nature of their care planning activities with clients, their families, and with other disciplines. Let's look at some areas.

Does the nursing carried out reflect a focus on tasks and routines rather than on individualization of care? (See contrasts of job descriptions for a night nurse in one institution and a primary care nurse in another, pp. 290-291.)

Do assignments and priorities show greater concern for protection and support of the staff than for the clientele?

Is conformity to policies and procedures valued over the needs and rights of clients?

How are the values of accountability and a degree of professional autonomy balanced within the care planning system?

Is cost effectiveness valued to the point that staff are used at the appropriate level of skill in assessment-diagnosis, in prescription of nursing care, in implementation and evaluation of care, in related staff development?

Is the expertise of the nursing staff, in relation to knowledge about a client's readiness to cope with the demands of living in his home setting, being used by the Utilization Review Board as they make decisions regarding appropriate length of stay in institutions?

Are priorities of planning for health care associated with client needs or with the traditional hierarchical status of the discipline making the plan? Practically speaking, if nursing care is more important to a client's well-being at a point in time, do nursing plans assume priority of attention even though a physician may be in attendance?

Do prescribed nursing therapies carry as much weight as prescribed medical care with the nursing staff when both are important to client well-being?

How important are clients and their families seen to be in nursing care planning? Specifically, what expectations are set for consistently involving them at an appropriate level within their expertise in planning? How much in evaluation of the plans and the care given?

How much consideration is given to values held by the client? Is any effort made to determine what they are? When they are known, is any effort made to regard them? When are they overridden?

How does the nature of the clientele shape the beliefs about strategies of nursing care planning, e.g., the one-visit transients, the residents of institutions for the mentally retarded, the residents of nursing homes?

In health care settings where clients flow through the clinic into in-house units and then back to ambulatory care again, what provision is made to support the belief about the continuity of care?

All of these questions and others need to be dealt with in terms of the specific values of nurses and nursing leadership before drafting the section of the philosophy which deals with the place of nursing care planning in the nursing system. It is wise to look at the implications of the beliefs before they are written, if a philosophy is to be worth more than the paper it is written on. It is wise to look at the working philosophy as it is manifested in the choices and behavior of everyday nursing to find the real values that are influencing care.

With nursing care planning systems it is important to be realistic—about staff skills in planning, about current case loads, about the nature of the clientele. At the same time, it is exciting to be creative. Often an explicit statement of a valued belief initiates action and the impossible becomes possible.

OBJECTIVES OF THE NURSING DEPARTMENT AND THE CARE PLAN SYSTEM

Out of the philosophy grow the objectives that will translate values into working reality. With the current trend toward management by objectives, these are becoming increasingly important to evaluation and identification of progress in organized nursing services, whether these "departments" are large or quite small. Even individuals can function with management by objectives and be more purposeful in their development as well as more concrete in their evaluation of themselves over time.

These system objectives need to begin where the organization, the individual, and the staff are. Then they should set realistic concrete expectations for growth for the year, or other designated time period. Thus, if nursing care planning is in a ritualistic, unskilled state—where "the letter of the law" of care planning rather than its spirit of care planning is the current state of affairs—then objectives for the year may well deal with attitudes, learning the value of nursing care planning, demonstrating it to other disciplines, developing the basic skills, the needed vocabulary, and increasing the speed as well as beginning the necessary modification of relationships between nurses and other disciplines required by the collegiality of mutual care planning.

In settings where these goals are already met, the objectives may be set at another level to outcomes that depend upon the foundation of skilled, predictable nursing care planning. For example:

To guide and facilitate the implementation of a nursing audit:

Provide	educational programs for individual units.
Develop	the criteria measures of an audit tool.
Test,	evaluate and revise the audit tool.
Explore	issues related to implementing the audit tool.

Just as in an earlier chapter we suggested that goals for clients should be realistic, achievable, and practical, this is equally apropos in setting goals for ourselves. Setting goals that have a reasonable degree of opportunity for achievement within the designated time frame makes it seem much more worthwhile to try for them. Most nurses are rather idealistic, committed persons who want to grow and to give good care. All nurses are subject to human frailties and therefore need the same care in setting goals that they direct to their clients. It pays to take good care of ourselves too. And, success breeds success, so plan for growth of system or self, one achievable goal at a time.

POLICIES AND THE CARE PLAN SYSTEM

Although policies are usually considered as written protocols, both written and unwritten policies do carry weight and should be considered in relationship to the care plan system. Written policies might set the expectation that,

"Every in-house patient will be bathed each day and each bed will be changed."

Unwritten policy may dictate that this skin scrubbing and bed changing will be completed by 11 A.M. Data from nursing assessments may indicate that daily baths are not appropriate for a particular client, or that rest is more important after a particularly restless night than having a bath. We know of nurses who knuckled under to the written and unwritten policies of the system to conform to the group norms rather than meet the documented needs of the client.

Policy may dictate that nursing assessments and care plans are not a part of the legal record; thus on readmissions, nurses may have to "reinvent the wheel" of the data base and previous nursing management while their medical colleagues can pull the old record and start where they left off to continue the data base and the care. We know of some nurses who tried to maintain their own file of assessments and care plans in a cardboard box on the unit, since the record room would not keep this information with the client's permanent file. That effort died in a few months. Furthermore the "nonlegal," nonpermanent care plan status says something about how important or how binding the system considers nursing care plans to be.

The policy may be that only nurses may prepare and pass medications or transcribe doctors' orders, and so professional nurses spend their expensive time in critical but mechanical, minimally direct client care instead of increasing the interaction between the presumably most skilled and knowledgeable professionals on the nursing staff and the clients. Does this seem reasonable? Is this cost effective use of personnel?

Consumers of health care complain that nurses at entry points to the health care system pay more attention to paper than to people. Note the title on the night nurse job description "11-7 Desk Nurse," p. 290. Is it policy that this nurse nurses the desk?

In public health agencies, policies often state that only one visit may be made to the home of a client without a doctor's order. This results in medical needs rather than health needs dictating the nature of nursing care which the client encounters. And ask school nurses about the policies that govern their nursing care.

On the other hand, policies may direct that a *nurse* will see clients for initial assessments on clinic visits or on admission. They may require review and updating of nursing plans at specified intervals. They may give emphasis to individualized recording rather than ritualistic charting. They may indicate where the buck passing stops in accountability for nursing diagnosis and prescription. They may set expectations that a nurse will undertake the care planning for those "difficult clients" rather than rotate assignments, *but* they may also specify the nature of the support system that the nurse is to have.

Policies, written and unwritten, are important to the survival of care plan systems as well as to their development and maturing. Why not begin a campaign to write down the unwritten policies on a unit or in an institution that influence nursing care planning? (They could be anonymously done in case there are some sacred cows among them.) Then they could be examined for their impact on the nursing care plan system in whatever its stage of development and decisions could be made as to whether these unwritten laws are productive or not. The same can be done for written policies.

BUDGET AND CARE PLAN SYSTEMS

Budget is a strong enabling force in the viability of nursing care plan systems. In health care systems, as in any other service-oriented business, time and people are money. Nurses cost more than nonprofessional nursing staff. Budgets can be developed that are so short on professional nurse funding that any systematic planning for the nursing care of individuals and groups is impossible. In fact, several nursing strikes in recent years have had staffing for safe, adequate nursing care as the crucial issue for negotiations. You can't plan health care, medical or nursing, if the staff is spread so thinly that only the highest priority emergencies and the passing of medications can be accomplished.

Budget items are needed not only for the nursing staff to do the nursing planning, but also for staff development and for research on cost effectiveness of the nursing care. In addition, planning of nursing care is going to be proportionately more costly if the higher paid nursing professionals who should be directing their knowledge and skills to assessment, diagnosis, and management of health problems are saddled with the technical, clerical tasks of transmitting orders on the various parts of the system for implementation.

Equipment too, could be used more efficiently in the transmission of segments of the nursing care plan. "Bell boys," pocket signaling devices, are used in some systems to keep hospital or community nurses in closer touch with their clients or other personnel without having to expend extra effort to do so. Carbonized forms for transmission of prescriptions to other parts of the system save time. Conveyor systems for supplies and records save steps. Dictaphone systems can be used for communication of assessments, progress notes, referrals. We know of at least one nurse practitioner who has a case load of several hundred clients, yet who does not have a dictation tie-in to the system comparable to those used by the physicians, nor is there adequate secretarial help.

Skilled nursing care planners—either among nurses or nurse practitioners, can offer their attention and skills to larger case loads if the less expensive support systems are used. Traditions of both nurses and most health care systems will need to undergo some changes before either body is really comfortable with this change, however. Nurses will have to see their capacity for planning for larger case loads, and will have to learn the skills of efficiently using technical assistance rather than doing for themselves. But systems, too, will have to change, particularly when the status of nursing care planning in some institutions (prestigious ones among them), is so very low. We know of an outstanding institution in which the nurses can have access to the Kardex for nursing plan rounds at such times as the ward clerks (or head nurse) are not busy transcribing the plans of medical care. So both attitudes and equipment are involved for the nurse and the agency.

It is, of course, true that an adequate budget for support systems will not guarantee an adequate nursing care plan system. It is equally true, however, that an inadequate budget can prevent its development. Budget cuts can also stifle flourishing care planning systems.

STAFFING AND CARE PLAN SYSTEMS

Some employers of nurses are seeking interest and skills in care planning as well as other proficiencies among their applicants; some are not. Some set expectations of care planning as part of their employment interview; others do not. And, as these expectations by employers are set more frequently, nurses and those who prepare them, will be pressured to raise the levels of performance and expectations regarding assessment-diagnosis and prescriptive skills in nursing.

Once nurses are hired, the staffing patterns come into play. Adequate time for the professional nurse to do the assessment-diagnostic-prescriptive and evaluative activities will not guarantee that they will be done, but not providing for the time can assure that even the prepared nurses will not be able to do them consistently and systematically. Further, staffing patterns which do not permit nurses to be accountable over time for a case load, tend to foster a sense of shift-based accountability for getting the work done, on this shift. And, while it will include the well-being of the clientele, the focus becomes the *well-being on this shift*. More than that is both possible and necessary. This is not to say that a cadre of float nurses skilled in this difficult form of nursing should not be used to cover emergency vacancies. The suggestion is addressed to those nursing systems whose pride is in knowing that their nurses are prepared to move to any unit at any time—and usually do. This is cost effective in "filling the slots," but penny wise and pound foolish in developing accountability for continuity of nursing care. Rewards from the system in such a setting are given for the ability to move, not to plan ahead for one's case load and be accountable over time for planning effectively for the complex patients who so easily fall into the cracks when everyone is accountable and no one person is. Planning for continuity requires investment of thought and energy, which will be enhanced if there is confidence that the planner will be there to see the results of her efforts. While staffing for continuity cannot assure planning, too much emphasis on mobility is certain to remove motivation for planning. Patterns of prolonged accountability will not develop.

Another factor in care planning related to staffing is the ratio of nurses to nonprofessionals in institutional settings and of nurses to doctors and nonprofessionals in ambulatory care settings. One staffs for cost effective use of skills. This means keeping people functioning in their premium areas of competence (except for the "down time" for regrouping that all professionals seem to need periodically during the work period). Thus, if a viable care planning system is desired or required by accreditation, nurses prepared to plan need to be hired; and the staffing should not channel them into activities that take them away from their clients or that do not contribute to their care planning productivity.

> For example: In some settings a nurse is expected not to bathe clients. Yet the activity of bathing may be used to permit needed observation, build trust for more sensitive data gathering or risk-taking in subsequent activities. It may be a time when touch is accompanied by other prescribed nursing activity.
>
> Transporting a client may be a highly skilled nursing activity or just pushing a wheelchair with a person in it. In the case of the latter a nurse should not be doing it. We know of a nurse practitioner who goes from her clinic room to the waiting area to escort her clients back to her office. She wants to see them as they wait—the man she placed on Aldomet, who is drowsing at 10 a.m., the man on Guanethidine whose wife is along and seems to want to see the nurse too, the gait and pace as they walk to the office, the signs of inability to cope with the exertion of walking. All these data become readily available in the short walk.

In other words, no activity is off limits as long as it contributes to nursing assessment-diagnosis and treatment of the client. An opposing example would be the use of nurses to substitute for days-only or weekdays-only schedules for members of other departments—pharmacy, lab, dietary, records, as the perennial "gofers" in ambulatory settings (go for this, go for that)

Staffing to support the nursing care planning system means either hiring skilled nursing planners or training them on the job. It means staffing for the support system of technical, clerical personnel and equipment as well as personnel to man the other departments so that nurses have the opportunity to plan care, then, holding the nurses accountable for doing so.

JOB DESCRIPTIONS AND STAFF EVALUATION CRITERIA IN THE CARE PLAN SYSTEM

If the previous factors are the general enabling ones, job descriptions, staff performance, and evaluation criteria are the specific influences. Here the job seeker, the newly employed nurse, the old timer have the guide for their practice. It makes concrete and visible the intangibles of the philosophy. It directs priorities. It identifies areas of performance where rewards or penalties are given.

Job Description

If the job description states that the registered nurse is the accountable person for the assessment, planning, and management of the nursing care given to her case load—this is reality. When the assigned nurse fails to do it or to delegate it appropriately, that nurse is accountable. When it is done and the outcomes are successful, the nurse and participating colleagues and staff are given appropriate recognition.

If the job description indicates that the nurse will facilitate and upgrade the ability of nonprofessionals on the service to contribute to the data base, to implement and evaluate care, then this too becomes a responsibility to be worked in, as the nurse assigns care, models behavior, makes rounds, and so forth. Such a job description would seem to be quite different from one we might derive from the observed behavior of nursing personnel in some settings where the instructions must be:

> All nursing personnel, regardless of preparation, are to function as interchangeable units.

Aides take histories, nurses copy orders, ward clerks counsel family members, licensed practical/vocational nurses function as charge nurses or team leaders. In fact, job descriptions that result in cost effective care need to specify uses of personnel at appropriate levels of skill. It is very expensive to have nurses underused, and very risky to have aides overused.

289

Let's look at another common behavior in institutional settings—that of doctor's rounds. If the job description indicates that nurses will:

> accompany doctors visiting clients in order to—contribute knowledge of nursing aspects of care, report on delegated medical responsibilities carried out together with the nursing adjustments made, seek coordination of medical and nursing plans for health care, assist the physician in tests and treatments with the goal of enabling the client to "live more effectively" before, during, and after the procedure,

this would certainly structure nursing behaviors on rounds or in assisting with procedures differently than a job description which read:

> Accompany physicians on rounds, report observations of client's response to disease, dx and rx. Assist with procedures.

To show you how a job description can set the tone and expectations of what will be rewarded in a system let's look at two that illustrate remarkable contrasts in their approach to the role of the nurse. One focuses on what needs to be done, the other on areas of responsibility of the nurse. One focuses on tasks and routines, the other on activities, relationships with clients and staff, and professional responsibilities. One focuses on units of time, the other does not. See how you would view your job differently if this were how it were described to you.

11-7 Desk Nurse

11:00 p.m.	Count narcotics Receive report and make out night work sheet Make out census sheet

11:20	Make rounds with the aides with Kardex—quietly
	    Check vital signs on critical patients
	    Check Posey Belts
	    Remove water from NPO patients and notice if all signs are up

12:00	Check medication cards with Kardex and set up all night meds Make out hold breakfast list (3 copies) Make out the x-ray slips
12:15	Pass midnight meds
12:30	Open charts Insert new sheets for doctors orders and nurses notes, filling out the headings Draw the midnight lines Check doctors orders and transcribe to appropriate forms Chart as needed
1:00 a.m.	Rounds
1:20	Finish charts and complete night report for business office
2:00	Rounds Pass specimen bottles—check requisitions and lids

Between 2 and 3 a.m. take coffee break (30 min. permitted)
Check assigned time in kitchen

Order drugs

3:00 Rounds. Take TPR on all elevations of 99° and above
Make postop checks
Update diet lists, TOR lists and Treatment lists

5:00 Collect specimens and take to lab
Send diet list to kitchen
Send x-ray list to x-ray

6:00 Make out new I&O sheets for 7-3 shift and pass
Collect the 11-7 I&O sheets and record
Sign off charts any time after 6 a.m.
Check doctors' orders for being taken off
Turn on the hall lights

6:30 Make rounds
Pass 7 a.m. medications and chart

7:00 Give morning report. State room number, name, doctor's name and diagnosis; then state other information.[1]

Now contrast the approach of the following job description. Think about how you would prepare to function in this role regardless of the shift you were working.

The primary care nurse:

Contributes to creation of a system in which all patients are assigned to a primary care nurse.

Makes available to the nursing staff information about each of her patients and his illness.

Communicates her plans and goals to other nursing personnel in such a way that these personnel can follow and carry out plans in the absence of the primary nurse.

Coordinates routine care and treatment activities for her patients as well as the diagnostic tests and special tests prescribed by the physician.

Arranges nursing care conferences.

Communicates plan of care through Kardex plan of care.

Communicates the nursing process through the Problem-Oriented Chart.

Assures that the patient understands health care options.

Allows patient to make decisions regarding his health care.

Maintains an awareness of cost to the patient.

Utilizes appropriate resources in assuring her knowledge of patient's condition.

Continues the development of her professional knowledge.

Attends interdisciplinary rounds.

[1] Anonymous job description shared by a registered nurse.

Assesses the patient and family through the admission interview, observation, and physical examination to determine physical care needs, the lifestyles, need for education and emotional needs and goals of the patient.

Identifies problems and creates a plan of nursing care involving the patient and the family in the plan.

Provides care to the patient during the time she is working.

Assumes major responsibility for patient-family teaching, with other personnel participating in the areas of repetition and evalution.

Prepares the patient *and* the family for operative procedures or diagnostic tests and procedures, *and* provides support during and after the procedure.

Evaluates outcome of plan through observation and nursing audit.

Informs the family that she is their Primary Nurse and what that means.

Communicates with the patient and family throughout the hospitalization. This may be for health teaching, information gathering, emotional support, discharge planning, etc.

Involves patient and family in the nursing care plan.

Involves patient and family in care conferences when appropriate.

Attends physician rounds, communicates with the physician and is present when the physician sees the patient.

Communicates with others caring for her patients, for example, through giving suggestions, comparing patient reactions, sharing evaluations of the patient, and correcting health care practices which interfere with health care goals.

Arranges interdisciplinary conferences.

Communicates relevant information to other members of the health team through direct communication, through problem-oriented records or through the patient's problem list.

Writes summaries on the clinical record, to communicate pertinent information at the time of transfer or discharge.

Refers appropriate problems to dietician, social worker, family, inhalation therapist, occupational therapist or physical therapist, etc.

Prepares family for discharge and arranges for appropriate referrals and follow-up care.

Assists the patient and family in developing long- and short-term goals.

Provides support and teaching for family members who are assising in the care of the patient.

Solicits information which will assist in assessing effectiveness of nursing care, e.g., through discussion with patient and family member, through follow-up phone calls or through post hospitalization questionnaires.[2]

[2] Working Draft of "Major Activities Relating to the Elements of Primary Care." 12/27/74. Seattle: University Hospital, University of Washington, Unpublished, pp. 3–4. Mimeographed.

Job descriptions in which nurses are accountable for nursing functions to the level of their expertise and assigned area/level of responsibility are the crux of a viable care planning system. They form the basis for recruitment, hiring, staff development, counseling, job relationships and evaluation.

Evaluation Criteria

Out of the job description and the philosophy of nursing emerge the criteria for evaluation of nurses' performance. In terms of the nursing planning component, one may set criteria on several variables.

How much consistency does the nurse show in doing systematic assessments, recording the data base, developing a stated plan of care, sharing or obviously using criteria for evaluation?

Is the speed with which the process is carried out appropriate to the nature of the clientele and the work load? Are priorities well set?

How clearly does the nurse communicate in verbal and written form the elements of the plan to others who share responsibility? Is the language used appropriate to the listener? (e.g., physician, client, nurse colleagues, LPN's aides, LPNs?)

Do others seem to enjoy participating in the nursing care implementation of this nurse's plan? Do they give feedback that they learn from it? Are their contributions effectively acknowledged? Do they feel that their potential for participation is upgraded in the course of contacts with the nurse and the planning process?

How well does the nursing plan articulate with those of other health care workers? Is the nursing component an influence on the plans of others? Does it carry appropriate weight?

Do clients seem to cope with the challenges more effectively because of the nurse's intervention—in their eyes, in the eyes of the nursing staff, from the physician's point of view? Do clients and families acknowledge the usefulness of the nurse's planning with and/or for them?

Do the criteria for evaluation of client response show use of knowledge? Are they logical? Observable?

Are the nursing diagnoses made by this nurse respected by other nurses, by nonprofessional nursing personnel, by the client when they know of them, by physicians? Are they regularly seen on the "problem list?"

Are the nursing prescriptions based on knowledge of the underlying mechanisms of the presenting situation? Are they practical? Do they take client abilities and resources into account? Do they take the realities of the health care system into account? Are they clearly communicated? Are they creative?

Do staff identify this nurse's care plans and activities as contributing to their development because it leads to professional/personal growth?

A complete evaluation of a nurse would encompass other areas, of course;

however, since our concern in this book is with care planning, we have limited ourselves to this. On the other hand we wish to assure the reader that we are aware of other needed expertise for nurses as well.

If motivation theories are correct, behavior is shaped by rewards—verbal, nonverbal, monetary, recognition, status, and so forth. It is also shaped by negative feedback: reminders of omission, anger over risky or costly mistakes, being passed over for promotion, being assigned to "Siberian" territories of the agency, loss of respect. It follows then that *if* rewards are consistently given for planning and excellence in planning; and *if* negative freedback is given for failure to plan or for stereotyped, inadequate, or inappropriate planning, then the activities of the nursing process of planning, implementation, and maintenance of care plans should improve. This will be particularly true if there is genuineness and consistency in the leadership's concern for the spirit of nursing care planning rather than only the mechanics. An assessment on every chart is the "letter"; the "spirit" is a nursing data base that is being used in the delivery of appropriate nursing care. Nurses quickly recognize which pattern nursing leadership is seeking and requiring.

Evaluation of personnel, recognized or unconscious, is carried on daily—by peers, by immediate supervisors, by colleagues in other disciplines, by clients, and by others. Within the nursing discipline or department, primary nurses, team leaders, head nurses, clinical coordinators, and so forth should be clear in their criteria for evaluating dimensions of the use of the nursing process as well as the communications and activities that emerge for this pattern of thinking.

This leads to the important subject of the *climate* surrounding evaluation of the skills of care planning. The nursing profession has been quite overtly critical of itself and the colleagues within it. Care planning as envisioned in this book is a very "public" behavior. It exposes the planner to the scrutiny of other nurses and, with the advent of problem-oriented records, to the critiquing of other disciplines as well. Furthermore, many currently practicing nurses were trained to act by carrying out the decisions of others or making protocol-controlled decisions. Work settings have reinforced this "do as you're told—get the work done" mind set.

If care planning is risky for some nurses who are not prepared for this complex, analytic, decision making process, then threatening their self-concept even further by ruthless critiquing is not likely to produce much enthusiasm for learning and engaging in the activity. It might even block out the excitement and stimulation that learning and growing in the area of care planning can bring.

Ultimately, we want rigor in our critiquing to the end that nursing care plans become increasingly effective. However, we need to be judicious in our decisions about the timing and degree of rigor in our critiquing, adjusting it to the level and confidence of the planner. We are, after all, seeking to build positive attitudes as well as skills, not trying to discourage the less skilled planners.

This concern for the climate surrounding the learning and improvement of care planning performance rather naturally leads to a consideration of the staff development program. Certainly this is a major influence on the maintenance of a viable care planning system.

STAFF DEVELOPMENT AND THE NURSING CARE PLAN SYSTEM

Staff development involves all levels of nursing personnel. Given priorities, however, it would seem wise to give initial and continuing high priority to the quality and development of the professional nurse group and then to structure the staff development program and the clinical environment so that they in turn become accountable for the growth of the nonprofessionals in the care planning implementation skills at an appropriate level in day-to-day work relations, conferences, assignments, and evaluation encounters. Making the professionals responsible for the growth of nonprofessionals who work with them once again enhances the sense of accountability for care planning with another dimension of responsibility. It also brings home the knowledge that the care plan and its implementation are only as good as the persons who participate in both aspects; so, any nurse who wishes to give outstanding nursing care needs to be concerned about providing for the learning of her coworkers as well as her own.

Orientation

Orientation classes communicate the tone of the nursing leadership, the realism of its philosophy, and the weight it carries in the lifestyle of nurses in this setting. This is true whether the work setting is a clinic or office, where one nurse orients her replacement, or a huge hospital or community agency with a highly sophisticated orientation package. In the larger organization, the incoming nurses may bring with them a high degree of skepticism as to whether the philosophy of nursing reported in a session or handed out in a flyer is the kind you or hang on the wall or use in daily nursing care (particularly if they have heard the same unsupported pitch before).

For example:

> Nurses have told us of being rehearsed for accreditation visits where they were given questions they would be asked by the accreditors. When their own answers were "incorrect" they were told the proper and expected way to respond. They say that these are the same institutions where nursing care plans are whipped up in the few weeks preceding accreditation.

Nurses who have had such experiences are bound to be somewhat cynical if they come to a setting in which nursing care planning and the associated values are genuinely used and expected in daily client-coworker encounters.

Inservice or staff development nurses, unless they are truly in tune with the reality of the nursing lifestyles on the units, also suffer from a credibility gap.

Most new employees, even brand new graduates with all their vaunted idealism, have listened to a grapevine or two and believe that the party line and reality are miles apart. Therefore, the orienter does well to lace the philosophy with valid, *current* examples of how values and expectations regarding nursing care plans are actually being implemented on the units where the new employee will be working.

If new employees are to become cost effective contributors to the nursing care plan system in the least amount of time, a process similar to the nursing process needs to be applied. First, a data base of previous education, experience, and perceived skills needs to be gathered. For example:

In your previous experience, what constituted a *working* (not academic) care plan?

How long were they?

Where were they kept?

Who did them? RNs___LPNs___Aides___Others_____(specify) (check as many as appropriate)

In the end was any one person accountable for the NCP? Yes___ No___ If yes, who?

On what kinds of clients were assessments made?

Who did them?

Were assessments assigned (like baths or meds)?

Did the person who made the assessment do at least the initial planning? Yes___ No___

How much experience do you have in making nursing assessments?

On the average, how long does it take you to do a routine nursing assessment on a client who can verbalize?

What process do you use to rule out problems?

For you, what constitutes a nursing diagnosis?

In what way do you believe nursing diagnoses differ from medical diagnoses?

What has been your experience with nursing orders? Who wrote them?

How much weight did they carry? (E.g., was anyone obliged to carry them out?)

Illustrate a nursing order as you might write it.

In your experience, how have nursing care plans been maintained?
  The responsible nurse making planning rounds _____.
  Planning by team conference_____.
  Anyone with new input updates the plan _____.
In your experience, how do physicians learn about the nursing plan of care?

How is it incorporated into the medical plans?

In writing a progress note involving nursing content and nursing planning, how would you see this varying from the progress note written by the doctor on the case?

For nurses hired to work in emergency or intensive care units where physiologic survival and safety are primary considerations, an addendum to the questionnaire would be needed:

In emergency/intensive care units, effective living often focuses on survival and maintaining the integrity of vital organs and functions. More often than not, the data gathering and energies for treatment are directed toward the diagnosing and management functions a physician would do if especially prepared nurses were not available.
Given this focus, what areas, if any, for nursing assessment and management do you see beyond these?

How have you/could you incorporate the data gathering for the additional nursing areas you identified into the orientation and pace of activties in the ER__ ICU__ Recovery Room__ CCU__?

This data base on the care planning experience and thoughts of new nursing employees would give the inservice staff information needed to individualize the staff development program to the nurse, or more likely, to show the new employee how to use the offerings and resources to bring herself to the level of expertise expected in this work setting.

The orientation may address itself only to employee policies, to geographic/departmental tours or functions, or to administrative rules and regulations accompanied with the pious admonition, "Of course, we expect all our nurses to plan nursing care." But then care plan values will be judged for the importance they have been given within the orientation. All of us learn as much from what is not said on these occasions as what is. So, if care planning is important, watch the timing, placement and emphasis communicated about it in the orientation material and presentations.

Staff Development in Day-to-Day Nursing

The crucial environment within which the attitudes, skills, priorities, short cuts and the knowledge of nursing care planning will be taught and caught is on the work unit. The mere words of an orientation or inservice class are soon lost if the reality does not match. Furthermore, the cost effectiveness of the next inservice class may well be ruined by that loss of credibility. An inservice program can only be an adjunct to the learning in the clinical setting. Where there is active collaboration between the reality of care given and the inservice classes, then inservice makes possible new insights, plans, knowledge, cross fertilization of ideas and skills that would be hard to achieve on the clinical unit (because of distractions and restrictions of the environment). But, if one had to choose between the two for the greater opportunity for impact on learning, it would have to be the day-to-day work environment and the learning either incorporated into or made available there.

This places a tremendous responsibility for staff development on nurses in the work environment. Primary accountability for staff development undoubtedly rests with the clinical coordinator or head nurse (whatever the current title), but it cannot be accomplished by one person. The learning-teaching responsibility is every colleague's business if one looks at learning in the broad sense.

Nursing care planning is learned from the following typical everyday behaviors (some of these will result in positive learning, some in the opposite):

assigning baths, medications, temperatures and vital signs, but not admission assessments or case loads for nuring care planning over time

changing assignments daily and/or unpredictably so the sense of personal accountability is lost

taking a colleague along during an assessment to give you feedback on your performance (they may learn about assessments, and about risk-taking behavior while the assessor may learn something from another's perception of her assessment skills)

asking a less experienced nurse to critique your diagnosis and plan and then offering to return the help when it is desired (Again, there is the opportunity to learn about risk-taking behavior as well as critiquing.)

giving team assignment conferences that: consistently outline criteria for observation and expectations of feedback, that concisely indicate the data on which nursing diagnoses were reached and the rationale for prescribed actions:

    a. to illustrate the thinking component that precedes diagnosis and prescription

    b. to model the willingness to "go public" in one's thinking

    c. to invite critiquing

giving a colleague or nonprofessional enthusiastic praise for effective contributions to care planning by being careful to identify the specific skill that was outstanding

asking questions (that do not humiliate) when you feel that not all the data have been incorporated, that the differential diagnosis is not precise enough, the rationale not tight enough, the action not based on an understanding of the underlying mechanisms in the presenting situation

disagreeing with ideas as needed (without attacking the person who holds the ideas), and exploring other options

giving priority to talking about nursing in a well-organized, enthusiastic manner in the change of shift report as well as medical care or, in lieu of medical care, if the nursing aspects are the crucial ones

modeling enthusiasm for nursing planning and nursing's contribution to health care to clients, families, peers, administrators and other disciplines

making regular planning rounds that involve the client in his own care at an appropriate level, with or without other members of the staff

illustrating accountability by accepting praise for nursing orders that work and criticism for those that don't, letting others know that you expect to be held accountable for your plans

honestly sharing concerns about another nurse's nursing orders with that person if you are to implement them rather than ignoring them, subverting them, or complaining to other members of the staff

rotating the care of the "difficult" client so that no nurse needs to learn to assess his behavior and deal with the challenges the client feels he has and the coping behaviors he is engaging in with such poor pay off

OR

assigning such a client to a nurse over time so that someone has an opportunity to learn how to gather data on client-perceived challenges and goals, and to learn the possibilities for enabling that client to modify his behavior to cope more effectively; it may also mean that other staff learn how to give effective support to colleagues caring for such clients.

The list of learning opportunities to be offered is as endless as the skills, knowledge, values, and encounters for application. Thus, staff development for nursing care planning in the practical sense is a personal responsibility for every nurse—to herself, to her nurse colleagues, to clients and families (who ultimately become "the public"), to colleagues in other disciplines, and to administration. The skill of learning to make care planning work, together with an appreciation for its values comes in precepting with others and being preceptor to others in the clinical setting.

INSERVICE AND CARE PLANNING

In earlier times, and perhaps still in some places, inservice classes for nurses most often consisted of lectures by physicians on pathology and medical management, by pharmacists on new drugs, demonstrations of new equipment, or a discussion of policies and procedures for common emergencies. This pattern of ongoing education for a profession said something about us. It made us an "importing" rather than a partially self-sustaining and "exporting" discipline. No wonder there has been so little appreciation for nursing's knowledge base and expertise outside of implementation of medical and administrative aspects of health care. Other professions have been invited regularly to teach us and we have rarely returned the service. Times are changing. More nurses are teaching other nurses about nursing and seeing that there is much in nursing to be valued and learned, then passing on the knowledge and skills to other disciplines.

Nursing care planning itself suggests a host of areas for use in inservice education classes, day-long continuing education workshops, and college-based education on degree bound or non-matriculated options.

Diagnostic Concepts

Many nurses these days are working to develop diagnostic concepts related to common health challenges and effective daily living. Some of these diagnostic concepts commonly used by nurses include: addiction, anxiety, body image, dependency, frustration, grieving-restitution, hypoxia, immobilization, ischemia, loneliness, poverty, role ambiguity—incompetence or conflict, sensory deprivation or overload, sleep deprivation, stigma, trust, and so forth. Concepts such as these can and are being organized for diagnostic and therapeutic efficiency in terms of a consistent system of headings:

Title/definition	Label and overall description of the phenomenon
High risk populations or situations	Prediction of individuals, groups, ages, or situations in which the nurse should consider this diagnosis and seek data to rule it in or rule it out
Etiologic factors	antecedent, current or predicted events, current environment, changes or predicted changes in coping abilities and support system that could lead to the phenomenon
Signs and symptoms	subjective and objective data to be used in ruling in or out the phenomenon and making a differential diagnosis
Dynamics	underlying functions and mechanisms, life situation involved in the presenting situation and associated relationships

Prognosis	predicted direction/duration/possible-probable outcomes
Therapeutic regimen	rationale for and common guidelines for prescription of nursing actions and participation
Complications	intervening factors or undesired side effects
Evaluation	criteria by which the nurse and client can judge effectiveness of the nursing-client management and resolution or continuation of the presenting situation

Physicians have presented medical phenomena in a comparable format to enhance understanding of and participation in medical care. Nurses can present to their nursing colleagues and to other disciplines a complete, well-organized basis for understanding phenomena that lend themselves to nursing management. It may enhance *their* understanding of and participation in nursing care as well as our own.

Nursing Assessment Diagnostic and Prescriptive Skills

In the future, it may be expected that registered nurses should come with the salable skill of efficient, systematic, initial nursing assessments and ongoing assessment-diagnostic management skills. It is presently expected to some basic degree from every medical or dental school graduate. However, for some time to come, nurses who have not developed these skills will be continuing to work in our health care systems. Institutions and agencies may choose to teach and/or upgrade these skills on the job, or require applicants to do so through independent study or continuing education.

Once the basic nursing assessment knowledge and skill are developed, nursing assessments for specialty areas or the achievement of advanced levels of skill and flexibility in them may be added. Inservice may offer activities (not lectures) to increase sensitivity to cues in the client and the environment. Growing skill in the fine art of branching logic—that play-it-by-ear skill—is a blend of working knowledge, interviewing, and observation in an assessment-diagnostic activity that separates fine diagnosticians in any field from their run-of-the-mill colleagues. Like most skills, it cannot be learned in a classroom, but it can be augmented. It can be modeled, analyzed, and practiced in simulated situations and role playing. More knowledge can be attained and organized. The motivation to grow in the skill, as one sees what is possible, can be achieved in the classroom as well as in the clinical setting.

Vocabulary to describe findings precisely is always an ongoing need, as is the ability to translate nursing diagnoses and therapy into the languages of other disciplines. Inservice may start the ball rolling with interdisciplinary panels or client-nurse participants discussing and modeling the lack of shared meaning and techniques for learning to speak a shared language.

Care conferences comparing and critiquing nursing management can achieve two objectives. They can increase the knowledge about nursing management of particular phenomena and about critiquing values, behavior, and skills. The latter can be enhanced if the one doing the critique will step out of the role following a presentation and describe how she prepared for the critique and the ways in which she decided to present the ideas for consideration. A discussion of the risks to the person who critiques is helpful, too, since she is as much at risk as the one being critiqued—both are exposing their capabilities.

Consultation roles in nursing have been growing within work settings and beyond them. What does it take to be an effective consultant? How can one facilitate cost effective, personally useful consultation? How does one prepare for a consultation visit? How does one most effectively brief the consultant on the situation under study? This may seem like a fringe area to nursing care planning, but formally and informally, it will be of increasing importance as nursing care planning systems develop. If nurses truly take their places as colleagues in the health care system, they will be consulting more not only within the nursing discipline, but also with colleagues in other disciplines as well. We will need to be ready. We will need to be competent.

Continuing Education

Continuing education is being seen as a lifelong obligation of all health professionals. Nurses can and should insist that subjects offered enhance their nursing care planning skills and knowledge even as they may address medical or other related areas.

Summary

Thus, whether in orientation, in day-to-day informal teaching-learning interactions and encounters on the clinical unit, nursing care planning—its underlying knowledge and skills, the problems associated with accountability, and coordination of the planners, the finesse of appropriate involvement of clients and their families—all these are the substance of professional development for practicing nurses. The learning experience can occur on the job, in continuing education, and in degree-bound advanced education. It is, however, an essential, ongoing area of obligation for learning that concerns the new practicing nurse and the veteran alike.

RECORDS AND THE CARE PLANNING SYSTEM

Any nurse can make a plan of care on a blank sheet of paper, but nursing care planning systems require records so that information, decisions, actions, and outcomes are predictably locatable. The record system or style gaining momentum in the 1970s is that of problem-oriented records. They have been developed and promulgated primarily by physicians or persons attuned to the medical model. Thus, nursing again finds itself working to find a way to enter a medically oriented health care system developed to the point of computerization. Actually, the problem-oriented record system has been a boon as well as a challenge, because it is forcing even the most unbelieving nurse to think in terms of the nursing process. How else can they get the clients' nursing problems into the problem list? How else to get the challenges to daily living and coping resources into the overall data base? How else can nurses think, if they too must S-O-A-P[3] problems in order to record them?

Many problem-oriented record systems are labeled POMR—Problem-Oriented Medical Records. This offers nurses an easy way out—they may record in terms of medical data, diagnoses, and prescriptions. But an increasing number are choosing to push for a POHR—Problem-Oriented Health Record, in which all health workers contribute to an integrated record. No doubt there are and will be stresses on everyone, on physicians, as they see their efficient medical records "cluttered up" by non-physician types and on nurses, as they attempt to communicate nursing diagnoses and prescriptions at a sufficiently scientific level to be an accepted and respected contribution. The advent of problem-oriented record systems certainly does give incentive to nurses and nursing to clarify the territory of health care for which they are assuming accountability and to upgrade the quality of their recording performance in that area so that it is not omitted as the system matures and solidifies. Individual nurses and groups of nurses need to be unified and supported in their entry into integrated record systems.

But whether because of the prodding by an integrated problem-oriented record or not, a nursing care planning system does need the support of a record system that meets several criteria. It must legitimize and give prescribed space for the nursing data base in the client's legal record. It must offer space on the official client record for nursing diagnoses and prescriptions. This is particularly important in chronic care settings where effective living is often more closely tied to nursing management than to medical management.

Routine tasks and observations are only one dimension of nurses' recordings. Beyond this, nurses must be accountable for *recording progress* that extends over shifts and days. These recordings must be made in terms of nursing diagnoses and goals as well as effectiveness or ineffectiveness of prescribed nursing care. Client progress should reflect perceptions of each group of involved health workers, whether these forms are integrated or not. Nursing as a constant contributor to *every* client (more than all other nonmedical health care workers), must be expected to document client progress in coping with everyday living. Forms, protocols, regulations and policies regarding recording should incorporate nursing's recordings as rigorously as that of any other health discipline.

[3] Subjective — *Objective* (data) — Analysis — *Plan.*

NURSING CARE PLANS AND RELATIONSHIPS WITH NON-NURSING DISCIPLINES AND DEPARTMENTS

Because nursing touches so many other aspects of health care and the health care workers who deliver it, any changes in the practice of nursing tend to have implications for others as well. This is particularly true in acute care institutional settings where every day and every client bring together the goals and actions of multiple departments. Almost every other department in a hospital encounters nursing daily.

If nurses and the nursing department seriously address themselves to helping the client to manage the demands of daily living as effectively as possible during hospitalization (instead of primarily seeing that the required medications, tests, and treatments were accurately accomplished), this change in emphasis could pose adjustments and problems for other departments. The reader might try to imagine what kinds of changes would occur in clinical settings with which they are familiar if nursing were to take concerted action to address themselves to such a goal. Even deviating from the carrying out and recording of medical care to the extent of adding nursing concerns to the medical plan and trying to incorporate these into records and client care seems to cause difficulties enough and this represents only a partial change. Let's examine a few situations.

> A hospital nurse, in evaluating the status of a severely depressed 42-year-old male with a leg amputation, was concerned because the planned nursing approaches were ineffective for this client. She initiated contact with the psychiatric nurse clinician on the medical/surgical unit for a more skilled assessment of the client's behavior and some consultation as to approaches that could be incorporated into the nursing care. The orthopedic surgeon, on seeing the consultation note written by the nurse clinician, referred the matter to the Hospital Administrator. The result was that a policy was issued that nurses could not consult with nurse clinicians about their clients without a doctor's written order.

> A group of physicians in another hospital were developing plans for implementing Professional Standards Review Organization protocols as indicated by federal legislation for Medicare patients. These physicians, with administrative support, assumed that the evaluation of the quality of care received by clients was to include nursing as well as medical care. Therefore, they set about to develop the criteria for evaluation of nursing care, assuming that evaluation of quality of nursing care was the prerogative of the physician group. Presumably, this decision was based on the assumption that physicians are as expert in nursing as they are in medicine.

It is a recognized fact that it is important for hospital administration to cater to the wishes and demands of physicians, since the medical group bring the revenue to the institution by admitting patients to the institution that pleases them the most. Thus hospitals, the second largest industry in the United States, function primarily to provide a work setting for physicians.

When *individual* nurses modify their nursing lifestyle, they negotiate overtly or covertly with physicians to incorporate these changes into their role relationships. But when a *whole nursing system* begins to engage in nursing care planning it means that the nursing system must engage with the medical system. This requires negotiations at the system level as well as at the individual level. The nursing care planning system will be a pretty anemic one if it is not articulating openly and legitimately with the medical care planning system as well as with other disciplines. The nursing directors have particular responsibilities, both in requiring accountability in care planning from the nurses, and in setting standards for excellence, but they also have responsibility in negotiating with departments and disciplines so that true effectiveness in nursing care planning can take place.

LEADERSHIP STYLES IN NURSING DEPARTMENTS AND CARE PLANNING SYSTEMS

The implementation of the nursing care planning system, the collegiality required within the nursing discipline and between nursing and other disciplines has implications not only for nurses engaged in the care planning, but also for the leadership in this discipline and department. The climate created by the leadership style in the work setting significantly influences the implementation of nursing care plan systems. If administration supports a purely hierarchical model, it pretty effectively rules out collegiality on a systematic basis, allowing only for individually negotiated collegial roles. Upper and middle management in organized nursing departments must be concerned about their own role model of interdisciplinary collegiality and policies that affect this for the staff.

Beyond this, however, is the *intra*departmental leadership style. Autocratic leadership styles with mandates and predeveloped forms and protocols that are handed down from on high have tended to result in nursing care planning being done *for the system,* not for the well-being of the client and the professional growth of the staff. The letter of the law tends to become more important than the spirit. We have seen care planning systems continue in such a setting, but there is frequently little joy in them.

We have also seen nursing care plan systems developed in which the staff at all levels was involved. The leadership style was democratic. Participation in the feasibility studies, tool development, experiments with aspects of the nursing process, with planning and its impact on relationships, were undertaken involving the staff. Participants felt creative, involved, growing. There was real enthusiasm. Here the growth and maturation of the system was slower, but the end product was not only a paper-type system, but a people-oriented system as well, encompassing all facets of nursing care delivery and staff development.

305

The following are some vignettes of leadership styles the authors have encountered in the development of nursing care planning systems. You can make a judgment as to the leadership style and its productivity.

A head nurse gives consistent praise for clean, orderly units, requires a problem on all patients on the Kardex, but never gives any praise for the quality of the care plan.

A head nurse, on a regular basis, consults with staff regarding their case load, their needs for support in management of the nursing care, their sense of achievement and problems. Evaluations reflect knowledge of the interest and competence of the nursing staff in nursing care planning.

At the head nurses' meeting, the director hands out a nursing assessment tool and informs the group that henceforth this tool will be completed on all newly admitted clients within 24 hours of admission by some member of the staff.

There is a highly competitive environment in an IC unit wherein nurses strive to be the "best nurse." Nurses who acquire particular client data are known not to share them with other nursing staff because it gives them an edge the others do not have.

The director of nursing in a small rural hospital who was trying to revitalize the philosophy of nursing began the process with the night shift by coming in and sharing the coffee break with the night personnel until she had a feel for the values that were important on their shift. Her concern was that permanent night personnel tended to be less considered in early steps of changes.

A director of a large teaching hospital is requiring that her associate directors spend at least a half day each week in direct client contact to keep them reality-oriented about client needs, care planning, and staff problems in these areas.

An associate director with staff development responsibilities, comes to work at 4 a.m. some mornings in order to make rounds with the night supervisor, spends time with the families of the seriously ill, checks on clients who need some special attention—all this to get a feel for the problems and staff development needs (in terms of care planning) on this shift, as they may differ from the other shifts.

Indeed, nurses in a variety of settings are exposed to leadership behaviors and styles among their middle and top management that either facilitate or bar their abilities to participate effectively in nursing care planning. The effects are sometimes insidious and unrecognized, but they are there. There are, of course, whole books written about administrative competence and leadership styles. Our goal here is to ask any nurse in a leadership role to look for behavior and role models being offered to staff as they relate to care planning. We would also suggest that staff look to behavior in the leaders to see where it can be used to enhance their care plan system, and where some negotiations need to be undertaken to seek modification so that it is a more productive force. Each of us, of course, is offering leadership and a role model to someone—it is wise to be aware of the impact it can have.

SUMMARY

Nursing care planning involves individuals; it also involves whole systems. It is the product of an individual nurse's effort and thought, but going beyond the accountable nurse and the involved client and family, it requires the participation of others—individuals and groups. Furthermore, at present, practicing nurses vary remarkably in their care planning inclinations and skills. Some have never been taught to value nursing management or the breadth of knowledge required to be proficient in the nursing assessment-diagnosis, prescription implementation, and maintenance involved. Others vary in their ability and speed. Thus, the supportive environment and the learning opportunities are crucial to this component of health care planning. It is a time and place for colleagueship among nurses, of fostering growth in ourselves and others rather than practicing one-ups-manship based either on educational qualifications or competence. What we all want is effective health care for our clients and the excitement of professional growth for ourselves and our careers. Only as we make this possible for ourselves and our nursing colleagues will there be an effective, viable nursing care planning system that will take its recognized and legitimate place with the planning of others in the health care system.

chapter Fifteen

The Profession and Nursing Care Planning

In previous sections of this book we have discussed nursing care planning as it relates to nurses, to the clientele, to colleagues in other disciplines, and to institutions and agencies. We have not yet considered the relationship between the professional association at all its levels and care planning activities of the individual nurse. While the influence is less obvious and less direct, it is a significant force. Current nursing practice and future developments are profoundly shaped by the decisions, policies and actions of nurses functioning as a collective entity within their professional organizations. As nursing's positions on issues are communicated to action-taking bodies within and outside of the profession, the practice of the individual nurse is often modified—and of course this includes care planning.

The relationship between the profession and the individual member is a two-way street. Practicing nurses must give realistic input to their association representatives so that they can represent accurately the current and future territory and status of nursing. It is from these positions taken by the organization that representations will be made to legislators, governmental agencies, other allied professional groups, the insurance industry, health care delivery systems, and others. In addition to influencing non-nursing groups, the policies and decisions of the profession exert a direct intraprofessional force on nursing practice.

Let us look at some ways in which nurses working together as a professional group have developed positions directly affecting nursing care planning. Then let us look at some of the issues that face the profession wherein nurses must give realistic input so that sound positions may be taken for the evolution of future nursing practice, particularly in the care planning sphere.

THE PROFESSION'S INFLUENCE ON CURRENT NURSING CARE PLANNING PRACTICES

Nursing's characteristics as a profession are directly related to nurses' care planning behavior. The definition of our unique professional contribution to society determines the focus of our care planning activities. Our code of ethics shapes the style with which we assess, diagnose, prescribe, implement, and evaluate our nursing care. Our professional standards serve as guidelines to individuals and systems in planning, implementation, and evaluation of their service. Nursing as a profession also engages in activities to insure the competence of its members and the safety of the consumer through control of entrance into the profession and continuing education.

As you look at these descriptions of current professional positions, consider how your practice is shaped by them. But think also of input you might give to shape future decisions of the professional organization.

Nursing as a "Unique" Contribution to Society's Health Care

In recent years the profession has been increasingly addressing itself to the component of health care that is *not* a delegated medical function. In the interim between the first and second editions of this book, the definition of this area has become increasingly clear. Nursing care planning has its own area of accountability to the public that is *in addition to* that of accountability through the physician for medical care.

Then, too, because the service has a particular focus, the body of knowledge that supports it is used differently from that of other professions. Nurses will use knowledge from a variety of disciplines to enable them to define and diagnose the challenges being encountered by their clientele as well as the coping abilities and resources which clients have available to them. Neither humanities, the physical and natural sciences, nor social sciences are outside the knowledge base nurses need. Thus, it is not the knowledge which is unique to the nursing profession but the relationships and the insight with which it is applied to the client's situation.

Eventually, with more explicit experience in using the knowledge base in this manner and with a better backlog of research, it would seem fair to predict that nursing's own body of knowledge will emerge. For example, much is being done in the area of cardiac and hemodynamic function in normal and post-myocardial infarction individuals at varying levels of activity. These findings will form a knowledge base for helping clients to cope more effectively with the demands of daily living and their desired lifestyle following heart problems. Cultural aspects of health-seeking behavior are being studied and used by nurses to determine effective means of making nursing care available to differing ethnic

309

groups. Health beliefs and their relationship to learning about one's illness and its therapeutic management are being studied and used in helping individuals make effective decisions regarding their health care. With increased clinical testing and utilization of these ideas, there is no question that nursing's body of knowledge will gradually emerge in sharper focus and be transmitted to both new and experienced nurses.

The definition, the focus, the accountability, and the emerging body of knowledge that will more substantially support competence in delivering nursing care are strong forces in current practice. They bid to continue to shape and improve our professional practice.

Nursing's Code of Ethics and Care Planning

The development of a code of ethics is another characteristic of a profession. Nurses, through the American Nurses Association, delineated and voted acceptance of the following Code of Ethics for Nurses. As you read each of the statements, reflect on its significance to nursing care planning activities and systems as we have described them in previous chapters and as you yourself carry them out.

1. The nurse provides services with respect for the dignity of man, unrestricted by considerations of nationality, race, creed, color or status.
2. The nurse safeguards the individual's right to privacy by judiciously protecting information of a confidential nature, sharing only that information relevant to his care.
3. The nurse maintains individual competence in nursing practice, recognizing and accepting responsibility for individual actions and judgments.
4. The nurse acts to safeguard the patient when his care and safety are affected by incompetent, unethical or illegal conduct of any person.
5. The nurse uses individual competence as a criterion in accepting delegated responsibilities and assigning nursing activities to others.
6. The nurse participates in research activities when assured that the rights of individual subjects are protected.
7. The nurse participates in the efforts of the profession to define and upgrade standards of nursing practice and education.
8. The nurse, acting through the professional organization, participates in establishing and maintaining conditions of employment conducive to high quality nursing care.
9. The nurse works with members of health professions and other citizens in promoting efforts to meet health needs of the public.
10. The nurse refuses to give or imply endorsement to advertising, promotion, or sales for commercial products, services or enterprises. (ANA, 1968.)

Throughout the book certain concepts, skills, behaviors, ideals, and principles have been inferred or stated. To see how some of these concepts link up with the Code of Ethics, try matching the listed concepts taken from the book with the statements of the Code.

Accountability	Creativity	Philosophy of Care
Assessment	Diagnosis	Primary Focus of
Authority	Delegated Medical	Nursing
Client advocacy	Care	Privacy
Collaboration	Evaluation	Rights of Clients
Collegiality	Implementation	Rights of Nurses
Competence	Objectives of Care	Risk taking

The implementation of the Code of Ethics is currently being enhanced because nurses collectively in certain areas of the country are insisting that it be included in contract agreements at places of employment. And, of course beyond this, individual nurses are carrying out their nursing lifestyle in such a way as to give visible daily support to this code. Certainly, the nursing process, care planning, and implementation of care are influenced by the values in the current ANA Code of Ethics.

Professional Standards and Nursing Care Planning

The nursing profession also has both the right and the responsibility to delineate standards for practice, service organization, and education. This activity is one means by which the profession assures the public of the quality of its services. Individual nurse members working in concert through their organization have developed standards for general nursing practice, for nursing departments, and for education. These standards have been disseminated and are currently being implemented by nurses throughout the country.

How do these developed standards relate to the nursing care planning system? All of the standards developed for practice, service and education reflect a common definition of nursing and the scope of practice that forms the territory for nursing care planning. One cannot assess, diagnose, plan, implement or evaluate nursing care given to the client if one does not know the primary focus of nursing. Nor can one prepare and educate future practitioners in nursing without a clear map of the territory.

The ANA generic Standards of Nursing Practice delineate the nursing process —the assessment of client status, the plan of nursing actions, the implementation of the plan, and the evaluation. Sound familiar? Now examine each of the following seven generic standards and reflect on the congruence of these standards to the nursing care planning process and system described previously in the book:

STANDARD

1. The collection of data about the health status of the client/patient is systematic and continuous. The data are accessible, communicated and recorded.
2. Nursing diagnoses are derived from health status data.

3. The plan of nursing care includes goals derived from the nursing diagnosis.
4. The plan of nursing care includes priorities and prescribed nursing approaches or measures to achieve the goals derived from the nursing diagnosis.
5. Nursing actions provide for client/patient participation in health promotion, maintenance and restoration.
6. Nursing actions assist the client/patient to maximize his health capabilities.
7. The client's/patient's progress or lack of progress toward goal achievement directs reassessment, reordering of priorities, new goal setting and revision of the plan of care. (ANA, 1973.)

Growing out of the foundation of these generic standards of practice, specific standards have been developed and published through the ANA which reflect specialized areas of nursing practice. There are standards with specialized focus for psychiatric-mental health nursing, medical and surgical nursing, maternal child health nursing, community health nursing, cardiovascular nursing, geriatric nursing, orthopedic nursing, and nursing practice in the operating room. All of these standards, and more to come, are congruent with the concept of nursing process and its relationship to the care planning system. It is interesting to note that the nursing profession is the first among the health professional groups to officially proclaim their standards of practice.

Similarly, the standards and guidelines for nursing services in all kinds of institutions and agencies reflect an organizational system which enhances and supports the nursing care planning system within each work setting. Do you recall in Chapter Fourteen our discussion of the significance of budget, personnel policies, orientation, staff development programs, client-oriented philosophies, and other environmental factors? If you are experiencing some organizational obstacles to care planning and the care planning system in your work setting, then one can assume that the Standards of Nursing Services accepted by the profession are not being met.

Let's look at each of the standards and ask some questions. Your answers will reveal the extent to which nursing services in your work setting are meeting these standards, for your perspective. Note that these are only sample questions. Do not limit yourself to these. Begin to add your own as they relate to nursing care planning systems in your work setting.

STANDARD

1. *Nursing administration has a philosophy and objectives which reflect the purposes of the health care organization and give direction to the nursing care program.*
   How many of the staff know what the values are in the departmental

philosophy? How congruent are they with actual practice? When are they consulted?

Are objectives screened through the philosophy? Are objectives set with a time for achievement in mind and then updated? Are they consulted as guides to decision making? Do they influence priorities? Do they guide practice? Do they shape staff development?

Are nurses cognizant of the rights of clients and their families? (How do you know this?) Do you see and hear nurses serving as advocates for the rights of clients?

2. *Nursing administration has the responsibility and authority for the quality of nursing practice within the health care organization.*

What evidence have you seen of your nursing administration developing programs to assure safe, competent nursing care to the consumer?

What provisions are made for involving consumers in the formulation of plans of health care in order to provide for acceptability and continuity of nursing care?

How are nurses held accountable for the quality and quantity of nursing care provided to the consumer? Where does the buck passing stop in planning for the care of the individual client?

Are there stated goals on the nursing care plans? What evidence do you have that they are used as guidelines by all of those who share in giving of the care? In what ways are they used when recording of progress is noted?

3. *A nursing service has a designated leader who is a qualified, registered nurse and a member of the operational policy making leaders of the health care organization.*

What evidence do you have that the leader of the nursing department is interpreting and supporting nurses' accountability for the management of nursing care within the interdisciplinary health care system, with management, budget, the medical staff, the records department, with other departments?

4. *The nursing care program is integrated into the total program of the health care organization.*

What evidence do you have that nursing aspects of health care receive appropriate priority in the care given? How much voice does nursing have regarding the use of institutional resources? In the planning of diagnostic or treatment regimens how much is nursing consulted? On boards of utilization, are nurses giving data on client-family readiness to cope with life back in the home and community? Are admissions to institution decisions made in collaboration with informed nurses? Are medical-nursing rounds in institutions using a collaborative approach? Are nurses represented and articulate on PSRO committees and on other appropriate committees of the institution?

5. *Nursing administration determines the budget necessary to carry out the nursing care programs and administers the approved budget.*

313

Are the objectives of nursing care utilized in forecasting the nursing service budget? Do nurses have an opportunity for input into budget formation as it relates directly to the giving of nursing care to clients, to staff development options?

6. *A nursing service organization plan delineates the functional structure of the department and shows established relationships among nursing personnel and with other services.*

How does the organizational structure of your work setting reflect the philosophy and objectives of care (relationship between elements and positions)? What provision is made for direct lines of communication with other members of the health care team? How does the structure facilitate the accountability and authority of nurses to deliver nursing care to clients?

7. *The nursing administration has written personnel policies which assist in recruiting and maintaining a qualified staff.*

Where are the written personnel policies available in your work setting? How soon did you become aware of them? How do nurses participate in their formulation, evaluation, revision? How do they influence nurses' ability to plan care for the clientele? Do the job descriptions of nurses include care planning skills and responsibilities?

8. *Nursing administration shall detail guidelines for utilization of nursing personnel.*

In your work setting how is provision made for the effective utilization of nursing knowledge and skills in the provision of direct client care? How are nurses recognized and rewarded for superior clinical practice? How do staffing patterns enhance nursing care planning and provision of nursing care that reflects continuity? Are nurses serving equipment and records or is equipment serving nurses as they care for the clientele? Is there evidence that nurses feel effectivly used in the delivery of nursing care?

9. *The nursing administration provides programs for orientation and continued learning of nursing personnel.*

Did your orientation lead you to expect that you would be planning care for your clients? Did you learn about resources to facilitate your planning in this new setting? Do inservice classes stress the nursing aspects of planning care as well as medical or technological elements?

In what ways does the staff development program enable you to critique your performance in care planning (any element of the process), and find ways of experiencing professional growth in this aspect of your nursing?

10. *A nursing service has responsibility to participate in education of students in the health care field.*

Are nursing students and students in other disciplines seeing role models in nursing care planning? Do they have a chance to observe and participate in the staff nurse's activities of planning care? Can they critique it? Question? Try it out with the nurse's support? (Or, is nursing care planning done by the students and tolerated by the staff?)

How are nurses helping students to translate the model of care planning—assessment, diagnosis, prescribing, implementing, recording, evaluating that they learn in books and the classroom into the reality of the clinical situation. How are they learning the tricks of the trade? The nuances in assessment? The safe short cuts? The finesse of diagnosis? The data resources? The techniques of articulating nursing care planning with the medical plan and those of other disciplines? The art of realistically including the client in the planning process?

11. *A nursing service supports research in the health care field.*

What means are used to keep the nursing staff current on applicable research developments in the field? What efforts are made at researching elements of care planning and its applicability to the clientele in this setting?

How are nurses learning to participate effectively in valuing and implementing ongoing research of other nurses and persons in other disciplines that involve nursing?

12. *A nursing service evaluates its clinical and administrative practices.*

What regular evaluation of nursing care planning and outcomes is undertaken? How are the climate for and the facilities for care planning evaluated in terms of quantity and quality of care planning done? How are consumers used in this evaluation? (ANA, 1973.)

One can readily see that the Standards of Nursing Services are directly applicable to the viability and productivity of the nursing care plan system and the nurses as they are involved in it.

Other standards that relate to nursing care planning are those addressed to the education of nurses. These standards, too, reflect knowledge and skills to provide for effective care planning among future and present nurses.

All of these standards provide the basis for development of operational statements of criteria for evaluating specifically: the nursing care, the organizational system, and the educational system in any work setting. The care planning process is an integral part of each of them. They provide the profession's means of insuring quality of care to the consumer and quality of environment and education to the provider of the health care service.

Professional Competency and Care Planning

Society expects that a profession will monitor the competence of all its members. This expectation is implemented by the nursing profession in several ways, all of which influence the care planning process.

Admission to the profession. Through the national accreditation process, standards for educational institutions teaching nursing students are set. These accreditation procedures examine criteria used by schools in selecting students, and also examine the facilities, faculty, and processes used to prepare nurses to provide competent care. In recent years the teaching of the nursing process and care planning have received increasing attention.

Formal admission to the nursing profession and the right to call oneself a registered nurse is regulated by state law, but the examination and prerequisites of graduation from state accredited schools are nationwide. As with the accreditation standards, so the nurse-prepared NLN examination has tested with increasing frequency the skills and knowledge base associated with nursing care planning. Thus, any nurse who is legally admitted to practice has given evidence of beginning competence in these skills, to the extent that they can be measured on paper and documented in terms of graduation from a school. Since nurses are involved in accreditation standards, in creation of the test pool items, and in state accreditation of schools of nursing, obviously a two-way mechanism of nurses' influencing and being influenced in their practice of care planning is occurring. This relationship offers us the opportunity to upgrade these standards to improve care planning in order to provide better service to the public.

Nurses, through their association, helped to draft a model act for state laws which more precisely defines nursing and offers a broader scope of nursing practice to encompass and legalize the changing roles of nurses in providing increased emphasis on primary and ambulatory care. Within the last five years, thirty states have used that model to upgrade their nurse practice acts and, in turn, to upgrade nursing practice in their states.

It is obvious that these revisions in nurse practice acts are closely related to nursing care planning activities and systems. To check this out, take your own practice act and examine it for the following content related to care planning:

> How is nursing defined? How does this relate to your own practice in planning nursing care?
>
> What is the primary focus of nursing? How does this influence your decisions and priorities?
>
> Does your law indicate the nursing practice of making assessments and diagnoses?
>
> Is there provision for nursing prescription? Implementation of nursing prescriptions? Accountability for prescribing in the area of nursing care?
>
> Do nurses evaluate nursing care?
>
> Do nurses initiate health care?
>
> Can nurses delegate and supervise others in the giving of nursing care? (How does this relate to nursing care planning?)
>
> To whom are nurses accountable? Are there differing areas of accountability —to oneself, to the consumer, to the physician, to the employer?

If you are not certain whether your current law was built on the model act, make a comparison. Determine how the differences would influence your care planning practice. Your district and state associations, your hospital, or the agency or school library should be able to supply you with materials needed to make the comparison.

Continued Competence of Nurses

Currently, in most states the license of the nurse is renewed each year merely by payment of a fee. No evidence is required of continued competence, even though society expects the profession to insure this. With changes in health care knowledge and technology moving so rapidly, a basic education loses its viability in a remarkably short period of time. Thus, many health professions, nursing among them, are contemplating or enacting licensing laws that make renewal of licensure contingent upon evidence of ongoing upgrading of current practice through continuing education.

The nurses' association has vigorously supported continuing education during the career life of the nurse. Standards, guidelines, and, now, accreditation standards and mechanisms have been developed nationally. They are being implemented in many of the states. Currently in many, if not most states, these Continuing Education Recognition Programs (CERP), are voluntary programs at present with the probability that as continuing education offerings are developed to meet the demand, they will become a mandatory requirement for renewal of licensure. Nurses who have been active on the workshop scene are increasingly familiar with the demand for submission of objectives, course outlines, and evaluative criteria and procedures that truly upgrade their offerings. Certainly, the authors have seen it happening in their workshop travels with increasing frequency.

Our experiences with the nursing care planning process in all varieties of health care settings involving hundreds of practicing nurses indicates a continuing need for C.E. programs relating to assessment, diagnosing, prescribing, implementation, and evaluative skills in nurses. We see a need for practicing nurses to upgrade their knowledge base through reading and courses so that their rationale for diagnosis and prescription and their criteria for evaluation are soundly based. We also see the need for continuing education for leaders in nursing departments and faculty members as they develop and administer systems for the support of nursing care planning.

Recognition of advanced competency. In addition to the gate-keeping activities and the provision for continued growth in the profession, another force has been introduced that has added impetus for excellence in care planning as well as in other activities. This is the identification—the certification—of nurses with outstanding, advanced competency in an area of clinical nursing practice. Rigorous documentation that standards of excellence have been met precedes the awarding of this designation. Again, nurses have set these high standards and rules of evidence to guide their practice. And again, we see how it in turn feeds back to influence the nursing lifestyle.

Certainly this professional recognition of outstanding performance offers incentive to nurses to develop their capabilities fully. These capabilities and standards are, of course, closely involved with the nursing process, the knowledge base, and care planning skills appropriate to the special clinical area.

Evaluation of Care Given

For a profession, it is not enough to evaluate the practitioner; the final criterion is the quality of the service rendered and the outcome. Thus, we see nurses involved in the evaluation of health care actually renderd to the client. To this end, nurses are seeking placement on the Professional Standards Review Organization (PSRO) Boards and Commissions. We see nurses increasingly learning how to participate effectively in peer review and seeking mechanisms by which to incorporate this into everyday practice. There are Nursing Audits. Increasing attention is being paid to "Quality Assurance." Of course, only as the nursing component—the nursing diagnosis, the appropriate prescriptions—is truly established and some norms are documented can relevant criteria be determined and applied. And these, of course, bring us right back to that essential element of the nursing process, the nursing knowledge base and the documented nursing care plan. It becomes the crux of evaluation of nursing care which is planned and delivered.

Summary

Perhaps our biases are showing, but it is difficult for us to see that our professional quality of care can proceed without the foundation and core of the nursing process and plan, whether we are addressing ethics, standards, or member competence. It becomes the substance of development and improvement; it is the target of the ethics and standards of evaluation.

THE PROFESSION AND THE FUTURE IN CARE PLANNING

So far in this chapter we have addressed ourselves to the activities already being undertaken by the profession to insure the provision of safe, competent nursing care to consumers and to identifying the relationship between these ethical codes, standards, and review procedures and the care planning process. But one of the characteristics of a profession that keeps it exciting to its members is its dynamic state. There are always more questions than answers, more issues crying for our best creative efforts. And so it is with the nursing profession and nursing care planning. There are some issues that have emerged because of a more precise definition of nursing, because of the assumption of colleague status with accountability for a particular dimension of health care and because of a definitive area for diagnosis and health care management. These issues are being addressed by individual nurses, but, because they involve the entire profession and our relationships to other professions and agencies as well, they must be addressed by the profession as an entity and be communicated to other national or state bodies by representatives of the profession speaking for the constituency.

Defining Nursing's Territory of Care Planning Accountability

Until recently, the shifts in the territory of nursing have always been an extension into that of medicine—into medical and diagnostic treatment areas. Certainly, nurses moving into physician assistant roles and some nurse practitioners indicate a continuation of this pattern. But, with the definition of nursing as something other than delegated medical functions, the profession must increasingly communicate the boundaries and norms of this nursing territory to closely related disciplines, to consumers of nursing care, to legislators, to insurance companies, to employers of nurses, and to nurses themselves.

Development of a Nursing Diagnostic Taxonomy

Another issue that is receiving attention from the profession as a separate entity is the development of a classificatory system for nursing diagnoses. For any unified approach to nursing diagnosis and for communication of nursing diagnoses to take place, some recognized body must coordinate and expedite, and eventually communicate the diagnostic taxonomy and classification system. Computerization of diagnostic classifications has been occurring for some time in the health field. The articulation or integration of nursing diagnoses into the system is another issue to be faced.

Incorporation of the Nursing Contribution into National Health Care Plans

Provision for some form of National Health Insurance and the concomitant increase in federal control of health care dictates that nursing must have individuals representing the profession who will ensure that nursing's contribution to health care is identified, recognized, and made financially feasible in the national health care plan. There is no doubt that individual nurse's care planning is profoundly influenced by laws of this nature. Resolutions defining the profession's position have been passed and machinery for translating these ideas and values into reality are ongoing.

FINALE

All these pages of professional ethics and activities may seem far-fetched in a book on the nursing process and nursing care planning systems addressed to the practicing nurse. What we have been trying to show is that today it is not enough for the professional nurse to concern herself with the planning of care for a current case load. Developments within the profession, within the city and state or province, and in the nations' capitals are currently shaping, and will predictably influence, future practice.

The nurse who wishes to practice as a professional has no option but to wade into the larger scene. There is the obligation to contribute reality-based data to the decision making process—to be certain that the broadest perspective, the sharpest perspective, and the most accurate one is available to the professional body before decisions and policies are set. Once the actions are taken within or outside of the profession, even then the professional nurse's task is not complete. The new approaches, the new influences, the regulations, the systems must be tested and the feedback process continued.

If professional nursing was ever a routine eight-hour job, that is certainly a thing of the past. Today it is demanding, dynamic, creative. It is a career and a lifestyle worthy of our best efforts.

REFERENCES

American Nurses' Association, "Code for Nurses," Adopted by House of Delegates. Dallas, Texas, May, 1968.

American Nurses' Association, *Standards for Nursing Services*. Kansas City, Mo.: The Association, 1973.

American Nurses' Association, *Standards of Practice*. Kansas City, Mo.: The Association, 1973.

Index

Sensory data, 137–138
  and cues, 56, 70
  goals, 188
  input, 165–166, 248–250
Sexuality, 138
Shifts, 306
  change, 273–275
  and communication, 273–274
Skill and dexterity, 167, 191–192
  evaluation, 242
Sleep patterns, 138, 159, 177–178
Smoking problems, 90–92
Staffing
  and accountability, 221, 223–224
  and assessment, 101, 104
  development, 295–300, 313, 314
  evaluation, 256–258
  and nursing care plan, 287–289, 305
  ratios, 288
Strength, 165, 186–187
  evaluation, 236–238
Stressors, 147
  and coping, 149–151, 154–156
  and diagnosis, 15, 161–162
  and treatment, 163–164
  unusual, 148–149
Subjective data, 12, 15, 97
  and assessment, 125, 127, 134, 135–136, 142
  and cues, 55, 66
  and evaluation, 242–243, 245, 248, 251
  and inferences, 56
Support systems, 139–140, 167
  evaluation, 246–247
  family, 270
  goals, 192–193
  and strength, 237
Surgery, 127, 278
  as stressor, 148, 171–172

Taxonomy, 168, 176–177, 186
  diagnostic, 319
  and knowledge, 239–241
Team nursing care, 255–256
  and care plan reporting, 275–277
  conferences, 298–299
Terminal patients, 9–10, 43, 142, 185, 254
Therapists, 7, 8
Third party payors, 104
Time
  and nursing order, 216–218
  and rounds, 256
Tuberculosis, 47, 205–206
Turning schedules, 216, 220

University of Oregon Medical School Hospital, 44–45
University of Washington, 39–42

Values, 24–53
  and goals, 197, 202
  institutional, 51
  and patients, 49
Verbalization, 97, 209
  and assessment, 119–120
  and cues, 55, 66–69
  of diagnosis, 169
  and nursing orders, 214–216, 219
Veterans Administration hospitals, 57
Vocabulary
  cues, 57, 61, 64–65, 72, 74, 75
  and nursing, 168, 176–177, 214–216, 301

Wards, 42–48
Weight Watchers, 237
Wortman, Paul, 85, 89